Examination Medicine

6th edition

Nicholas J Talley

MD, PhD, FRACP, FRCP (London), FRCP (Edin), FAFPHM, FACP, FACG, AGAF
Professor of Medicine and Epidemiology, and Consultant Physician, Mayo Clinic,
Jacksonville, Florida and Rochester, Minnesota;
Visiting Professor, University of Sydney, Nepean Hospital, Penrith

Simon O'Connor

FRACP, DDU, FCSANZ
Cardiologist, The Canberra Hospital;
Clinical Senior Lecturer, Australian National University Medical School, Canberra, ACT

CHURCHILL LIVINGSTONE

ELSEVIER

Sydney   Edinburgh   London   New York   Philadelphia   St Louis   Toronto

ELSEVIER

Churchill Livingstone
is an imprint of Elsevier

Elsevier Australia. ACN 001 002 357
(a division of Reed International Books Australia Pty Ltd)
Tower 1, 475 Victoria Avenue, Chatswood, NSW 2067

National Library of Australia Cataloguing-in-Publication Data

---

Talley, Nicholas Joseph.
Examination medicine: a guide to physician training/
 Nicholas J. Talley, Simon O'Connor.
6th ed.
ISBN: 978 0 7295 3911 1 (pbk)

Includes index.
Bibliography.

Physical diagnosis.
Medical history taking.
Internal medicine.

O'Connor, Simon.

616.0754

Publisher: Sophie Kaliniecki
Developmental Editor: Sabrina Chew
Publishing Services Manager: Helena Klijn
Editorial Coordinator: Lauren Allsop
Edited by Caroline Hunter, Burrumundi Pty Ltd
Proofread by Kerry Brown
Index by Max McMaster, Master Indexing
Internal design and typesetting by Pindar New Zealand
Cover design by Stan Lamond
Printed in Australia by Ligare

£45.99

Examination
Medicine

6th edition

15/7/10

£45.99

RC 71

£24.99

Contents

Foreword

Hippocrates knew this: 'The life so short, the
craft so long to learn.'

The autumn months through to early winter are a beautiful time of year in Australia,
with remarkable changes in our flora and relief from increasingly hot summers
and the bushfire period. For most people this period creates a good feeling, but for
some the reduction in daylight hours and colder temperatures engenders a more
melancholic mood—similar feelings are usually experienced at this time of year by
FRACP candidates, this being the period that begins with the 'high' of success in
the written examinations followed by an inevitably anxiety-producing phase as the
clinical examination approaches. Thank heavens, then, for a text like this that provides
candidates with a succinct and important source of information to assist them through
this difficult time.

This edition rightly begins with sections describing the Royal Australasian College
of Physicians' approach to basic physician training. This is a time of major change
within the College, with continual endeavours to improve its training program in a
less threatening manner without compromising standards. The early chapters describe
some of these endeavours, and the College should be congratulated on these efforts,
even though the reforms are probably happening slower than many would like. I
suspect that it is unlikely that the current mode of clinical examinations will change
substantially in the next few years. As such, this text will remain invaluable for every
candidate undertaking the clinical examinations.

This edition builds on its successful original format and approach to long- and
short-case examinations. At times the detail may be more than is required to master
the average long- or short-case examination, but this is only an advantage to future
learning. Indeed, this text can help us in our day-to-day work as physicians and is
not one to be discarded when the examination is complete. Some of the simplified
classifications of important diseases and their relevant investigations and management
are set out in a clear tabulated format that becomes an easy reference for all of us
at any stage of our career. Exam candidates may be interested to know that it is not
uncommon to see examiners carrying this text with them during the week of clinical
examinations. Indeed, examiners share some of the same anxieties as the candidates
(doing a 'blind' neurological short-case examination in front of a professor of
neurology was certainly one of my anxiety-producing moments). Yet this serves to
reassure candidates that there has been a significant change in the conduct of the exam
in recent years so as to make it as fair as possible, and what the examiners find when
seeing long and short cases 'blind' on the day is what is examined.

Registrars and examiners are not the only ones using this text. Medical students
find it valuable, too, even though it is pitched at a level higher than their required
knowledge. This goes to the heart of learning to be a physician—namely, that it is a
lifelong process, one that begins in medical school and then progresses through the
training period of resident and registrar life and continues into consultant physician
life. The 'best' physicians are those who have the capacity to continue to learn, who
know their limitations, adopt a holistic approach to patient care and are able to help
their patients by prioritising and managing their medical and social issues. Not

surprisingly, these are the facets of learning that are tested in the long-case examination and are well-addressed in this text.

More-experienced candidates (not that one wants to earn this title) will know that at times the information in this text is more than is required in the real exam and some of the supposed common long cases are not all that common in the actual exam. Nevertheless, a good text will err on the side of including more than is required, rather than leaving out important components of learning. Many of the mnemonics used in the chapters will facilitate recall, although some may not be politically correct!

There is no doubt that the FRACP clinical examination period remains a difficult time in the lives of many doctors and their families. It is pleasing that the College is striving to find more relevant and less imposing methods to assess both the competency and performance of doctors wishing to enter advanced physician training. This is by no means an easy task but is one that must be achieved. The rewards of getting past this barrier are great. Like any job, being a physician has its ups and downs but it is a career in which no two days are the same, where the subject matter is continually changing, where there is wonderful opportunity to engage with a wide variety of junior and senior colleagues, and where we have the privilege to be able to help others on a day-to-day basis.

Professor Mark Brown
Professor of Renal Medicine
St George Hospital and University of New South Wales, Sydney

Preface

It is now almost 25 years since the first edition of *Examination Medicine* appeared. There have been many changes in medical practice and in the Royal Australasian College of Physicians certifying (Part One) examination over this period. We are delighted that previous editions of this book have proven very helpful for senior medical students, Australian Medical Council examinees and postgraduates preparing for specialties that require a detailed knowledge of general medicine and physical examination techniques. We hope that this sixth edition will continue to assist candidates sitting for the FRACP examination. This examination remains a significant hurdle; indeed, we would argue that it is the most rigorous of its kind in internal medicine anywhere in the world, and all who pass (and most will, thanks to the excellent preparation offered through the College) are much better clinicians for the experience.

The clinical examination is now being attempted by a record number of candidates, which has caused considerable logistical difficulties for the College. More than 600 sat the test in 2009 and it is now held in almost every large and middle-sized hospital in the country. The increased number of candidates has led to discussion about the need to consider holding the exam twice a year. The second examination could be offered to candidates who fail their first attempt at the clinical by a small number of marks, the idea being to reduce the numbers sitting the exam in the following year. Other solutions are being canvassed for this difficult logistical problem, so you can expect yet more changes in the near future.

There continues to be vigorous discussion within the College about transformation of the examination process in the future. The short case is viewed by many as an entirely artificial way to assess a candidate's interaction with patients. For this reason, its contribution to the total mark has been reduced, and it is possible to pass the overall exam despite relatively poor marks in all four short cases. Supporters of the short case believe that a person entering advanced training in a subspecialty should know how to comprehensively examine all the systems of the body and synthesise the data properly in a limited time, which the short case teaches. This debate is likely to continue for some time, but it remains our view that the short case will probably survive.

This edition of *Examination Medicine* has been carefully updated to reflect modern medical practice and the realities of the exam. It is important to remember that we have set out an approach to the long and short cases; you will need other resources to learn all of internal medicine and we offer a list of useful learning materials for you to consider. Candidates should build on the approaches suggested here to develop their own systematic methods. Some examiners have complained (perhaps unfairly!) that all candidates examine, for example, the hands in much the same way. Be guided by this book, your teachers and fellow candidates, and then create your own methodological approach that you can apply with success every day in clinical practice.

Nicholas J Talley
Simon O'Connor
Jacksonville and Canberra
October 2009

Acknowledgments

The following specialists have been kind enough to review the text. We are very grateful for their advice and comments:

- Patrick Manning BHB, MBChB, MMedSc, FRACP, Consultant Endocrinologist, Dunedin Hospital, Dunedin, New Zealand and Associate Professor of Medicine, University of Otago, Dunedin, New Zealand
- Stephen Clarke MBBS PhD FRACP FAChPM, Senior Staff Specialist, Medical Oncology, Concord Hospital, Sydney and Professor of Medicine, University of Sydney
- Jack R Wall MD, PhD, FRACP, FRCPC, Professor of Medicine, University of Sydney and Consultant Endocrinologist, Sydney West Area Heath Service, Nepean Hospital, Penrith
- Nerida Paterson BMed (Newcastle), Dip RACOG, Senior Lecturer, University of Newcastle, New South Wales
- Lilijana Mikuletic MBBS (hons), BMedSc (hons), MPH, DCH, DipO&G, general practitioner and Clinical Associate Lecturer, Faculty of Medicine, University of Sydney

The publishers and authors would also like to thank Professor G Buirski, Director of the Department of Medical Imaging, The Canberra Hospital, for granting permission to use some of the X-rays and scans from The Canberra Hospital X-ray library. In addition, many of the ECG tracings are from *Practical Cardiology* 2nd edn (Elsevier, 2008) and were originally contributed by Dr George Nikolić.

An historical note

The problem is not so much how to test
candidates but how to test examinations.
J Parkhouse, Lancet 1971; i: 905–906.

Internal medicine at the beginning of last century was still in its infancy. It was practised largely on an empirical basis. Therapeutics was very limited. Surgery was a more popular specialty, partly because of its greater efficacy in treating many diseases. There were consultant physicians in Australia, but medicine was mainly practised by the family doctor.

In 1930 some leading physicians formed the Association of Physicians of Australia. It aimed to foster expansion of scientific knowledge of medicine in Australia and New Zealand. It also allowed physicians to meet socially. It was an exclusive organisation—only physicians who held honorary appointments at teaching hospitals were eligible to join.

However, non-members began to lobby for the formation of a college. Eventually, after considerable opposition from members of the Association, the Royal Australasian College of Physicians was legally incorporated in 1938 (the title 'Royal' was conferred by King George VI). The inauguration ceremony occurred, with great pageantry, in the Great Hall of the University of Sydney. Sydney was chosen for the headquarters because the Royal Australasian College of Surgeons had previously been established in Melbourne.

Since its beginning, the Royal Australasian College of Physicians has been responsible for maintaining the standards of training and practice of medicine and paediatrics. This was originally achieved by conducting an examination known as 'the Membership'. The College set two major prerequisites for this test:

1. The candidate had to be a graduate of three years' standing or more from an acceptable medical school.
2. Two Fellows of the College must vouch for the candidate's integrity and character.

No limits were set on age or experience, no attention was given to previous training, no standard was defined for the examination and few guidelines were laid down. Although this was a rather subjective test, Censors carried out their obligations well, as is obvious from the high standards of internal medicine practised in Australia and New Zealand today. The Membership examination consisted of two papers of essay questions and a clinical and oral examination. Multiple-choice questions were introduced only in 1967.

With the growth of technology and medical knowledge, the College began to coordinate the flourishing specialty associations and societies. By 1968 the need for a change in the evaluation of physician trainees had become apparent. In 1976 the Membership examination was replaced by the Fellowship examination. After considerable discussion within the College, it was decided that the emphasis should be on training, rather than examination. To this end, the FRACP (Part One) examination was established as an early examination to admit candidates to advanced training. Candidates successful in this Part One examination would then have three or four years of supervised training in general medicine or a subspecialty, and in most cases no further examination would be required. An advanced trainee would be elected a Fellow after the required time of supervised training in accredited terms, if the supervisors' reports were satisfactory.

In this the College decided on a different course from the Royal Australasian College of Surgeons, which requires candidates to sit for an examination at the end of advanced training before election to Fellowship. The actual training emphasis of the Colleges still remains different.

The FRACP examination is now held at centres in Australia and New Zealand. The examination system has its critics. The pass rate for the FRACP is low; on average in the past only 40% of candidates passed both the written exam and their first attempt at the clinical examination. Changes to the format of the clinical examination have increased this somewhat in recent years. In the United Kingdom, the MRCP (UK) also has a low pass rate. In an editorial in *Lancet*, it was suggested there are only two possible reasons for a low pass rate in the MRCP: either the training is of poor quality or the examination is of poor quality, and the College is directly or indirectly responsible for each (*Lancet* 1990; i:443–445). The Royal Australasian College of Physicians has tried to tackle some of these issues in recent years, but vigorous debate on the method of examination continues.

There is no doubt, however, that physician training remains very popular. More than 600 candidates presented themselves for the clinical examination in 2009, many more than the number attempting the examination in the mid-1990s.

The objectives of the Royal Australasian College of Physicians remain the same as they were at its inception. Essentially the College strives to promote the study of the art and science of medicine, and to encourage research and dissemination of knowledge, as well as *to promote and ensure the fitness of persons desirous of qualifying for membership of the College*. This book deals with strategies to enable candidates to satisfy the strict examination requirements of the College.

Abbreviations

ABP	ambulatory blood pressure
ABVD	adriamycin, bleomycin, vinblastine and dacarbazine
ACE	angiotensin-converting enzyme
ACTH	adrenocorticotrophic hormone
ADP	adenosine diphosphate
AF	atrial fibrillation
AFB	acid fast bacilli
AHI	apnoea hypopnoea index
AICDs	automatic implantable cardioverter-defibrillators
AIDS	acquired immunodeficiency syndrome
ALL	acute lymphocytic leukaemia
ALT	alanine aminotransferase
AMA	antimitochondrial antibody
AMC	Australian Medical Council
ANA	antinuclear antibody
ANCA	antineutrophil cytoplasmic antibody
anti-LKM1	anti-liver and kidney microsomes type 1
AP	anteroposterior
APC	activated protein C
APD	automated peritoneal dialysis
AR blocker/ARB	angiotensin II receptor blocker
AR	aortic regurgitation
AS	aortic stenosis
ASAP	Australian Self-Assessment Programme
ASCA	anti-*Saccharomyces cerevisiae* antibodies
ASD	atrial septal defect
ASH	asymmetrical hypertrophy
ASMA	anti-smooth muscle antibody
AST	aspartate aminotransferase
ATP	antitachycardia pacing
AV	atrioventricular
B2-GP-1	beta2-glycoprotein-1
BCG	bacille Calmette-Guérin
b.d.	twice a day
BiPAP	bilevel positive airways pressure
BMD	bone mineral density
BMI	body mass index
BMS	bare metal stent
BNP	B-type natriuretic peptide
BPPV	benign paroxysmal positional (positioning) vertigo
CABG	coronary artery bypass graft
CAD	coronary artery disease
CAPD	continuous ambulatory peritoneal dialysis
CCP	citrullinated cyclic peptide
CEA	carcinoembryonic antigen

CFE	Committee for Examinations
CIDP	chronic inflammatory demyelinating polyradiculoneuropathy
CKD	chronic kidney disease
CML	chronic myeloid leukaemia
CMV	cytomegalovirus
CNS	central nervous system
COP	cryptogenic organising pneumonia
COPD	chronic obstructive pulmonary disease
COX-2	cyclo-oxygenase 2
CPAP	continuous positive airways pressure
CPT	Committee for Physician Training
CREST	calcinosis cutis; Raynaud's phenomenon; (o)esophageal involvement; sclerodactyly; telangiectasia
CRH	corticotropin-releasing hormone
CRP	C-reactive protein
CRT	cardiac resynchronisation therapy
CT	computed tomography
CVP	cyclophosphamide, vincristine and prednisone
DAF	decay-accelerating factors
DC	direct current
DES	drug-eluting stent
DEXA	dual-energy X-ray absorptiometry
DIC	disseminated intravascular coagulation
DIP	distal interphalangeal
DLCO	diffusion capacity for carbon monoxide
DLE	discoid lupus erythematosus
DMARDs	disease-modifying, antirheumatic drugs
DOT	direct observed treatment
DPE	Director of Physician Education
DPT	Director of Physician Training
dsDNA	double-stranded DNA
DVT	deep venous thrombosis
EBV	Epstein-Barr virus
ECG	electrocardiogram
ECOG	Eastern Cooperative Oncology Group
EF	ejection fraction
EIA	enzyme immunoassay
EMG	electromyogram
ENA	extractable nuclear antigen
EPG	electrophoretogram
EPS	electrophysiological studies
ES	educational supervisor
ESR	erythrocyte sedimentation rate
FAP	familial adenomatous polyposis
FBC	full blood count
FET	forced expiratory time
FEV1	forced expiratory volume in one second
FFP	fresh frozen plasma
FHH	familial hypocalciuric hypercalcaemia
FS	fractional shortening
FSH	facio-scapulo-humeral
FSH	follicle-stimulating hormone
FVC	forced vital capacity

G6PD	glucose-6-phosphate dehydrogenase
GGT	gamma-glutamyl transferase
GH	growth hormone
GI	glycaemic index
GM-CSF	granulocyte-macrophage colony stimulating factor
GORD	gastro-oesophageal reflux disease
GPI	glycosylphosphatidylinositol
GTHs	general teaching hospitals
GVHD	graft versus host disease
HAART	highly active antiretroviral therapy
HBV	hepatitis B virus
HCC	hepatocellular carcinoma
HCV	hepatitis C virus
HDL	high-density lipoprotein
Hib	*Haemophilus influenzae* type b
HIV	human immunodeficiency virus
HLA	human leucocyte antigen
HMG-CoA	hydroxymethylglutaryl coenzyme A
HMSN	hereditary motor and sensory neuropathy
HNPCC	hereditary non-polyposis colon cancer
HPL	human placental lactogen
HPO	hypertrophic pulmonary osteoarthropathy
HSV	herpes simplex virus
HUS	haemolytic uraemic syndrome
HZV	herpes zoster virus
IBD	inflammatory bowel disease
ICD	implantable cardioverter-defibrillators
IDL	intermediate-density lipoprotein
IEPG	immunoelectrophoretogram
IGF-I	insulin-like growth factor I
ILD	interstitial lung disease
INR	international normalised ratio
IPF	idiopathic pulmonary fibrosis
IPH	idiopathic pulmonary hypertension
IPI	International Prognostic Index
IRTC	Independent Review of Training Committee
IVP	intravenous pyelogram
JVP	jugular venous pressure
KUB	kidneys, ureters, bladder
LA	left atrium
LAD	left anterior descending
LAHB	left anterior hemi-block
LAM	lymphangioleiomyomatosis
LBBB	Left bundle branch block
LCAT	lecithin cholesterol acyltransferase
LDH	lactate dehydrogenase
LDL	low-density lipoprotein
LH	luteinising hormone
LIMA	left internal mammary artery
LNAT	learning needs analysis
LV	left ventricle/left ventricular
LVEDD	left ventricular end-diastolic dimension
LVH	left ventricular hypertrophy

LVOT	left ventricular outflow tract
LVPW	left ventricular posterior wall
MAC	*Mycobacterium avium* complex
MALT	mucosa-associated lymphoid tissue
MCP	metacarpophalangeal
MCTD	mixed connective tissue disease
MCV	mean corpuscular volume
MELD	model for end-stage liver disease
MEN	multiple endocrine neoplasia
MGUS	monoclonal gammopathies of uncertain significance
mini-CEX	mini-Clinical Evaluation Exercise
MKSAP	Medical Knowledge Self-Assessment Program
MR	mitral regurgitation
MRI	magnetic resonance imaging
MS	multiple sclerosis
MSF	multi-source feedback
MSI	microsatellite instability
MTP	metatarsophalangeal
MV	mitral valve
MVP	mitral valve prolapse
NAFLD	non-alcoholic fatty liver disease
NAP	neutrophil alkaline phosphatase
NASH	non-alcoholic steatohepatitis
NEP	National Examination Panel
non-STEMI	non-ST elevation myocardial infarction
NSAIDs	non-steroidal anti-inflammatory drugs
NSTEACS	non-ST elevation acute coronary syndrome
NYHA	New York Heart Association
OAT	Open Artery Trial
OTPs	overseas-trained physicians
PA	plasma aldosterone
PA	posteroanterior
PAH	pulmonary arterial hypertension
p-ANCA	perinuclear antineutrophil cytoplasmic antibodies
PAP	pulmonary artery pressure
PBS	Pharmaceutical Benefits Scheme
PCH	pulmonary capillary haemangiomatosis
PCR	polymerase chain reaction
PDA	patent ductus arteriosus
PDA	professional development advisor
PET	positron emission tomography
PIE	pulmonary infiltrate and eosinophilia
PIP	proximal interphalangeal
PNH	paroxysmal nocturnal haemoglobinuria
PPD	purified protein derivative
PPI	proton pump inhibitor
PRA	plasma renin activity
PREP	Physician Readiness for Expert Practice
PTH	parathyroid hormone
PTLD	Post-transplant lymphoproliferative disease
PTTK	prolonged partial thromboplastin time with kaolin
PUO	Pyrexia of unknown origin
PVD	peripheral vascular disease

PVOD	pulmonary veno-occlusive disease
PY1	Postgraduate Year 1
RACP	Royal Australasian College of Physicians
RAD	right-axis deviation
RBBB	right bundle branch block
RDW	red cell distribution width
REM	rapid eye movement
RLS	restless legs syndrome
RIMA	right internal mammary artery
RNP	ribonucleoprotein
RV	right ventricle/right ventricular
SAAG	serum-to-ascites albumin gradient
SAC	Specialist Advisory Committee
SAM	systolic anterior motion
SE	supplementary examination
SIAT	Significant Incident Analysis Tool
SLE	systemic lupus erythematosus
STEMI	ST elevation myocardial infarction
SVC	superior vena cava
SVGs	saphenous vein grafts
SVT	supraventricular tachycardia
TB	tuberculosis
TIA	transient ischaemic attack
TIPS	transjugular intrahepatic portosystemic shunt
TNF	tumour necrosis factor
TNM	tumour node metastases
TOE	transoesophageal echocardiography
TPHA	*treponema pallidum* haemoglutination test
TR	tricuspid regurgitation
TSH	thyroid-stimulating hormone.
TTP	thrombotic thrombocytopenic purpura
TZDs	thiazolidinediones
UKPDS	United Kingdom Prognosis in Diabetes Study
UTHs	university teaching hospitals
VC	vital capacity
VDRL	venereal disease research laboratory
VF	ventricular fibrillation
VLDL	very-low-density lipoprotein
VSD	ventricular septal defect
VT	ventricular tachycardia
VVI	ventricular-ventricular inhibited
WC	ward consultant
WCC	white cell count
WPW	Wolff-Parkinson-White

Chapter 1

Basic training requirements

> I would live to study, and not study to live.
> *Francis Bacon (1561–1626)*

There is nothing more exciting than working as a consultant physician! Colleagues will turn to you for advice on how to diagnose and treat complex cases. You will change the lives of your patients for the better. To become such a respected professional, you must first complete basic physician training. The requirements for basic training, after which a trainee may sit the Royal Australasian College of Physicians' (RACP) written and clinical examinations, are set out on the RACP website (**www.racp.edu.au**) under the link to the Basic Training Portal. Basic trainees must register with the College and will have access to this extensive program. Only an outline of the information available to trainees is given here.

As of 2009 many remarkable new acronyms have been introduced to basic training (see Table 1.1) and the training program has been amended. Although it remains to be seen how practical this new and complicated scheme will be, trainees should not be put off by it: basic training will still teach clinical medicine and instil the key skills needed to become a first-class physician, as well as promoting a lifelong love of learning medicine and helping patients.

The new training program has the overall title of *Physician Readiness for Expert Practice* (PREP) and it includes basic training as well as the three or more years of advanced training. The College describes the principles of training as:
- learner-centred
- workplace focused and assessed
- competency-based
- a blended working environment.

The basic training period is now closely supervised by the College via the Director of Physician Education (DPE; previously the Director of Physician Training, DPT) and the educational supervisor (ES), along with the candidate's own self-evaluation through his or her *learning plan*. This process is known as a *learning needs analysis* (LNA).

Trainees have access to the *Significant Incident Analysis Tool* (SIAT), which provides online support for both 'good and bad' learning experiences. They should also be helped by the introduction of *multi-source feedback* (MSF). Using MSF, trainees must ask a number of people to assess them, including the educational supervisor, ward consultants (WCs), senior nurses, junior medical staff and allied health professionals. Trainees must undertake at least one MSF encounter per year involving a minimum of six assessors.

TABLE 1.1	The garbled soup of College acronyms
CPT	Committee for Physician Training
DPE	Director of Physician Education
DPT	Director of Physician Training
ES	Educational supervisor
IRTC	Independent Review of Training Committee
LNA	Learning needs analysis
Mini-CEX	Mini-Clinical Evaluation Exercise
MSF	Multi-source feedback
NEP	National Examination Panel
PDA	Professional development advisor
PREP	Physician Readiness for Expert Practice
PY1	Postgraduate Year 1
RACP	Royal Australasian College of Physicians
SAC	Specialist Advisory Committee
SIAT	Significant Incident Analysis Tool
WC	Ward consultant

In addition, trainees will have the help of a *professional development advisor* (PDA), who reports to the Director of Physician Education about the trainee's development and MSF results. The ward consultant is also expected to be involved in active teaching, supervision and support of the trainee, as well as to provide advice to the educational supervisor and information sheets for the educational supervisor and Director of Physician Education.

For the trainee's idle moments, another recent innovation is the *mini-Clinical Evaluation Exercise* (mini-CEX). The mini-CEX requires trainees to examine a patient in their own hospital while being watched by an assessor. The trainee will be guided to a specific aspect of history-taking or examination, or both. Before the trainee examines the patient, the trainee and assessor spend some time discussing what should occur. The trainee then spends 15–20 minutes with the patient and another 10–15 minutes afterwards with the assessor again to discuss the performance. The idea is to simulate a normal clinical encounter in which a targeted history and examination are taken and performed.

Physician training has always depended on voluntary (and largely unpaid) help from senior colleagues such as consultants and senior registrars. This help ranges from informal teaching during ward rounds to formal long- and short-case practice sessions and various supervisory roles. Physician training could not work without this assistance. Both trainees and physicians benefit from this close association, personally and professionally. The new physician training should, if anything, strengthen these bonds.

The College requires three years of basic training after the intern year (PY1) in Australia or New Zealand. It consists of at least 36 months of supervised training across the breadth of internal medicine in both general medicine and the other medical subspecialties ('core' training), which must involve the continuing care of medical patients in approved hospitals. Approved hospitals are listed on the College's website. There are four categories of training hospitals: level 3 hospitals—previously called university teaching hospitals (UTHs); level 2 hospitals—previously called general teaching hospitals (GTHs); level 1 hospitals—generally regional hospitals; and secondment hospitals. Trainees must spend at least 12 months in a level 3 hospital and at least three months in a general medicine term. Only six months may be spent in a single subspecialty. Up to three months of this time may be undertaken in each of coronary care, relieving, emergency medicine, nuclear medicine, psychiatry, dermatology or an approved secondment post, but the total time spent in these combined cannot exceed six months. A DPT is appointed in each hospital with an accredited training scheme and he or she is responsible for supervising basic training. The DPT's approval is required for each rotation.

Accreditation of terms that are suitable for basic training are now looked at more critically to ensure adequate levels of supervision and support for trainees, and some hospitals have lost their accreditation. This applies especially to hospitals that receive resident medical officers on secondment. Up to three months of core training may be carried out in a single approved secondment post. It is important to check with the RACP Department of Education if there is any doubt that the terms are acceptable. Basic training requirements are now so strict that careful negotiation with the hospital for suitable training terms from the beginning of basic training is the only way to ensure that it is possible to sit the examination in the minimum time.

The College details the sequence of steps involved in entry to the Fellowship (FRACP) with fees in 2009 as follows:
- Register as a basic trainee (postgraduation Year 2)—$1500 per year.
- Apply for FRACP examinations—written $2500; clinical $4000.
- Apply for approval of advanced training program—$1200 per year.
- Receive accreditation of advanced training.
- Apply for admission to Fellowship—$749.

The fees rise by about 10% each year. The cost of travel and accommodation must be added to the examination fees. Claiming these expenses as a tax deduction usually seems to be allowed.

The forms for registration as a basic trainee should be downloaded from the College website, and applications can be made online. Applications for approval of basic training must be made early in the year of training and signed by the DPT. Late applications for training and to sit examinations are sometimes accepted (subject to an extra fee), but not always. The exact dates by which all applications are required are set out on the College's website and must be taken very seriously.

The registration fee is paid annually during basic training and is the start of a physician's long financial association with the College. In exchange for this 'small fee', trainees receive regular information from the College. At the moment this includes the College journal, *Fellowship Affairs*, but not the *Internal Medicine Journal*.

Interrupted and part-time training are possible. Research may be accepted for part of non-core basic training. Trainees who have a higher degree (MD or PhD) may apply to have accredited one year of basic training or one year of advanced training.

All trainees are notified by post and by email when their applications are received and again when approval to sit the examination is granted. This second letter gives the times, date and place of the examination. The application to sit the examination is required in November of the prior year.

Success at the written and clinical examinations is *not* recognised as a specialist qualification. To be admitted to Fellowship of the College requires success in both examinations and completion of basic and advanced training. Once a trainee has completed three years of basic training, he or she can undertake a conditional year of advanced training. During the year the examinations must be successfully completed for the year to be accredited. If the trainee does not pass the examinations, the year cannot count towards advanced training. All advanced training in general medicine or a subspecialty must be approved by the appropriate Specialist Advisory Committee (SAC) and by the Committee for Physician Training (CPT). There is no longer any exit examination.

In some cases, exemption from the written examination may be granted. This usually applies to those with postgraduate physician training and overseas qualifications—for example, Membership of the Royal College of Physicians (MRCP) of London or Edinburgh, the Diploma of the American Board of Internal Medicine (ABIM), Fellowship of the Royal College of Physicians (FRCP) Canada or the Master of Medicine (Singapore). The appropriate application form for exemption can be obtained from the College. Approval is not automatic, but rather is at the discretion of the CPT. Exemption from the clinical examination will occasionally be given to highly qualified senior people who trained overseas.

Each year of advanced training is assessed by a supervisor—usually one of the consultants for whom the trainee works during the year. The supervisor submits a report on the trainee's performance during the year and a recommendation about accreditation of part or all of the year's training. Unsatisfactory reports are rare. An advanced trainee who receives an unsatisfactory report is offered an interview with a member of the CPT and a representative of the appropriate SAC. This committee will also interview the trainee's supervisor. A report is then issued by the Independent Review of Training Committee (IRTC). This has replaced the old verification interview. The report and recommendation are considered by the CPT, which makes the final decision. The emphasis for advanced trainees and their supervisors is very much on addressing problems with performance during the year, through regular meetings. Supervisors are encouraged to discuss any problems they perceive with a trainee *before* the end of the year and to suggest ways of improving performance.

Advanced training requirements are very different for the various subspecialties and details can be obtained from the College.

Determination to pass both sections of the examination at the first attempt is an important part of preparation. The first section is the written examination and the second section is the clinical viva-voce (live-voice) or 'viva' test. In December 2004 the College announced that candidates who pass the written examination must pass the clinical examination within five years, otherwise they have to re-sit the written examination before sitting the clinical examination. So a candidate who is successful in the written examination in 2009 has until 2013 to pass the clinical examination. It may be possible to defer sitting the clinical examination for a year, under certain circumstances, but a pass must still be obtained within five years. This change to the rules is retrospective and applies even to candidates who have passed the written examination but then failed the clinical examination and failed the written at the second attempt.

An exemption from the written examination entitles the candidate to sit the viva.

The written examination is held only once every year, in March, in each of the Australian capital cities and in four main centres in New Zealand. Past examination papers are available, usually from two years prior. They are an essential reference point for candidates.

A list of successful candidates is published at each hospital in which the written examination is held. Those who have failed the written examination are sent a feedback sheet indicating their performance in the various subspecialty areas. The DPT of each hospital is sent a list of the average marks for the candidates from that hospital in each subspecialty. Failure in the written examination means waiting a year to sit again.

The clinical examination can be attempted only by candidates who have been successful in the written examination. The viva is held only once each year, in July or August, in a number of cities in rotation. This rotation forms the basis for the unofficial 'FRACP See Australia Travel Plan'. Experienced candidates know this tour well. In

Australia, clinical examinations are held in the major centres (Sydney, Melbourne, Brisbane or Adelaide) as well as 'less major' centres (Hobart, Canberra, Newcastle, Perth, Darwin, Cairns, Wagga Wagga, Geelong and others). In 1989, for the first time in living memory, the viva was postponed in Australia for two months because of a pilots' strike. Such events cannot be relied on to give more time for preparation.

A pass in the viva counts as a pass in the year that the examination was sat. A supplementary examination (SE), or 'post', is offered to fewer than 5% of the candidates who encountered some major disaster during their examination, such as sickness on the day of the examination, or a patient who was too sick to allow proper examination or had a heart attack during it; the 'post' is held about three weeks later.

The practice of putting up viva results in one location on the day of the examination has now been reintroduced. Currently, results are posted at 5 pm at a location to be advised; it is usually at the site of the examiners' meeting. A list of successful candidates in the viva examination is also published in the national press within a week. Notification by mail occurs a little later.

Successful candidates receive a letter of congratulation. Unsuccessful candidates receive an offer to arrange an interview with a College examiner to discuss the reasons for failure. The case notes and marks for each short and long case, which are made by the teams of examiners during the 10-minute period provided for discussion of a candidate's performance, will be available to the candidate and the member of the Committee for Examinations who is providing the advice. Candidates who have been given a 'post' can obtain this information very soon after the examination; for the others it will be available somewhat later. The College no longer sends a detailed critique of the candidate's performance from the notes.

There is no limit to the number of times candidates may sit the entire examination. Some persistent individuals have sat many times (the record, we believe, is 11—and the candidate passed). More than 85% of those who continue to sit do eventually get through, if they have the stamina. The pass rates for the last few years are published by the College and summarised in Table 1.2.

For further information, write to one of the following:
Department of Education
The Royal Australasian College of Physicians
145 Macquarie Street
Sydney NSW 2000 Australia

Department of Education, New Zealand Committee
The Royal Australasian College of Physicians
Kevin Chambers, 16 The Terrace
Wellington 1 New Zealand

TABLE 1.2 Past examination pass results		
	Sat	Passed
2009 viva	604	n.a.
2009 written examination	698	430 (62.0%)
2008 written examination	508	380 (74.8%)
2004 written examination	500	346 (69.2%)
2003 written examination	475	320 (67.4%)
2003 viva	446	287 (64.3%)
2002 viva	425	259 (60.9%)

The future

There has been much discussion within the College and between the College and the Australian Medical Council (AMC) over the past few years about transforming physician training. As a result, a more formal syllabus will probably be introduced within the next few years. This may be followed by changes to basic training, including *formative* and *summative* assessments that contribute to the candidate's mark. Currently, these assessments must be undertaken but they do not contribute to the candidate's mark in the written or clinical examinations. Although the clinical examination is often regarded as too subjective to be fair, it still has much support and is very unlikely to be abandoned in favour of a purely written examination, as is used in the United States.

There is also likely to be the addition of more problem-oriented short cases in the future. The 'stem' or introduction given to the candidate will in these cases be more in the form of a problem (e.g. this patient has gained weight, or this patient has had a problem with dropping things, or this patient has neck pain etc.). The candidate will then have to decide what examination to perform rather than being directed to a particular body system.

Chapter 2

The written examination

No man's opinions are better than his
information.

Paul Getty (1960)

The examination format

The written examination is a screening examination to select candidates for further testing. There are two papers, which are held on the same day. The written examination is an objective multiple-choice examination, with five choices in each question.

The first paper (Paper 1) is set with an emphasis on medical sciences and relevant basic science. It contains 70 questions to be answered in two hours. These are all 'A-type' questions—that is, of the five alternatives given, only one is correct. Marks are not deducted for wrong answers and therefore it is no longer possible to score a negative mark for the total question. An incorrect or omitted answer will score zero. This is meant to encourage candidates to attempt to answer all questions. There is evidence that 'A-type' questions discriminate better between candidates than other formats. The second paper (called, not unexpectedly, Paper 2) contains 100 'A-type' questions to be answered in three hours. Again, each correct answer gains a mark and an incorrect one scores zero.

Although most candidates report that the time limit is sufficient for the completion of Paper 1, this is not the case for Paper 2, which is considerably more rushed. Some candidates have reported difficulty completing Paper 2 in the time allowed. The questions in Paper 2 are clinical scenarios and often contain long preambles, which may include a clinical history and the results of numerous investigations. They can be spread over several paragraphs. The clinical application questions are designed to include tests that a practising clinician must be able to interpret. Various X-ray films (including chest radiographs, computed tomography [CT] and magnetic resonance imaging [MRI] scans), blood films (actual photographs or reports, or both), photographs of urinary sediments and histopathology slides (e.g. renal biopsies) may be included. Photographs (both black-and-white and colour) are usually of high quality. Interpretation of biochemistry results (e.g. liver function tests) is also examined. Normal values are always supplied. The 2009 examination had rather shorter preambles than in recent years, perhaps because of candidates' complaints regarding having insufficient time to complete the paper.

A pencil is provided at the test, as well as a well-used eraser. It is advisable, however, to bring a pencil sharpener, a spare soft B pencil and a good eraser—particularly if you are indecisive.

The marking system is complex. All questions are approved by a test committee. About one-third of the questions on each paper come from previous papers. These are questions that have been found to be particularly discriminating.

There is, unfortunately, no predetermined pass mark. All candidates' papers are first scored. Any question that most candidates get wrong is examined carefully for degree of difficulty and ambiguity and may be eliminated. The best questions discriminate between 'good' and 'bad' candidates and each question is analysed statistically to determine whether it meets this standard. Then various statistical methods are employed to separate candidates into two groups. The exact pass mark is set at approximately 2.5 standard deviations below the mean mark for Australasia, in such a way that the cut-off falls in a gap between clusters of candidates. Approximately 60–70% of candidates are in the 'good' group, and these people pass. This means that one must aim to be better than at least 35% of the other candidates to be successful. The pass mark is not set according to the number of places that are available in the clinicals. It is expected that about two-thirds of candidates will continue to pass the written examination each year.

The examination used to be held in winter, when experienced candidates could be spotted in the centre of Sydney equipped with coats, scarves and thick woollen socks (for some reason the examination room at the University of Sydney was not heated). This problem has been solved by changing the date of the examination to March.

Approaching multiple-choice questions

By the time most candidates sit this examination, they will have had considerable experience with multiple-choice questions. However, it is worth stating a few relevant points:

- Ensure that you estimate in advance the amount of time you have for each question.
- The questions are complicated and each question tests several items of knowledge. The correct answer may be a number of steps removed from the initial statement. This means that it is important to read each question with great care; noting or underlining the salient points may be helpful, and do look especially for negatives and double negatives. Most candidates find that their first carefully considered answer is more reliable than a change of mind on later review of the paper.
- It is worth remembering that the words 'always' and 'never' do not often apply in medicine. The word 'recognised' means that an association has been described, whereas 'characteristic' implies that the given factor is important to the condition and essential to the diagnosis.
- It is always better to guess at an answer when the question is obscure rather than to leave it out entirely.
- To avoid coming to the end of the paper and finding an unexpected unfilled space on the answer sheet, keep a constant check that question and answer numbers match.

Preparation for the written examination

The College does not provide a curriculum for the written examination but recommends the use of any major textbook and some journals (see the Further Reading section at the end of this book). We recommend concentrating on the latest edition of a standard textbook (e.g. the most recent edition of *Harrison's Principles of Internal Medicine* or the *Oxford Textbook of Medicine*); it is a most satisfactory method of preparation. The *Medical Knowledge Self-Assessment Program* (*MKSAP*) of the American College of Physicians is also very useful. It contains brief up-to-date accounts of most areas of internal medicine. It clearly indicates the currently fashionable topics on which questions are likely to be set and has a comprehensive series of multiple-choice questions (and excellent critiques) based on the text. However, only some of these questions are of a similar standard to the written examination questions.

In addition, the College regularly produces its own self-assessment questions—the *Australian Self-Assessment Programme* (ASAP). None of these questions is ever likely to appear in the examination paper, because the ASAP is primarily educational and therefore tends to have a bias towards positive responses, unlike the written examination.

There is great value in practising multiple-choice questions. Sample questions from past papers are available from the College. These are taken from papers that have been used in recent years. Currently the Committee for Examinations also releases, every second year on the College website, complete copies of written examination papers that were set two years previously. Some of the old released questions usually appear in the current examination paper. The College has a large bank of questions that are adjusted annually. The Written Examination Committee adds new questions and updates and improves old questions.

Many hospitals conduct their own trial examinations, with questions written by staff. Also available on the market are books of multiple-choice questions based on other postgraduate examinations such as the MRCP, but these are of less value.

Many candidates find that practising multiple-choice questions in a study group of three or four to discuss the various options is very helpful.

The College recommends a number of general medicine journals that candidates should read regularly. These currently include (roughly in order of usefulness):

- *Lancet*
- *New England Journal of Medicine*
- *Annals of Internal Medicine*
- *British Medical Journal*
- *Internal Medicine Journal*
- *American Journal of Medicine.*

We recommend concentrating on editorials and review articles. Study of specialist journals is not required.

Each year, postgraduate institutions hold courses on various topics, which some candidates find helpful. A course of lectures lasting 34 weeks (one night per week for 17 weeks per year over two years) is available for candidates in Sydney. Short but comprehensive courses are also available in Australia (e.g. at the Royal Prince Alfred Hospital, Sydney) and New Zealand (e.g. in Dunedin) and can be particularly useful for revision.

The comprehensive lecture series given by the Victorian State Committee of the RACP, running over 40 weeks of the year and held once a week in the evening for three hours, is now videoconferenced widely across Australia. The series covers the entirety of the syllabus in one year. This is particularly useful for trainees in regional centres. Details can be obtained from the RACP Department of Education.

A number of audio programs are available on medical topics. The Audio Digest Internal Medicine programs are available in many libraries and provide updates of topics, but are mostly from a North American perspective and of somewhat patchy quality. The American College of Physicians sells recordings of Board Review Courses in Internal Medicine that provide excellent summaries of recent topics.

In summary, here are a number of conventional but important suggestions for the written examination:

1. Be well rested and avoid travelling long distances on the eve of the examination. Make sure you know where the examination centre is situated.
2. Be familiar with the format of the paper and know how much time to allow for each question.

3. Work through the paper at a leisurely, deliberate pace and return to troublesome questions at the end. Inspiration may well come from other questions.
4. Rely on first careful impressions and do not change an answer if in doubt.
5. Check every tenth question or so to be sure that answer numbers match the question numbers.

Have a short rest after the written examination, but then begin work for the 'viva' examination, as time between the two parts of the examination is limited.

Chapter 3
The clinical examination

This is a very testing part. It is more difficult than
the written test.
Nick Talley and Simon O'Connor (1986)

The examination format

The clinical examination consists of two sessions (morning and afternoon), each
comprising two parts (one long case and two short cases), and now takes up a whole
(rather exhausting) day. There is evidence that lengthening a clinical examination
improves its reliability and the College believes that the changed format has certainly
done that.

Candidates are notified of the starting time of the ordeal after their success in
the written examination. Be on time for the clinical examination: it runs to a strict
timetable and no allowances can be made for late arrivals.

On the day

For half of the candidates the first session begins with a long case. At the appropriate
moment, each candidate is escorted to the patient by a 'bulldog' (a term derived from
the name of proctors' attendants at the universities of Oxford and Cambridge). The
bulldog is usually a resident medical officer working at the examining hospital who
has an interest in sitting the clinical examination. The bulldog introduces the candidate
to the patient and then leaves. If ever you have the opportunity to work as a bulldog,
you should take it: there is no better way to come to understand what is expected of
candidates in the exam.

There are never any examiners in the room during a long case. The time is limited
to 60 minutes with the patient. A five-minute warning is given after 55 minutes. At
the end, the candidate is escorted by the bulldog from the patient's room to a chair
outside the examiners' room. Ten minutes are allowed for candidates to pull themselves
together and get to the examination room. A glass of water or weak orange juice is
usually offered at this stage. If not, do ask for a drink if you need one.

A bell then rings and the candidate is taken in, seated and introduced to the
examiners. Try to appear self-possessed (even if weak at the knees), but don't give an
air of nonchalance (e.g. by slouching in your chair).

As a rule there are two examiners in the room, but there may be three (one an
observer only) and there may be a bulldog sitting in as well. One examiner will be a
member of the Committee for Examinations (CFE) or National Examination Panel
(NEP), and the other will be an experienced examiner who is a local physician, perhaps
even the DPT. Local examiners and NEP and CFE members undergo 'calibration'

exercises before they examine. Even experienced examiners are not allowed to examine unless they have been 'calibrated' that year. Immediately before the examination, all the examiners interview the long-case patient 'blind'; that is, without reference to the patient's case notes. This ensures that the history is up to date, helps gauge any difficulty in terms of the patient's ability to give a history and enables the examiners to assess the physical signs.

The examiners assess the candidate's ability to take a detailed history and complete the examination. They also assess the candidate's ability to identify the patient's active problems and to recognise priorities for investigation and management. The examiners are interested in seeing whether the candidate recognises the effect of the patient's disease on the patient and his/her family.

The examiners mark the candidate's performance in each of these domains according to set key criteria. It would be wise for candidates to examine these anchor statements carefully—they are available on the College website or from the DPT at each hospital. Concise, standard questions will usually be asked. Only two examiners will ask questions—one 'leads' the discussion and the other follows near the end for 5–7 minutes. For reasons of fairness, it is unusual for specialists to 'lead' the examination of a candidate on a patient with problems in their own field. Examiners will not lead if they know the patient or the candidate. Twenty-five minutes are spent with the examiners, presenting the case and discussing diagnosis and management. The discussion period is critical to passing (or failing).

At the end of the time a bell will ring and the candidate is taken to begin the short-case examination. There are a few minutes available, however, for drinking weak orange juice. Many candidates ask the bulldog's opinion of their performance. We believe this to be an unwise policy, since the resident medical officer is usually junior to the examinee and so often gives an incorrect assessment.

The candidate is then introduced to the short-case examiners. The examiners for the first short case are never the same as those who examined for the long case, but you may see the long-case examining team for your second short case. Again, one examiner in each team will be a member of the CFE or NEP. Fifteen minutes are allowed for the first short case; a second short case is then examined after a 5- or 10-minute break. The new examination system does not allow for more than two cases per session. This, and the extension of time to 15 minutes for each case, means that examination of each patient is a little less rushed. However, the result of this extra time means that there is a greater opportunity for the examiners to ask questions related to the physical findings. The examiners assess five domains during the short-case examination: the way the candidate approaches the patient, the thoroughness of the candidate's examination technique, the candidate's accuracy of detecting physical signs, the candidate's ability to offer a diagnosis on the basis of the findings and the candidate's ability to use investigations to support the physical findings. Examining centres have also been told to have X-rays, CT scans, MRI scans and electrocardiograms (ECGs) available for discussion. The key criteria and the skills that are required to achieve a satisfactory standard are available from the College or the DPT.

The other half of the candidates do this routine in the reverse order.

After lunch the second session begins, and this time the order of the short and long cases is reversed for each candidate. There is no longer provision for extra short cases for candidates who are thought to be borderline.

The marking system

The mark required to pass the examination is 40. Each long case is worth 21 marks and each short case is worth 7 marks—so the total mark possible is 70.

The mark awarded for each short case is out of 7 as follows: 1, very poor performance; 2, well short of expected standard; 3, short of expected standard; 4, expected standard;

5, better than expected standard; 6, much better than expected standard; 7, exceptional performance. In 2006 part marks were introduced for the short case, so now for both the long and short cases the scoring system incorporates positives and negatives (part marks) between 1 and 7, giving a 19-point scale. The use of part marks helps some candidates who are very close to a pass overall. For example, if the examiners agree that a candidate's performance was better than a 4 but not deserving of a 5, a 4+ is awarded, while if the candidate's performance was much better than a 4 but not deserving of a 5, the mark will be a 5–. When the marks are added up at the end of the day, 4+ for example will be 4.33 and 5– will be 4.67. Once a 'raw score' out of 7 is awarded, it is weighted; the long-case scores are multiplied by three.

The examiners try very hard to be fair. Each candidate's performance is discussed at the end of each long- and short-case session. Each examiner scores independently: if there is disagreement about a mark, this is discussed and a consensus mark is chosen. If the examiners cannot agree, the NEP member has the final say. Examiners record any special considerations that may have caused difficulties for the candidate (and flag the assessment sheet with the infamous 'red dot') so that these can be considered later by the executive, if necessary. The Chief Examiner of the day (always a member of the CFE or NEP) is responsible for collecting the marked score sheets and dealing with any red dot matters. The examiners do not know the candidate's marks in other sections of the exam (including the written examination), and therefore they do not know the effect of their own mark on the candidate's overall success or failure. The examiners see the same short case four times with four candidates. They give a mark at the end of each session and cannot change this after assessing the other candidates' attempts at the same case. The examination is not meant to be competitive. This means that every candidate can pass if the required standard is achieved.

Rather than trying to pass candidates (as at undergraduate level), the examiners are trying to evaluate the true standard of each candidate. Examinees must prove to the College that they are 'good enough'—that is, they must demonstrate that they have mastered the material and have reached the required standard. The standards are very high, but the College emphasises to the examiners that the standard is that which is required for a person to enter advanced training and not the standard expected of a consultant physician. The rationale for this approach is that trainees who are likely to begin training in a subspecialty should know how to examine all the systems of the body properly and have a sensible approach to the management of medical problems outside their specialty.

Overseas-trained physicians (OTPs) are examined on one long case in their subspecialty area. The standard expected in this case is higher (i.e. at specialist or consultant physician level rather than end-of-basic-training level).

To achieve uniform standards, the CFE has been constantly working on improvements. Senior members of the CFE examine more often with less-experienced examiners. The CFE also holds regular formal calibration exercises, in which all examiners view videotapes and mark a candidate's performance. A general discussion is then held to try to develop a uniform approach. There is no doubt that problems continue, as it remains difficult (if not impossible) to judge ability accurately in such a short period and the calibration is far from perfect; however, the CFE is working towards eliminating obvious mistakes.

The overall pass rate (for the written *and* viva examinations) in any one year in the past was about 40%. The eventual pass rate after success at the written examination and over four vivas (the old system) approached 85%. Under the new system, the pass rate has increased to 65% or more for the clinical year, although more recent results were better than this, thankfully.

The mini-CEX

In 2008 the *mini-CEX* was introduced for basic trainees in their final year; eventually, it will be used in all years of basic training. This is quite separate from the clinical examination and although it has to be performed, it does *not* count towards marks in the formal clinical examination. The trainee undertakes three or four mini-CEX exams a year, usually in the trainee's own hospital and marked by the DPT or a suitably trained delegate. Each exam lasts 20 minutes and is a cross between a long and short case. The trainee is introduced to a patient and given a clinical problem; for example, 'Mr Smith has had problems with dyspnoea for a year and has noticed a recent deterioration in his symptoms. Please take a relevant history and examine him.' The trainee is expected to ask directed questions about the symptoms and then examine the relevant system or systems of the body. This is all observed by the examiner. The trainee then presents the findings and a differential diagnosis, and suggests investigations and possible treatment.

Preparation for the clinical examination

> For one mistake made for not knowing,
> ten mistakes are made for not looking.
>
> *JA Lindsay*

The clinical examination aims to test not only clinical ability but also attitudes and interpersonal skills. For most candidates a successful approach to the viva depends on seeing a large number of long and short practice cases. It is usually too late to start practising these cases after passing the written examination; preparation should start at least several months beforehand.

To practise for the long cases, try to set aside a regular time each week. Most physicians, if approached, are only too willing to test-run candidates. Being exposed to many different examiners is desirable—this will help iron out mistakes and provide practice in answering different types of questions. Although most teaching hospitals have a training scheme in which long cases are examined by consultants or senior registrars, this is not enough. It is difficult to quote numbers, but we believe 50 formal long cases (across all disciplines) in which different specialists and senior registrars act as examiners represent the bare minimum requirement for preparation. Remember also that each time a patient is admitted to hospital, practice can be gained in the long-case technique—this turns overtime into useful preparation time. Practising cases is also critical in order to be able to cope with management issues in Paper 2 of the written examination.

Practice for the short cases is also important. More examinees used to fail these than the long cases, although this has changed now that the long cases are receiving more emphasis. It is valuable to have senior colleagues, as well as peers, take you on short cases. Travelling to other hospitals to practise is also worthwhile, because you have to examine in strange surroundings while being watched by unfamiliar examiners—it also relieves the boredom somewhat. The best practice examiner is the one who frightens candidates a little but does not demolish them when they make an error. Seek out constructive criticism. For example, many candidates practise in pairs, each person taking turns to be the examiner. Practising being an examiner helps you to appreciate the bad habits that annoy the real examiners.

Equipment is always provided at the hospital where the examination is held. However, it is important to take the following:

1. a familiar stethoscope that you have used for a long time; do not buy a new fancier stethoscope the day before the test—it takes time to get used to a new instrument

2. a hand-held eye card—obtainable from OPSM for a moderate charge and essential for cranial nerve or eye examinations (see Ch 15)
3. a red-tipped hatpin—you can buy a plain one and paint the top with nail polish; this is invaluable for visual field testing (see Ch 15)
4. paper and pens.

It is debatable whether candidates should take in their own bags of instruments. Many favour bringing their own ophthalmoscope and pocket torch (with fresh batteries in both). Others also like to have cotton wool, neurology pins (an unused one for each case) and spatulas, as well as tuning forks (256 Hz and 128 Hz) and a patella hammer, which is too much to carry in the pockets. This has led to a trend for leather briefcases to house all the equipment (see Fig 3.1). However, the occasional difficult examiner has been known to complain about this! There is a story about one candidate's briefcase, which was filled with such elaborate equipment, including an inverted cardigan for testing dressing apraxia, that his examiners spent their time inspecting the contents rather than watching him examine the patient (not a recommended approach!).

1. Eye charts
2. Buttons and long patella hammer (underneath)
3. Stethoscope
4. Torch
5. Tape measure
6. Tuning forks
7. Ophthalmoscope and auriscope
8. Hatpins (red and white)
9. Jar with lid (containing key for key grip assessment)
10. Disposable neurology pins
11. Cotton wool
12. Spatula
13. Cotton buds and spare patella hammer
14. Carefully shaped foam inserts

Figure 3.1 A candidate's bag

A few more cautionary tales:
• Candidates who have just bought their bags have been known to forget the combination number needed to release the lock at the critical moment in the exam when the bag has to be opened.

- One candidate placed her open bag on the sink in the examination room for her first case, only to have the bag flooded with water when one of the examiners leaned closer to watch the examination and accidentally turned on the tap above the sink.

HINT BOX
1. Remember your bag lock combination number.
2. Do not place your bag on a sink.

During practice sessions, it is always a good idea to place equipment in the same pockets each time. In the exam, you do not want to be fumbling at this crucial time—it will only create a poor impression. Consultants, other than cardiologists, carry their stethoscopes or put them in their coat pocket; rarely do they place them around their neck. This seems a sensible policy for aspiring consultants also. Candidates who do carry a briefcase into the test (and many neurologists carry one everywhere) can usually place it on the patient's bedside table and leave it open so that its contents are easily accessible.

Some candidates take beta-blockers on the day of the test to remain calm. An interesting story from the *Lancet* highlights this very situation. A Scottish physician refers to a British censor who had the habit of counting the temporal pulse of candidates: if he found that the pulse rate was less than 60 beats/minute, he would take this fact into account when giving his mark (Bamber MG 1980 Dope test for doctors. *Lancet* ii:1308). We are unaware of a similar practice in Australasia. However, candidates intending to use these drugs should give themselves a dose during a practice session. One doctor who did not do this learnt to his horror during the actual examination that beta-blockers caused him severe bronchospasm (he failed).

Nervous individuals with a tendency to sweat can have problems. One candidate (now a professor) who was balding and wore glasses, found that, during times of intense stress, rivers of sweat rolled down from his forehead to fog up his glasses and wash them from his nose. His solution was antiperspirant (unscented of course) applied to the forehead (he passed).

Dress is important. The medical establishment is well known for its conservatism, and the nonverbal messages that your appearance gives should not be forgotten when dressing. Traditionally, men and women wear a conservative suit and men a noncommittal tie. Other important considerations for men are having short tidy hair, a neatly trimmed beard if you cannot bear to shave it off, and a neutral smell. Dress formally, with care to project an air of quiet efficiency. White coats are never worn. However, being well dressed is no guarantee of success. There is a story of two male candidates, wearing grey suits and with recently cut hair, who were viewing with satisfaction a third examinee whose long hair was tied neatly in a bun and who was dressed in a flowing Kaftan-like garment—they felt their own success assured with such competition. However, it turned out that they were unsuccessful and their colleague passed.

Preparation is the key to success. Like an Olympic athlete, obtain plenty of sleep in the week before the ordeal; take no alcohol or tranquillisers in the 48 hours before it; and do not study during the final 24 hours. Make sure that you eat something before the examination and avoid taking a long trip to the examination city on the morning of or the night before the test.

Chapter 4

The long case

In what manner are the examiners elected? Are
they elected by the profession or any part of the
profession whose interests are equal to those
of the whole and are they responsible to the
profession at large for their conduct?
Neither the one nor the other.

Lancet 1824; i:20

When the examiners discuss a long case with a candidate, they are expecting to find out how the candidate would manage the patient and his or her problems. They want to know whether the candidate has a practical grasp of what is required in consultant practice. Candidates are expected to have a mature and sensible approach to the patient and his or her problems. It may help to picture yourself as the physician taking over the care of a new patient. Practising long cases trains candidates to be better clinicians.

Careful allocation of time with the patient in the long case is vital. The exact proportions will depend on the case itself but, as a rough guide, spend 25 minutes on the history-taking, 15 minutes on the examination and the rest of the time preparing discussion and reviewing vital facts with the patient. Nothing is more important than ensuring you leave enough time to put your thoughts in order.

Candidates favour many different systems for recording long case details (as an aid to memory). There are two we recommend. One is to use a small pad that can be held comfortably in the hand and the pages turned unobtrusively. The other is a small card system. One side is used for the history and the other for the examination findings; a second card (if necessary) is used for relevant investigations, management and short lists of facts you may wish to mention. Obviously, numbering each side is important so as not to mix up the order of presentation. These cards are usually provided to candidates who want them at the examination site. Mixing up the cards can be a disaster. One candidate was sitting, preparing to enter the examination room, when the side door opened and a puff of wind blew the cards out of her hands. She was then ushered straight into the examination room with the cards in random order. She began the long case badly and failed.

Candidates who do not want to rewrite the whole long-case presentation before facing the examiners (time is often a problem) may find it helpful to number the paragraphs with a red pen in the order in which they wish to present the story.

Many examination centres provide manila folders. These are large enough for candidates to be able to write out one whole long case on one folder.

The history-taking and physical examination

Once you have said 'How do you do?' to the patient at the beginning of the long case, we suggest initially following the steps outlined below. These may help you rapidly ascertain the patient's major problems so that you can direct further questioning more easily.

1. Explain to the patient that this is a very important examination. Gain the patient's interest and support. This is a test of bedside manner.
2. Ask the patient what is wrong. If he or she says 'Am I allowed to tell you?', look confident and firm and say 'Yes, of course'. Candidates are entitled to all the information the patient can offer.
3. Ask why the patient is in hospital this time (i.e. is he or she an inpatient or outpatient?) and, if relevant, the presenting symptoms when he or she was admitted. A number of patients are brought in specifically for the examination and will have no acute medical problems.
4. Ask early on what medications the patient is taking. This will give you valuable information about both current and past problems.
5. Ask the patient about any recent tests, again to obtain clues about the current problem.

In the majority of long cases, the patient has a chronic illness about which he or she may be very well informed. It is sensible to make use of this knowledge, but remember the trap that patients may be biased in their opinions and give (inadvertently) false information. Having established the main diagnosis early, confirm this with specific questioning. On finding symptoms not fitting the diagnosis, decide the likely possibilities and follow up with further questions. Never blindly believe the patient.

Next, enquire about other problems. Most long-case patients are chosen because they have multiple medical problems. An example might be an elderly woman with pulmonary fibrosis as her major presenting illness who also has significant ischaemic heart disease and chronic kidney disease and peptic ulceration secondary to aspirin use. It is a terrible experience to discover another major illness only minutes before the end of the time. List all the important diseases chronologically and obtain full details about each one. Organise to present the most important (i.e. often the current) problem first, followed by the others in order of importance. Some healthy scepticism about the patient's opinion of the diagnosis is usually warranted. A history of exotic previous illnesses without a history of appropriate investigations or treatment for such conditions should prompt a careful retaking of the history.

It is important to appreciate the great amount of detail the examiners will expect about the patient's past history. A lot of time needs to be spent on this. Failing to uncover a medical problem from long ago that the examiners found when they saw the patient counts against the candidate. Remember that the patient's history is often well rehearsed after the examiners and perhaps another candidate have taken it.

If the patient has an illness that can become suddenly severe or life-threatening—for example, asthma or insulin requiring diabetes—ask whether there is an *action plan*. That is, does the patient know what to do or whom to contact if he or she becomes suddenly worse? All patients should be asked about their immunisation status, including influenza, hepatitis A and B, and pneumococcus.

Do not forget the social history. This is especially important because the examiners (and society) are keen to have caring specialists who are fully aware of the complete social environment of their patients. The examiners will expect great detail here as well. Always ask about:

- *occupation*—now and in the past
- *adequacy of income*—particularly if the patient is on a pension
- *current housing arrangements*—e.g. renting, mortgage
- *ability to cope* at home and the quality of life if this is a chronic disease problem—the activities of daily living (ADLs) should be assessed
- *mobility*—particularly the number of steps that need to be climbed at home and at work, and on which floor of the building the patient lives

- *hobbies*—e.g. contact with animals, chemicals or dusts
- *marital status* and number of children
- *sexual problems*—particularly ask about erectile dysfunction in men (e.g. diabetic patients)
- *place of birth*
- *overseas travel* in relationship to the illness.

A family history must also be taken. This sort of information is easy to obtain and fills in discussion time neatly, but disaster can threaten if the candidate does not know it. The most important aspects should be outlined in your initial presentation and the rest kept in reserve to be unleashed if the examiners show an interest.

As you examine the patient, always ask when the examiners came, what parts they examined and whether any comments were made about the signs. One candidate was told by his patient that, during a fundoscopic examination, the examiner had said: 'What an interesting Roth's spot!' However, this is no substitute for a thorough examination.

Even though you should spend most time on the relevant systems, remember that sometimes unexpected signs will crop up, such as a large breast mass, gross papilloedema or an abdominal mass. The examiners always have in front of them a list of the signs and have always gone to the trouble of checking that, in fact, these signs are present. You will be expected to have found all the important signs, so be thorough. Any very equivocal findings should probably be ignored. Ask the bulldog for the results of the urinalysis and rectal examination; you are not expected to perform these personally. Also, don't forget to take the patient's blood pressure at some stage and check for a postural change, if at all relevant (e.g. diabetes mellitus).

At the end of the history-taking and physical examination, always ask the patient: 'Is there anything else you think I should know?' Amazingly important information is often volunteered at this point. Then ask yourself: 'Could this be anything else?' and 'Can I tie all the multisystem problems into one disease?'

During the 20 minutes or so remaining, decide what type of case it is—that is, is it a *treatment* problem or a *diagnostic* problem, or both? Sort out the active from the inactive problems. Draft your introductory statement; for example, 'I saw Mrs J Smith, a 30-year-old woman, who presents for the treatment problem of active rheumatoid arthritis and also for the diagnostic problem of jaundice'.

Next, mentally rehearse presenting the history and examination concisely and clearly. Your concluding statement should reiterate the problems (in order of importance). It is usual to end the presentation by requests for relevant investigations. Always formulate a differential diagnosis, even if the history and examination lead to a definite diagnosis. Create a list of the findings on history and examination that support (or refute) the diagnoses considered. If a positive diagnosis cannot confidently be made, try to decide on the most likely diagnosis.

The discovery of a major problem with a particular long case (e.g. a patient with obvious dementia) shouldn't lead to panic. By recognising the problem, fully examining the patient and having a plan of management (finding reversible causes, eliciting from relatives the social set-up etc.), you will pass. One candidate who was faced with a demented patient in the long-case examination became angry and complained bitterly to his examiners. He failed.

Occasionally there are other difficulties, such as language problems (usually the candidate is supplied with an interpreter) or the patient becomes ill during the time (cardiac arrests have occurred). Be sure to inform the bulldog of any difficulties—people will go out of their way to be fair in such circumstances. The examiners will usually make a note of any such problems on their scoresheet, so that this can be taken into account by the executive later on. The lead examiner will ask the candidate as the first question if there were any problems with the patient during the case.

The presentation

Your whole presentation to the examiners should take 10–12 minutes. Leave out any irrelevant detail—padding the presentation never impresses. Avoid repetition, for example mentioning various medications as a part of the history of a particular system and then later as part of a long general list. Also, remember never to use abbreviations when presenting (e.g. do not use JVP for jugular venous pressure or MCP joint for metacarpophalangeal joint).

The examiners are only human too: sometimes they are hungry, tired or just bored after previous presentations (particularly if yours is the last long case of the afternoon). Show interest and enthusiasm while speaking. Do not read your notes in a monotone. The notes are meant to be a memory aid. Ideally, the long case should be a discussion between consultants, with the candidate being a respectful junior colleague. The examiners only rarely interrupt during the presentation. At the end they may try to clarify a particular point. Sometimes they direct the candidate to a particular line of discussion.

It is likely that the examiners will want to discuss the patient's active problems. These should be the areas of management that you are best prepared for. It is very unsatisfactory for examiners to feel that they have not been told all the major problems, and what the management plan for each problem is, by the end of the discussion. At the end of your presentation and before discussion of management, the examiners may ask some questions to clarify aspects of the history or examination findings. This should be no cause for alarm. After this you are usually given the opportunity to outline a plan of management or the examiners may ask specific questions. Examining styles differ, but you should strive to direct the discussion tactfully. Being allowed to do this is usually a good sign, but not being allowed to control the discussion is not necessarily a bad sign.

When appropriate, ask for one or two important investigations relevant to the problems, rather than for a string of routine tests. *A reason should be given for ordering every test.* For a diagnostic problem it may be useful to ask for the results of previous investigations. Any mentioned test may have to be discussed in detail with the examiners. We suggest that you write down the results you are told (it is embarrassing to have to ask for the figures to be repeated). Don't ignore any information that is given; for example, if the haemoglobin value is normal, comment on this and explain how it helps. Remember not to touch X-ray films or criticise the quality of the material shown. Pathological specimens are not shown in the clinical examinations.

Always prepare answers to the obvious lines of question and try to think like a consultant physician who is in charge of the patient's care (and hypothesise that the patient is a close relative of the examiner!). If there is a diagnostic dilemma, consider the tests you want and how positive and negative results will support or refute your proposed diagnoses. In a management case, prepare an outline of the suggested treatment and be able to justify it. Always set management goals for all key therapeutic interventions. The examiners may ask about theoretical aspects of the condition. Most often, they will concentrate the testing of factual knowledge in areas that are necessary for the formulation of adequate management decisions or interpretation of test results. You should think about these areas beforehand. Always consider whether the patient's current treatment is justified and whether the diagnosis previously made is consistent with the history and examination; it may not be. Do not be afraid to contradict the current management if there is clear justification.

A common series of questions for many long cases involving chronic diseases includes aspects of how you would discuss the illness and the prognosis with the patient. The examiners might ask: 'What would you tell Mrs Smith about her prognosis and likely future treatment?' and 'What would you advise her about the safety of future pregnancies?'

The examiners will not usually ask hypothetical questions unrelated to the patient being discussed. If you are answering well, the line of questioning may change or the depth may become overwhelming. Do *not* be frightened to say, in the latter situation, 'Sir [or Madam], I don't know', when asked a very difficult question. Obvious wild guesses will be detrimental. If the examiner persists in asking a question, it usually means he or she is trying to establish a basic fact. Talk sensibly around the topic—often a supplementary question will result in recall of the appropriate information. With an especially difficult issue it is reasonable to say you would consult the literature or an appropriate subspecialist for advice. Remember that examiners are instructed to avoid making snap judgements or failing candidates because of one small mistake.

You must be able to discuss sensibly anything that you mention in a viva, so don't casually allude to rare diseases that you know nothing about (e.g. kala-azar as a cause of massive splenomegaly).

The long-case rationale

The long case is a test of the candidate's ability at history-taking, physical examination, interpretation of findings and construction of a diagnosis (and differential diagnosis), and approach to management (investigation and treatment). Important and common long cases are presented in some detail in the next chapters. The list in Table 4.1 is not exhaustive but gives an idea of the range of possible cases. Most (but not all) are discussed in Chapters 5–13—some other relevant aspects are dealt with in Chapter 15.

TABLE 4.1 Common long cases
Cardiovascular long cases (Ch 5)
1. Ischaemic heart disease (p 25)
2. Infective endocarditis (p 32)
3. Congestive cardiac failure (p 37)
4. Hyperlipidaemia (p 45)
5. Hypertension (p 50)
6. Cardiac arrhythmias and atrial fibrillation (p 59)
7. Heart transplantation (p 54)
8. Valvular heart disease (p 32)
9. Revascularisation (p 30)
10. Pacemaker or implantable cardioverter-defibrillators (ICD) (p 64)
Respiratory long cases (Ch 6)
1. Bronchiectasis (p 71)
2. Lung carcinoma (p 73)
3. Chronic obstructive pulmonary disease (chronic airflow limitation [p 79])
4. Tuberculosis (p 104)
5. Interstitial lung disease (p 87)
6. Pulmonary hypertension (p 91)
7. Sarcoidosis (p 97)
8. Cystic fibrosis (p 101)

(Continues)

TABLE 4.1 Common long cases (Continued)

Respiratory long cases (Ch 6) (continued)

9. Sleep apnoea (p 84)

10. Lung transplantation (p 110)

Gastrointestinal long cases (Ch 7)

1. Peptic ulceration (p 113)

2. Malabsorption (p 116)

3. Inflammatory bowel disease (p 120)

4. Colon cancer (p 125)

5. Chronic liver disease (p 127)

6. Hepatitis B (p 133)

7. Hepatitis C (p 134)

8. Liver transplantation (p 137)

Haematological long cases (Ch 8)

1. Haemolytic anaemia (p 141)

2. Myeloproliferative diseases, e.g. polycythaemia rubra vera (p 151), idiopathic myelofibrosis (p 155) and essential thrombocythaemia (p 156)

3. Lymphomas (p 157)

4. Leukaemia (p 156)

5. Multiple myeloma (p 165)

6. Thrombophilia (p 147)

7. Bone marrow transplantation (p 170)

8. Breast cancer

Rheumatological long cases (Ch 9)

1. Rheumatoid arthritis (p 175)

2. Ankylosing spondylitis

3. Systemic lupus erythematosus (p 181)

4. Antiphospholipid antibody syndrome (p 190)

5. Scleroderma (p 192)

6. Systemic vasculitis (p 186)

Endocrine long cases (Ch 10)

1. Thyrotoxicosis

2. Hypothyroidism

3. Panhypopituitarism

4. Cushing's syndrome

5. Acromegaly (p 210)

6. Addison's disease

7. Phaeochromocytoma

8. Paget's disease of the bone (p 205)

TABLE 4.1 Common long cases (Continued)

Endocrine long cases (Ch 10) (continued)

9. Diabetes mellitus (p 213)

10. Hypercalcaemia (p 203)

11. Osteoporosis (and osteomalacia) (p 197)

Renal long cases (Ch 11)

1. Chronic kidney disease (chronic renal failure) (p 223)

2. Renal transplantation (p 231)

3. Nephrotic syndrome (see Table 11.2)

Neurological long cases (Ch 12)

1. Multiple sclerosis (p 235)

2. Myasthenia gravis (p 238)

3. Guillain-Barré syndrome (p 240)

4. Transient ischaemic attacks and 'funny turns' (p 242)

Infectious disease long cases (Ch 13)

1. Pyrexia of unknown origin (PUO) (p 247)

2. Human immunodeficiency virus (HIV) infection (p 250)

Types of long case

The cases in Chapters 5–13 are written as a guide to dealing with the long-case examination and are not meant to replace textbook descriptions. To pass you must really know and understand your general medicine. Remember that usually several problems occur in the one case. A patient with an unusual diagnosis will often have one or more common problems as well.

The examiners will often ask whether you would like the results of appropriate investigations. Be prepared to interpret any results you have asked for. Electrocardiograms (ECGs), chest X-rays, and computed tomography (CT) and magnetic resonance imaging (MRI) scans may be shown to candidates. Echocardiogram tapes are not usually shown to candidates but you are expected to be able to interpret echocardiography reports. Some common examples are included in Chapters 5–13 and also in Chapter 15. At the end of each report is a comment that gives an idea of the sort of interpretation expected from candidates.

We wish you good luck in the examination, but remember that great preparation is the key to success, so please read on.

Chapter 5

The cardiovascular long case

A rule of thumb in the matter of medical advice
is to take everything any doctor says with a grain
of aspirin.

Goodman Ace (1899–1982)

Ischaemic heart disease

Patients with recent acute coronary syndromes, including myocardial infarction, are always available for long cases if required. Many patients with more exotic medical problems will also have ischaemic heart disease. The whims of the long-case examiners may lead to concentrated questioning about the ischaemic heart disease of a patient in hospital for the management of, say, renal transplant rejection. These patients are more likely to present management rather than diagnostic problems once they reach the status of long-case patients.

There have been important changes in the classification of patients with episodes of acute coronary ischaemia. These are based on electrocardiogram (ECG) changes and on the detection of markers of myocardial damage (troponins), which have prognostic as well as diagnostic usefulness for patients with chest pain. Patients with chest pain and raised troponin levels have had a myocardial infarction even if the creatine kinase level is not elevated. Those who present with chest pain and ECG changes of ST elevation have an ST elevation myocardial infarction (STEMI). Those without ST elevation are said to have a non-ST elevation acute coronary syndrome (NSTEACS), but once abnormal cardiac markers have been detected the diagnosis can be revised to a non-ST elevation myocardial infarction (non-STEMI). The diagnosis *unstable angina* is no longer part of this classification.

Patients with ST elevation benefit from urgent action to reopen the blocked coronary artery (angioplasty or thrombolytic treatment). Those with non-STEMI are usually treated medically in the first instance. The presence of abnormal cardiac markers indicates an adverse prognosis (increased risk of further infarction or death) and these patients benefit from early but not immediate intervention (angioplasty or coronary surgery) and from immediate aggressive anti-platelet treatment and anticoagulation with fractionated or unfractionated heparin. Non-STEMI patients who have ST depression on the ECG have a worse prognosis than those with T wave inversion or flattening. The concept of risk stratification is based on these factors and determines the urgency and type of treatment.

The history

1. Find out whether the patient has been or is in hospital because of a recent myocardial infarction or an acute coronary syndrome (previously called unstable angina) or

25

for some other cardiac or non-cardiac reason. The term 'unstable angina' may reasonably be used for a patient who has experienced the recent onset of angina, a change (for the worse) in the pattern of existing angina or episodes of angina at rest. The most unstable patients (those with an acute coronary syndrome) are those with chest pain and ECG changes at rest (see Table 5.1). Clearly, these may represent different pathophysiological states, varying from occlusion of a coronary artery and inadequate collateral flow to rupture of a lipid-rich plaque with thrombus formation. Ask about obvious precipitating factors, such as a gastrointestinal bleed or the onset of an arrhythmia. Questions need to be asked about the character of the chest pain and what precipitated the admission.

Remember that the diagnosis of angina can be suspected from the history but needs to be established by investigations—an abnormal ECG or exercise test at least. You should be suspicious of the diagnosis unless it has been confirmed by investigations. The most common differential diagnosis is gastro-oesophageal reflux disease (GORD). This can be difficult to prove without endoscopy (and, if normal, oesophageal pH testing), but an excellent response to a trial of a proton pump inhibitor (PPI) is very suggestive.

2. Detail the patient's current treatment. Oral medications will probably include:
   - aspirin
   - a beta-blocker or occasionally a calcium antagonist
   - nitrates (intravenous, oral or topical)
   - statin
   - an angiotensin-converting enzyme (ACE) inhibitor or angiotensin II receptor (AR) blocker (ARB).

TABLE 5.1 Risk stratification in patients with ischaemic chest pain at rest

Highest to lowest risk

1. ST elevation myocardial infarction
2. ST depression
3. T wave inversion
4. Non-specific ST-T wave changes
5. Normal ECG

- The risk is higher in each group if cardiac biomarkers (troponins) are elevated.
- The risk is higher in each group for patients with previous ischaemic heart disease or diabetes.
- The higher the risk, the more the benefit of aggressive treatment.

Management history

1. Acute coronary syndromes are managed with heparin and aspirin and often clopidogrel. An additional benefit is obtained with glycoprotein IIb/IIIa (platelet aggregation) inhibitors in non-STEMI subsets of patients (those with resting ECG changes, especially ST depression, and those with increased troponin levels and continuing symptoms).

   Thrombolytic treatment is not effective for NSTEACS. This is possibly because acute coronary syndromes are not a single pathological entity and also because a state of increased thrombogenesis may follow initial thrombolysis with these drugs.

   Most patients have early angiography (within 48 hours) with the intention of angioplasty to the culprit lesion if this is practical. Ask whether the patient knows details of what investigations or treatment were performed.

2. If the patient has had an infarct during this or previous admissions, find out about the management, which may have included primary angioplasty or thrombolysis, and treatment of complications such as arrhythmias, cardiac failure, further angina and embolic events.

3. In many hospitals a comprehensive cardiac rehabilitation program will have been offered to the patient. Ask whether this has been helpful and ask about the hospital staff's explanations to the patient about his or her condition and prognosis. Also ask questions about the effect of this illness on the patient's life and work.

4. Next ask standard questions about risk factors in addition to age and male sex. Remember that risk factors are of vital importance to long-term prognosis, but add little to the likelihood that undiagnosed chest pain is ischaemic. Risk factors include:
   • previous ischaemic heart disease
   • hyperlipidaemia
   • diabetes mellitus (the increased risk in these patients is as high as that in non-diabetics who have already had an ischaemic event)
   • hypertension
   • family history (in particular, first-degree relatives with ischaemic heart disease before the age of 60; 92-year-old great-uncles with heart trouble do not count)
   • smoking
   • use of oral contraceptives or premature onset of menopause
   • obesity and physical inactivity
   • high serum homocysteine levels, which may have been measured if the patient has premature coronary disease and few other risk factors—levels in the top population quintile increase coronary risk twofold; trials of treatment (mostly with folate), however, have been negative and routine treatment is not recommended
   • long-term use, in high doses, of cyclo-oxygenase 2 (COX-2) inhibitors or other non-steroidal anti-inflammatory drugs (NSAIDs) (which should be stopped)
   • erectile dysfunction (which often precedes symptomatic ischaemic heart disease and is a marker of endothelial dysfunction).
   Remember that the presence of multiple risk factors is more than additive.

5. Then find out whether risk factor control has been successful. Remember the important results of recent secondary prevention trials.
   (a) Aggressive cholesterol lowering to below a level of 4 mmol/L of total cholesterol is now considered appropriate for patients with established coronary disease.
   (b) There is some evidence that statins have beneficial effects beyond their effect on cholesterol levels (pleotrophic effects).

6. Find out what investigations the patient can remember.
   (a) An echocardiogram may have been performed to assess ventricular function and possible complications of infarction, such as a pericardial collection, a left ventricular thrombus, mitral regurgitation or a ventricular septal defect (VSD).
   (b) An exercise test, a sestamibi or thallium scan or a stress echocardiogram may have been performed to assess ischaemia or myocardial viability.
   (c) Cardiac catheterisation is perhaps the most memorable of the investigations for ischaemic heart disease.
   The patient may know how many coronaries are abnormal and whether angioplasty was performed. Ask whether a drug-eluting stent (DES) was used

and for how long dual anti-platelet treatment was recommended. Remember clopidogrel, and probably most PPIs, use the same metabolic pathway in the liver and if used together may result in a loss of anti-platelet benefit.

7. Complications such as acute mitral regurgitation or an infarct-related VSD are usually treated surgically but have a relatively poor prognosis. All complications are less common if early coronary patency has been achieved.

The examination

Examine the cardiovascular system (p 263).

1. Note the presence of intravenous treatment. This might include heparin, nitrates, inotropes, vasopressors or antiarrhythmic drugs.
2. Record the blood pressure.
3. Look for signs of valvular heart disease, cardiac failure, rhythm disturbances (e.g. atrial fibrillation, frequent ectopic beats) and murmurs suggesting mitral regurgitation or a VSD caused by an infarct.
4. There may be spectacular bruises at venepuncture or femoral puncture sites if the patient has had thrombolytic treatment. Abdominal wall bruising suggests subcutaneous low-molecular-weight heparin therapy, and a bruise (sometimes very large) over one of the femoral arteries suggests cardiac catheterisation or angioplasty. More general complications include a stroke owing to embolism from the heart.

Management

It is best to concentrate on discussing the management of the presenting problem. If the patient has only recently been admitted with an infarct, this means a discussion of thrombolysis and primary angioplasty.

1. Candidates should have some knowledge of the major thrombolysis and angioplasty trials.
   (a) These have shown that early treatment has improved mortality. Treatment up to 12 hours after the onset of an infarct is worthwhile.
   (b) The indications and contraindications to the use of these techniques need to be well understood. The major differences between streptokinase and the fibrin-specific drugs (tPA [alteplase] or reteplase) are important. Streptokinase is much cheaper. Alteplase and reteplase have been shown to produce a small survival advantage, probably because they are more effective in opening occluded vessels, but have a slightly increased risk of causing cerebral haemorrhage. Alteplase is the drug of choice for patients who have had a previous dose of streptokinase more than a few days before. This is because antibodies to streptokinase develop within a few days and may cause an allergic reaction to a second dose, thus reducing its effectiveness.
   (c) Alteplase is given as a bolus followed by an infusion and reteplase is given as a double bolus injection with a 30-minute interval.
2. Urgent coronary (primary) angioplasty, if available, is of proven benefit and has been shown to reduce mortality compared with treatment with thrombolytic drugs.
   (a) The advantages, theoretical and real, include definite reopening of the infarct-related artery in more than 90% of patients (compared with <60% of patients given thrombolytics), normal flow in the infarct-related artery in most cases, dilatation and stenting of the offending (culprit) lesion and often removal of clot, very low risk of stroke and shortening of hospital stay, often to only three days.

(b) Patients are treated with potent anti-platelet drugs: aspirin, clopidogrel and often with one of the platelet aggregation inhibitors, abciximab or tirofiban.

(c) There is now trial evidence that transport of patients to a hospital where this procedure can be performed is preferable to treatment with thrombolytic drugs, if transport time is less than 2–3 hours.

(d) Rapid transport to the catheter laboratory is important and the 'door to balloon' time should be less than 90 minutes when angioplasty is available in the hospital to which the patient presented.

3. If the history has suggested complications resulting from the infarct, these will have to be discussed. Common complications include:
  • ventricular arrhythmias
  • bradyarrhythmias (especially following an inferior infarct)
  • cardiac failure
  • further ischaemia or reinfarction.

  It is important to have planned an approach to the management of these problems.

Investigations

These are aimed at assessment of the infarct size, complications and presence of further ischaemia:

1. **left ventricular function**—echocardiogram, left ventriculogram
2. **complications**—echocardiogram for valvular regurgitation, left ventricular thrombus, infarct-related VSD
3. **further ischaemia**—exercise test, sestamibi stress test, cardiac catheterisation.

Long-term treatment

1. Early revascularisation is of proven benefit for high-risk patients with acute coronary syndromes (ST elevation, troponin elevation).
2. Prognosis is improved with aspirin, beta-blockers and, for large infarcts (ejection fraction <40%), ACE inhibitors and beta-blockers (e.g. carvedilol, bisoprolol and extended-release metoprolol).
3. Patients with three-vessel disease and significant left ventricular damage or with left main coronary artery stenosis benefit prognostically from coronary artery bypass surgery even if their symptoms have settled on medical treatment. Those with tight proximal (before the first diagonal branch) left anterior descending lesions probably also benefit from surgery or angioplasty.
4. Epleronone, an aldosterone antagonist, is indicated for patients with cardiac failure following an infarct.

Secondary prevention

1. Control of cardiac risk factors is even more important once the presence of coronary artery disease has been established. It should be a routine part of the management of these patients.
2. Dietary advice for weight and lipid reduction may be indicated. Lipid-lowering drug treatment with a statin should be introduced for all patients who can tolerate it. Total cholesterol should be reduced to less than 4.0 mmol/L (aim for the LDL to be below 1.8 mmol/L).
3. Patients should be encouraged to take part in a cardiac rehabilitation program, if this is available, where advice about safe exercise, weight reduction and changes to dietary and smoking habits can be encouraged.

Revascularisation

For some long-case patients with ischaemic heart disease the emphasis will be on revascularisation (coronary surgery or angioplasty). These procedures are so common that many patients with other presenting problems will have had them.

The history

Similar information to that outlined in the ischaemic heart disease long case is required.

1. Careful questioning about risk factor control, both before and after surgery or angioplasty, is very important. The patient should know whether he or she has ever had an infarct and may know whether there was significant left ventricular damage.
2. Find out what procedure (or procedures) the patient has had and whether there has been complete relief of symptoms.
3. If coronary artery surgery was performed, ask how many grafts were inserted and whether internal mammary or other arterial (e.g. radial artery) conduits were used. It may be possible from the history to work out whether surgery was performed to improve symptoms or prognosis (e.g. three-vessel or left main disease), or both.
4. The patient will probably know how many vessels were dilated if angioplasty was performed and whether stents were inserted. The patient may know whether bare metal stents (BMS) or drug-eluting stents were used. Ask whether the angioplasty was performed in the setting of a myocardial infarction or acute coronary syndrome. Find out for how long clopidogrel was prescribed.

The examination

Examine the patient as for the ischaemic heart disease long case.

1. Note the presence of a median sternotomy scar. Patients who have had a left internal mammary artery (LIMA) graft often have a numb patch to the left of the sternum. This may be permanent.
2. Look at the sternal wound for signs of infection; osteomyelitis of the sternum is a rare but disastrous complication of surgery. Look and feel for sternal instability. Sternal wires are often palpable.
3. Examine the arms for the very large scar that results from radial artery harvesting.
4. Examine the legs for saphenous vein harvesting wounds. Infection and breakdown of these wounds are more common than for the sternal wound.

Management

Surgery

Use of the left internal mammary artery to graft the left anterior descending (LAD) coronary artery has been routine for more than 15 years. Other arterial conduits are used less often, but 'all arterial revascularisation' is performed routinely in some centres or where saphenous vein grafts (SVGs) are not possible (previous coronary artery bypass graft [CABG] or varicose veins in both legs and thighs). In these cases the right internal mammary artery (RIMA) may be used, usually to graft the right coronary, or the radial artery is used as a free arterial graft. The RIMA may also be used as a free graft attached to the aorta if that is necessary to make it reach. There is excellent evidence that LIMA grafts have a higher long-term patency rate (>90% at 10 years) than SVGs (50% at 10 years). There is less information about other arterial conduits.

In response to the increasing numbers of angioplasty procedures, surgeons have begun to perform fewer invasive bypass procedures. The most widely used alternative is the 'off-pump' LIMA graft to the LAD coronary artery. A median sternotomy incision is still used, but the LIMA is attached to the LAD coronary artery on the beating heart. A 'Y' graft from the LIMA to the circumflex and right coronaries can be performed using the RIMA attached to the LIMA. These operations avoid the need for cardiopulmonary bypass, speed recovery and possibly reduce the risk of intraoperative cerebral events. Minimally invasive bypasses are carried out in some centres. A series of lateral chest incisions are used as ports for surgery using thoracoscopic equipment. The technique is not easy and the chest wound, although small, is not necessarily less painful than a median sternotomy.

Angina may recur at any time after CABG. Very early angina suggests a technical problem, such as mammary artery spasm, thrombosis of an SVG, grafting of the wrong vessel or grafting of the correct vessel but proximal to the area of stenosis. Sometimes revascularisation may be 'incomplete' because one or more vessels were unsuitable for grafting—usually because of distal disease in the target vessel.

Recurrence of angina is more common if risk factors have not been aggressively controlled. Low-dose aspirin has also been shown to prolong graft survival. When angina recurs the patient usually describes symptoms similar in character to the old ones. Recurrent chest pain that is different from the old angina is less likely to be ischaemic.

Angioplasty

Angioplasty is now performed more often than surgery in many centres. It has not been shown to improve the prognosis for patients with stable angina. A number of studies have shown a similar outcome to surgery in patients with three-vessel disease, but at the expense of a higher number of repeat procedures. Diabetics were a subgroup with a worse outcome from angioplasty than from surgery.

Many angioplasties are performed to provide symptom relief for patients with one- or two-vessel disease. Increasingly, however, patients with acute coronary syndromes, and especially those with raised troponin levels, are treated with early angioplasty. There is now good evidence that this group of patients has an improved prognosis (fewer deaths and fewer large infarcts) and a shortened hospital stay when treated aggressively with angioplasty.

The majority (>90%) of dilated vessels are now stented, which has made a considerable difference to the risk of acute closure of the artery or the need for urgent surgery (now a rare event). It has also reduced the clinical restenosis rate (i.e. recurrence of symptoms and angiographic evidence of >50% loss of luminal diameter) from almost 40% to 10%.

Dual anti-platelet treatment with aspirin and clopidogrel has made subacute stent thrombosis a rare event (<1%). Clopidogrel is ideally given for 48 hours before angioplasty and for at least four weeks afterwards; six months to a year is often recommended for patients who have had an acute coronary syndrome.

For patients treated for an infarct or acute coronary syndrome, a loading dose of 300–600 mg of clopidogrel is given, and six months to a year of dual anti-platelet treatment is often recommended.

If a drug-eluting stent is used, one year of dual-platelet treatment is now commonly recommended because of concerns about delayed healing and a risk of late stent thrombosis (about 1% per year).

For primary angioplasties or complicated angioplasties (large dissection or large burden of thrombus), the potent platelet aggregation inhibitor abciximab (a receptor antibody) may be used as a bolus, followed by infusion for some hours. This drug is very effective in preventing closure of the vessel, but is expensive. Abciximab and tirofiban (which is a small molecule platelet aggregation inhibitor) are very valuable drugs for the management of acute coronary syndromes with angioplasty. Tirofiban has a shorter half-life than abciximab but should be used for at least 24–48 hours before intervention unless it is started in the catheter laboratory with a double bolus dose.

Primary angioplasty of the infarct-related artery is the recommended treatment for STEMI if it can be performed in an experienced centre and if there will not be more than 90 minutes additional delay compared with the use of thrombolytic treatment. It results in a lower mortality and shortened hospital stay.

The 'open artery hypothesis' suggests that having a patent artery after an infarct is an advantage (possibly because of its effects on remodelling). For this reason occluded arteries may be opened and dilated even late after an infarct, especially if the patient has evidence of persisting ischaemia. However, the Open Artery Trial (OAT) did not show benefit when routine reopening of the infarct-related artery was performed more than 48 hours after the infarct in the absence of evidence of ischaemia.

Restenosis remains a problem after angioplasty. It is very unusual after six months. It is more common in diabetics, in calcified and complex and long lesions, and in dilated vein grafts. A combination of these factors can result in a restenosis rate of more than 60%. Treatment is usually by redilatation and insertion of a drug-eluting stent.

Drug-eluting stents have dramatically reduced the incidence of restenosis. The currently available stents have either paclitaxel, everolimus or sirolimus bound via a polymer to the metal surface of the stent. These antineoplastic drugs are eluted for about a month and prevent the migration of smooth muscle cells into the lumen of the vessel that is the cause of restenosis. Very low restenosis rates of a few per cent have been obtained in trials, even when diabetics are included. These stents also seem to be effective in preventing further restenosis when used in a restenosed bare metal stent. Drug-eluting stents are very expensive—about four times the cost of bare metal stents—and the usual indications for their use include long lesions in small vessels, redilatation of restenosis and diabetes. They are not used for patients who may need a surgical procedure within the following six months to a year because of the risk of stopping anti-platelet treatment during this period.

Stents do not set off metal detectors and patients can safely have an MRI scan within a month.

Infective endocarditis

Patients with infective endocarditis stay in hospital for weeks, so they are often available for long cases. The disease presents diagnostic, plus short-term and long-term management problems. Cases combine cardiological, microbiological and immunological problems. The diagnosis is usually known to the patient. An intravenous infusion containing antibiotics is a valuable clue.

The history

Ask about:
1. details of presenting symptoms (e.g. malaise, fever, symptoms of anaemia)
2. symptoms suggesting embolic phenomena to large vessels (e.g. brain, viscera) or small vessels (e.g. kidney, with haematuria or loin pain)
3. recent dental, endoscopic or operative procedures—a precipitating event is identified in only about 5% of cases (the time between procedure and diagnosis may be up to three months); remember that *Streptococcus bovis* endocarditis is associated with colonic cancer and these patients all deserve a colonoscopy!
4. use of antibiotics for prophylaxis, either before an invasive procedure or for rheumatic fever, or both
5. a past history of rheumatic fever
6. a history of other heart disease or heart operations, especially valve replacement
7. a history of intravenous drug abuse, particularly for its association with tricuspid and pulmonary valve infection

8. antibiotic allergies
9. how the diagnosis was made—including the number of blood cultures and the use of transthoracic or transoesophageal echocardiography (TOE)
10. management since admission to hospital, including the names of the antibiotics used, the duration of treatment and whether the possibility of valve replacement has been discussed
11. a history of other major diseases, particularly those associated with immune suppression, such as renal transplantation or steroid use.

The examination

1. Start by examining for the peripheral stigmata of endocarditis.
   (a) **Hands:**
     - clubbing (a late sign)
     - splinter haemorrhages
     - Osler's nodes on the finger pulp (these are always painful and palpable, are probably an embolic phenomenon and are rare)
     - Janeway lesions (*non-tender* erythematous maculopapular lesions containing bacteria on the palms or pulps, which are rare).
   (b) **Eyes:** Roth's spots in the fundus, conjunctival petechiae.
   (c) **Abdomen:** splenomegaly (a late sign).
   (d) **Urine analysis** for haematuria and proteinuria.
   (e) **Neurological signs** of embolic disease.
   (f) **Joints** (occasionally resembles rheumatic fever pattern).
2. Next examine the **heart**. Assess for predisposing cardiac lesions. These are, in order:
   (a) Acquired:
     - prosthetic valve (mechanical)
     - mitral regurgitation, mitral stenosis
     - aortic stenosis
     - aortic regurgitation
     - prosthetic valve (tissue)
     - repaired mitral valve
     - mitral valve prolapse with mitral regurgitation.
   (b) Congenital:
     - bicuspid aortic valve
     - patent ductus arteriosus
     - ventricular septal defect
     - coarctation of the aorta.
   Remember:
   - an atrial septal defect of the secundum type is almost never affected
   - 20% of endocarditis patients have no recognised underlying cardiac abnormality
   - coronary stents and pacemaker leads do not appear to involve any risk of endocarditis.
3. Examine for the signs of cardiac failure. Look for signs of a prosthetic valve and for scars that may be present from previous valvotomy or repair operations.
4. Look for a source of infection and take the patient's temperature.

Investigations

1. **Three to six blood cultures** (at least) over 24 hours (98% of culture-positive cases will give positive results in the first three bottles).
2. **Full blood count and erythrocyte sedimentation rate (ESR).** Look for anaemia (normochromic, normocytic), neutrophilia, an elevated ESR, which

may be >100 mm/h and a raised C-reactive protein (CRP) level. The ESR tends to remain elevated for months, even when treatment has been successful, but the CRP level falls quite quickly and may be useful for assessing the effectiveness of treatment.

3. **Renal function.** A freshly spun urine sample will often show red cell casts.

4. **Chest X-ray film.** Look for left or right ventricular hypertrophy, increased pulmonary artery markings, Kerley's B lines, frank cardiac failure and valve calcification (lateral film). The onset of heart failure is a poor prognostic sign.

5. **ECG.** Atrial fibrillation in the elderly (particularly common) and conduction defects may occur, but are not specific.

6. **Echocardiography (see Fig 5.1) (2D and Doppler).** Vegetations must be larger than 2 mm to be detected. This procedure cannot distinguish active from inactive lesions. Vegetations are seen in approximately 40% of cases. They tend to occur downstream of the abnormal jet (e.g. on the aortic surface of the aortic valve in cases of aortic stenosis and endocarditis). Colour Doppler examination is a very sensitive means of detecting new valvular regurgitation, which may be an important sign of endocarditis. *Transoesophageal echocardiography* allows better definition of valvular involvement and is more likely to detect vegetations. Perhaps more importantly, it is much more likely to detect such complications as valve abscesses. It is now in routine use for the assessment of endocarditis.

7. **Serological tests.** These include tests for immune complexes and classical pathway activation of complement causing low C3, C4 and CH50 levels. The test for rheumatoid factor gives positive results in 50% of cases and that for antinuclear antibody in 20% of cases.

Notes

Organisms
Streptococci account for approximately half of these infections.

1. *Streptococcus viridans* (non-haemolytic)—usually presents subacutely. The names of the viridans streptococci are subject to frequent revision but current important types for endocarditis include *S. sanguinis*, *S. gordonii* and *S. mitis*.

2. *Streptococcus faecalis*—traditionally more common in older men with prostatism and younger women with urinary tract infections, but now in intravenous drug users.

3. *Streptococcus bovis*—associated with colon polyps and carcinoma.

4. *Staphylococcus aureus*—particularly in drug addicts; usually presents acutely. Note, though, that only a small minority of *S. aureus* bacteraemias are associated with endocarditis.

5. *Staphylococcus epidermidis*—more common in patients with recent valve replacement but can be a contaminant in blood cultures.

6. Gram-negative coccobacilli—rarely a cause; more common with prosthetic valves. The responsible organisms are called the HACEK group:
   Haemophilus
   Actinobacillus
   Cariobacterium hominis
   Eikonella spp.
   Kingella kingae

7. Fungi (e.g. *Candida*, *Aspergillus*)—particularly in drug addicts and immuno-suppressed patients.

Echocardiography Report

Reason for study: AR ?; endocarditis
Study quality: Good <u>Satisfactory</u> Poor

RV	18	(mm)	(N 10–26)
Sept.	10	(mm)	(N 7–11)
LVEDD	68	(mm)	(N 36–56)
LVESD	42	(mm)	(N 20–40)
LVPW	10	(mm)	(N 7–11)
Aorta	34	(mm)	(N 20–35)
LA	36	(mm)	(N 24–40)
FS	38	%	(N 27–40)
EF	67	%	(N 55–70)

Valves

Mitral	Mild MR
Tricus.	Mild TR
Aortic	Thickened, bicuspid
Pulm.	Appears normal

Doppler—2D
The left ventricle is dilated. The fractional shortening is in the normal range. The aortic valve is thickened and probably bicuspid. A mobile mass 2 mm in diameter is visible on the LV side of the valve and represents a probable vegetation.

Doppler—colour flow mapping
There is no aortic gradient. A large jet of aortic regurgitation is present, extending three-quarters of the way into the LV cavity. Mild-to-moderate MR is present. Mild TR. RV pressure = 28 mmHg.

Conclusions
Severe AR, probable vegetation, bicuspid valve.

Comment
The diagnosis of endocarditis cannot really be made on the basis of echocardiography alone. Even what appears to be a vegetation may be sterile. Nevertheless, a mobile mass attached to a valve in a patient with positive blood cultures makes the diagnosis of endocarditis almost certain.
   An abnormal echocardiogram adds weight to the diagnosis. It also enables detection of left ventricular enlargement, which suggests haemodynamic compromise. Serial echocardiograms allow assessment of the treatment of endocarditis and help with the decision about the timing of possible surgery.
   The underlying valve abnormality may be obvious. Here the aortic valve is congenitally bicuspid.
   More detailed analysis of the heart is possible with transoesophageal echocardiography, which is now routine in cases of endocarditis. It enables smaller vegetations to be identified, as well as complications such as valve ring abscesses.

Key
AR = aortic regurgitation; EF = ejection fraction; FS = fractional shortening; LA = left atrium; LVEDD = left ventricular end-diastolic dimension; LVESD = left ventricular end-systolic dimension; LVPW = left ventricular posterior wall; MR = mitral regurgitation; Pulm. = pulmonary; RV = right ventricle; Sept. = septal thickness; TR = tricuspid regurgitation; Tricus. = tricuspid.

Figure 5.1 Echocardiography report in a patient with possible infective endocarditis.

Causes of culture-negative endocarditis
Note: This diagnosis should be made with caution. It condemns a patient to prolonged treatment with intravenous antibiotics.

1. Previous use of antibiotics.
2. Exotic organisms (e.g. *Haemophilus parainfluenzae*, histoplasmosis, *Brucella*, *Candida*, Q fever).
3. Right-sided endocarditis (rarely).

Post-valve surgery endocarditis
Early infection is acquired at operation; late infection occurs from another source. This condition has a worse prognosis than native valve endocarditis.

Diagnosis

The diagnosis is usually a clinical one. The Duke criteria are often used to assist. Two major criteria, one major and three minor, or five minor criteria secure the diagnosis.

Major criteria
1. Typical organisms in two separate blood cultures.
2. Evidence of endocardial involvement: echocardiogram showing a mobile intra-cardiac mass on a valve or in the path of a regurgitant jet, or an abscess or new valvular regurgitation.

Minor criteria
1. Predisposing cardiac condition or intravenous drug use
2. Fever
3. Vascular phenomena or stigmata
4. Serological or acute phase abnormalities
5. Echocardiogram abnormal but not meeting above criteria

Treatment

Early involvement in the management by a cardiac surgeon in a cardiac surgical unit is usually indicated, particularly for staphylococcal infection.
1. Intravenous administration of a bactericidal antibiotic. If the organism is a sensitive *S. viridans*, give benzylpenicillin, 6–12 g daily for 4–6 weeks. If it is an enterococcus, at least 4 weeks of intravenous treatment are necessary and the choice of antibiotic depends on the organism's sensitivity. For prosthetic valves, 6–8 weeks of intravenous treatment is necessary.
2. Follow the progress by looking at the temperature chart, serological results and haemoglobin values.
3. The decision to go on to valve replacement is a difficult one; it is best made with the assistance of a cardiac surgeon who has been involved from the start. Indications for surgery include:
   (a) resistant organisms (e.g. fungi)
   (b) valvular dysfunction causing moderate-to-severe cardiac failure (e.g. acute severe aortic regurgitation)
   (c) persistently positive blood cultures in spite of treatment
   (d) invasive paravalvular infection causing conduction disturbances, or a paravalvular abscess or fistula (detected by TOE)
   (e) recurrent major embolic phenomena, although this is controversial (an isolated vegetation is not in itself an indication for surgery).

Factors suggesting a poorer prognosis

1. Shock
2. Congestive cardiac failure
3. Extreme age

4. Aortic valve or multiple valve involvement
5. Multiple organisms
6. Culture-negative endocarditis
7. Delay in starting treatment
8. Prosthetic valve involvement
9. Staphylococcal, Gram-negative and fungal infections

Differential diagnosis
1. Atrial myxoma
2. Occult malignant neoplasm
3. Systemic lupus erythematosus
4. Polyarteritis nodosa
5. Post-streptococcal glomerulonephritis
6. Pyrexia of unknown origin
7. Cardiac thrombus

Prognosis
Prior to antibiotic use, this was an invariably fatal disease. Currently, more than 70% of patients with endogenous infection survive, as do 50% of those with a prosthetic valve infection. Intravenous drug users have a good prognosis.

Prophylaxis
Confusion between rheumatic fever and endocarditis prophylaxis is rife. Rheumatic fever prophylaxis consists of long-term, low-dose antibiotic administration. Prophylaxis against endocarditis requires high-dose, short-term treatment only in patients with a very high risk, namely a previous episode of endocarditis, a prosthetic heart valve, a congenital heart malformation (unrepaired cyanotic heart disease, repaired cyanotic heart disease with residual defects or recent surgery within six months) or a cardiac transplant with valve disease. According to the latest 2007 American Heart Association guidelines, all other lesions no longer require prophylaxis.

Prophylaxis is also recommended according to the Australian (Heart Foundation) guidelines for:
• complex congenital heart disease, including patients who have had repair operations using shunts or artificial material and have persisting shunts (e.g. VSD repaired with Gortex, but with residual shunt)
• Aboriginal patients with any intermediate or high-risk lesion.

Prophylaxis regimens are as follows (recommendations from *Therapeutic Guidelines—Antibiotic*):
1. **Dental procedures (e.g. gum cleaning) or oral surgery**—amoxycillin 2 g one hour before the procedure. For patients unable to take oral antibiotics, ampicillin IV or IM just before the procedure. If the risk is high, give ampicillin and gentamicin as described below. For those allergic to penicillin, clindamycin 600 mg given orally one hour before the procedure is adequate.
2. **Gastrointestinal or genitourinary procedures:** no prophylaxis is recommended.

Remember that the effectiveness of antibiotic prophylaxis has not been proven. Patients need to be reminded of the need for good dental hygiene and regular dental review.

Congestive cardiac failure
This is a common therapeutic problem, but it may be a diagnostic problem. It is uncommonly the only major problem in a long case.

The history

1. It is important first to find out what may have precipitated episodes of cardiac failure. Precipitating problems include:
   (a) arrhythmias (especially atrial fibrillation)
   (b) discontinuation of medications (particularly important)
   (c) myocardial infarction
   (d) anaemia
   (e) infection and fever
   (f) thyrotoxicosis
   (g) anaesthesia and surgery
   (h) pulmonary embolism
   (i) high salt intake, drugs that cause salt and water retention (e.g. traditional NSAIDs, COX-2 inhibitors) or excessive physical exertion
   (j) pregnancy.
   Note: Chronic lung disease can be a cause of, or a precipitating factor for, right and left ventricular failure.

2. Then ask about the symptoms of left ventricular failure (e.g. dyspnoea, orthopnoea, paroxysmal nocturnal dyspnoea) and right ventricular failure (e.g. oedema, ascites, anorexia and nausea). Ask about symptoms of ischaemic heart disease (e.g. angina). These may help distinguish dyspnoea caused by lung disease from that caused by cardiac failure.

3. Enquire about the history of previous heart disease:
   (a) hypertension
   (b) ischaemic heart disease—infarcts, angina
   (c) rheumatic or other valve disease
   (d) congenital heart disease
   (e) cardiomyopathy
   (f) previous cardiac surgery (e.g. coronary artery bypass grafting, valve replacement or resection of an aneurysm)
   (g) cardiac transplantation.

4. Find out about coronary risk factors, in addition to age and male sex, including:
   (a) hyperlipidaemia
   (b) hypertension
   (c) smoking
   (d) diabetes mellitus
   (e) family history of early coronary heart disease
   (f) use of oral contraceptives or premature onset of menopause
   (g) obesity
   (h) physical inactivity.

5. Ascertain the risk factors for dilated cardiomyopathy:
   (a) excessive alcohol intake
   (b) family history of cardiomyopathy
   (c) haemochromatosis.

6. Ask what medications are currently being taken.

7. Ask what investigations have been undertaken—particularly echocardiography, stress ECG testing, nuclear studies and cardiac catheterisation.

8. Find out how the disease affects the patient's life and ability to cope at home (e.g. climbing stairs, sexual difficulties etc.). Remember to classify the patient according to the New York Heart Association (NYHA) guidelines.

NYHA classification	
I	Patients have disease but are asymptomatic
II	Angina/dyspnoea on mild activity
III	Angina/dyspnoea on moderate activity
IV	Angina/dyspnoea at rest

The examination

1. Perform a detailed cardiovascular system examination.
2. Look particularly for signs of cardiac failure, the underlying causes of the problem and any precipitating factors.
3. Look for a pacemaker or defibrillator box.
4. Note wasting as a result of cardiac cachexia.
5. Take the blood pressure lying and standing. Treatment with ACE inhibitors and beta-blockers often results in mild hypotension.

Investigations

1. **Chest X-ray film (see Fig 5.2).** Look for cardiomegaly and chamber size (e.g. left atrium), cardiac aneurysm, valve calcification, sternal wires suggesting previous cardiac surgery, signs of lung disease and pulmonary congestion.

Figure 5.2 Alveolar pulmonary oedema. When the pulmonary venous pressure reaches 30 mmHg, oedema fluid will pass into the alveoli. This causes shadowing (patchy to confluent depending on the extent) in the lung fields. This usually occurs first around the hila and gives a bat's wing appearance. These changes are usually superimposed on interstitial oedema. A lamellar pleural effusion (arrow) is seen at the right costophrenic angle where Kerley 'B' lines are also evident.

2. **ECG.** Look for arrhythmias, signs of ischaemia or recent or old infarction (see Fig 5.3), left ventricular hypertrophy and persisting ST elevation (aneurysm). Left bundle branch block is a common ECG finding in these patients (see Fig 5.4). The ECG is rarely entirely normal in a patient with heart failure.

Figure 5.3 Sinus rhythm. There are Q waves from V1 to V5. This is diagnostic of an extensive old anterior infarct, which is likely to be the cause of this patient's heart failure.

Figure 5.4 Sinus rhythm. Left bundle branch block (LBBB). The QRS complexes may widen further as heart failure progresses. LBBB is a common finding in heart failure but is not diagnostic.

3. **Electrolytes and creatinine levels.** To exclude hypokalaemia (as a cause of arrhythmia), hyponatraemia (which may indicate severe longstanding cardiac failure, a poor prognostic sign) and renal failure.
4. **B-type natriuretic peptide level (BNP; previously called brain natriuretic peptide).** Although there is doubt about the reference range, a definitely elevated level may help distinguish cardiac from non-cardiac dyspnoea. Since BNP falls when heart failure is treated, trials of monitoring BNP are underway as a means of assessing the adequacy of cardiac treatment.
5. **Haemoglobin value.** To exclude anaemia as a precipitating cause.

If the diagnosis is not already obvious, consider *dilated cardiomyopathy*. Investigations for this include the following:

1. **Echocardiography (see Fig 5.5).** This will show generalised or segmental wall motion abnormalities and reduced fractional shortening. An estimate of the left ventricular ejection fraction can be made. Segmental hypokinesia suggests that ischaemia is the cause of the cardiac failure. Doppler echocardiography will

usually show at least some mitral and tricuspid regurgitation in these patients. The presence of more severe valvular disease suggests a different aetiology for the cardiac failure. Serial echocardiograph measurements of left and right ventricular dimensions can be useful for following the patient's progress.

2. **A gated blood pool scan for the ejection fraction.** The right ventricular ejection fraction is normally >45% and the left ventricular ejection fraction is >50%. The scan will also show whether hypokinesis is global or segmental and to what extent the right ventricle is affected.

3. **Coronary angiography.** This is often necessary to exclude coronary artery disease.

4. **Right ventricular biopsy.** This may help determine the aetiology in selected patients.

Echocardiography Report

Reason for study: Assess left ventricular function, cardiac failure
Study quality: Good <u>Satisfactory</u> Poor

RV	13	(mm) (N 10–26)
Sept.	8	(mm) (N 7–11)
LVEDD	66	(mm) (N 36–56)
LVESD	49	(mm) (N 20–40)
LVPW	10	(mm) (N 7–11)
Aorta	22	(mm) (N 20–35)
LA	36	(mm) (N 24–40)
FS	26	% (N 27–40)
EF	50	% (N 55–70)

Valves

Mitral	Mild-to-moderate MR
Tricus.	Mild TR
Aortic	Thickened, not stenosed
Pulm.	Appears normal

Doppler—2D
The left ventricle is dilated. There is extensive antero-apical hypokinesis. The aortic valve is slightly thickened and there is mitral annular calcification. The mitral valve is not stenosed and there is no mitral valve prolapse.

Doppler—colour flow mapping
There is no aortic gradient; mild-to-moderate MR is present. MR jet to two-thirds of LA. Mild TR. RV pressure = 38 mmHg.

Conclusions
Severe segmental LV dysfunction; moderate MR.

Comments
This echocardiography report demonstrates the typical findings when a patient has cardiac failure caused by previous anterior myocardial infarction. The left ventricular dysfunction is not global (typical of cardiomyopathy) but involves the infarcted area. There is overall LV dilatation with an increase of the LVEDD. The FS is the percentage change in LV size from diastole to systole measured at the base of the heart. It can be in the normal range despite the presence of LV dysfunction, if the base of the heart is not involved.

The ejection fraction can be estimated from the LVEDD and LVESD measurements. There are a number of formulas, which are applied automatically by the calculation

---

Figure 5.5 Echocardiography report in a patient with cardiac failure caused by anterior myocardial infarction.

(Continues)

software of the echocardiograph machine. It is difficult to obtain an accurate ejection fraction, which is a volume change measurement on the basis of two 2D-image measurements. These calculated ejection fractions tend to have a higher reference range than those obtained by nuclear heart pool scanning. MR is almost always detected when moderate LV dysfunction is present.

Mitral annular calcification is a common finding in elderly patients; it can be associated with MR but not with mitral stenosis. The presence of left atrial enlargement suggests that the mitral regurgitation is not acute but can also be associated with hypertension.

TR is commonly found in patients with heart failure but may also be present in normal people. Interrogation of the regurgitant jet with continuous wave (CW) Doppler allows measurement of its velocity. This can be used to calculate the pressure difference across the valve. Since the pressure in the right atrium is usually close to 5 mmHg, the pressure in the RV can be calculated by adding 5 to the pressure difference. In this case the pressure difference across the valve is about 33 mmHg.

Key

EF = ejection fraction; FS = fractional shortening; LA = left atrium; LVEDD = left ventricular end-diastolic dimension; LVESD = left ventricular end-systolic dimension; LVPW = left ventricular posterior wall; MR = mitral regurgitation; Pulm. = pulmonary; RV = right ventricle; Sept. = septal thickness; TR = tricuspid regurgitation; Tricus. = tricuspid.

Figure 5.5 Continued

Treatment

1. Remove precipitating causes. Atrial fibrillation and other incessant tachycardias can be a cause of cardiac failure—tachycardia-induced cardiomyopathy. The prognosis is good if normal heart rate can be restored.
2. Correct underlying causes if possible (e.g. thrombolysis for an acute infarct or coronary artery bypass grafting or angioplasty for ischaemia) (see Table 5.2).
3. Control the failure.
   (a) Decrease physical activity (e.g. bed rest for the acutely ill patient).
   (b) Control fluid retention (e.g. by diuretics, low-salt diet, fluid restriction [1000–1500 mL for severe failure]).

   Patients should be advised to weigh themselves daily. An increase in weight of 2 kg or more over a few days is usually an indication of significant fluid retention. A temporary increase in the diuretic dose will often prevent a deterioration in symptoms.
   (c) Oppose inappropriate activation of the renin–angiotensin system.
   - ACE inhibitors are considered to be the drug class of choice for cardiac failure as they prolong life; symptomatic hypotension is the major side effect in cardiac failure. ACE inhibitors are indicated for all classes of heart failure, even for asymptomatic patients with left ventricular dysfunction. Every effort should be made to titrate the dose up to the maximum tolerated. The usual limitation is symptomatic hypotension.
   - AR blockers are indicated for patients intolerant (usually because of cough) of ACE inhibitors. The most common reason for the cessation of ACE inhibitors or AR blockers is deterioration in renal function (usually in patients with renovascular disease).
   - Renal function may improve again if the ACE inhibitor and diuretic doses are reduced and hypovolaemia is corrected. There is little therapeutic difference between the various ACE inhibitors.
   - Trials have also demonstrated some additional benefit when ACE inhibitors and AR blockers are combined. The treatment of cardiac failure involves polypharmacy. It is probably only the minority of patients

TABLE 5.2 Causes of ventricular failure

Left ventricular failure

1. Volume overload
   (a) Aortic regurgitation
   (b) Mitral regurgitation
   (c) Patent ductus arteriosus

2. Pressure overload
   (a) Systemic hypertension
   (b) Aortic stenosis

3. Myocardial disease
   (a) Ischaemic heart disease
   (b) Dilated cardiomyopathy—causes include:
       (i) idiopathic (most common)
       (ii) alcohol
       (iii) myocarditis
       (iv) familial (autosomal dominant)
       (v) peripartum
       (vi) neuromuscular disease (e.g. dystrophia myotonica)
       (vii) connective tissue disease (e.g. scleroderma)
       (viii) haemochromatosis
       (ix) sarcoidosis
       (x) drugs (e.g. doxorubicin)
       (xi) radiation
       (xii) diabetes mellitus—now a controversial cause.

Note: Restrictive cardiomyopathy and hypertrophic cardiomyopathy can be causes of heart failure.

Right ventricular failure

1. Volume overload
   (a) Atrial septal defect
   (b) Tricuspid regurgitation

2. Pressure overload
   (a) Pulmonary stenosis
   (b) Pulmonary hypertension

3. Myocardial disease
   (a) Cardiomyopathy secondary to left ventricular failure
   (b) Right ventricular infarction (rare)

who will be prepared to take an AR blocker as well as all the other drugs usually prescribed. The combination also seems to increase the risk of acute renal failure.

- Add spironolactone. This aldosterone antagonist improves survival in class III or IV patients. It may be especially useful for the management of ascites and peripheral oedema. Hyperkalaemia may be a problem for patients with renal impairment. Start with 12.5 mg per day. Epleronone is a newer aldosterone antagonist indicated for heart failure occurring soon after myocardial infarction.
- Asking the patient about the difficulties of compliance with a complicated drug regimen may be useful at this point.

(d) Oppose inappropriate increases in catecholamine drive.

- Give beta-blockers. Trials with carvedilol, bisoprolol and extended-release metoprolol have shown improvements in symptoms and mortality for this drug used in patients with class II–IV heart failure.
- The drugs must be introduced at a low dose (e.g. 3.125 or 6.25 mg b.d. of carvedilol or 1.25 mg daily of bisoprolol) and titrated upwards as tolerated to 25 mg b.d. of carvedilol or 10 mg daily of bisoprolol.

(e) Increase myocardial contractility (e.g. with digoxin).

Note: The use of digoxin in cardiac failure is no longer controversial. Recent trials have suggested an increase in symptoms if cardiac failure patients who are in sinus rhythm and on treatment with digoxin, diuretics and ACE inhibitors have their digoxin withdrawn. Digoxin mortality trials have shown no difference in mortality but definite improvement in symptoms (when used in combination with a diuretic and ACE inhibitor). Patients most likely to benefit have more severe heart failure, an S3 gallop, impressive cardiomegaly and an ejection fraction <20%.

(f) Intravenous inotropes (e.g. dopamine or dobutamine) may have a place in the short-term treatment of severe cardiac failure. Patients may be admitted for a 'dobutamine holiday' (a course of treatment with intravenous dobutamine, usually for about five days) and have improved symptoms for some months. Levosimendan is an intravenous drug that works as a calcium channel activator. A 24-hour course may improve symptoms and possibly prognosis. No effective oral inotrope is available.

(g) Control rhythm. Remember, cardiac failure has a poor prognosis. About 50% of these patients die suddenly of a ventricular arrhythmia. The detection of high-grade ventricular arrhythmias is an indication for an *implanted defibrillator*, which is associated with a proven improvement in prognosis. Routine use of these devices in patients with a low ejection fraction has been shown to improve survival, even when ventricular arrhythmias have not been recorded.

(h) Cardiac transplantation may now be offered to certain patients. The reduced availability of donor hearts and the improvement of many patients who would otherwise be suitable for transplant with beta-blockers have reduced the frequency of this procedure.

(i) Ventricular assist devices are sometimes used as a bridge to transplant in very ill patients. Survival for weeks or months is possible with these devices. Trials of entirely artificial hearts continue in small numbers of patients.

(j) Biventricular pacing or cardiac resynchronisation therapy (CRT) may be helpful for heart failure patients with very wide QRS complexes. The LV pacing wire is placed via the coronary sinus into one of the left ventricular veins. This complicated procedure enables both ventricles to be paced and dyssynchronous contraction of the ventricles associated with a very wide QRS to be corrected. About 70% of patients improve with the treatment. Although echocardiographic measurements of dyssynchrony are available, they have not yet been able to predict a response to resynchronisation treatment and the current guidelines allow their use for symptomatic patients with LBBB.

Diastolic heart failure (heart failure with preserved ejection fraction)

Most breathless patients with heart failure have abnormal left ventricular systolic function, which is characterised by dilatation and hypokinesis. Some cases of cardiac failure, however, may be caused by diastolic dysfunction. In such cases, the myocardium is stiff, often because it is hypertrophied and does not relax normally. The condition seems to be more common in elderly patients. Hypertension is a common cause. The diagnosis is difficult, but an echocardiogram will show preserved or increased systolic contraction without dilatation and there may be left ventricular hypertrophy and left atrial dilatation. Doppler echocardiography may show abnormalities of left ventricular filling caused by the stiffness of the ventricle. However, this is not easy to quantify and is very dependent on variations in preload and afterload.

The condition may have a prognosis as bad as that of systolic heart failure. Treatment is similar, but beta-blockers are used early and only small doses of diuretics should be required. At least in theory, digoxin should be avoided if the patient is in sinus rhythm. Every effort should be made to control hypertension.

Hyperlipidaemia

Hyperlipidaemia may be present in patients under investigation for vascular disease, pancreatitis, hypothyroidism or diabetes mellitus. It often presents both diagnostic and management problems.

The history

1. The patient should be able to indicate whether the main problem is vascular or not. If the problem is one of premature coronary artery disease, hyper-cholesterolaemia is the likely lipid problem. The most important inherited cause is *familial hypercholesterolaemia*, which is caused by a defective or absent low-density lipoprotein (LDL) receptor. The heterozygous form occurs in about one person in 500. As the transmission is autosomal dominant, the patient may know of first-degree relatives who have been affected. There may even be family members with the homozygous form. These people usually present with a tenfold elevation in serum cholesterol levels as a result of an increase in plasma LDL levels and have a myocardial infarction before the age of 20 years. People with the heterozygous form typically have myocardial infarctions in their 30s and 40s and have a two- to threefold elevation in cholesterol level. More than 80% of affected men and nearly 60% of affected women have had myocardial infarcts by the age of 60 years. Find out whether the patient has already had a myocardial infarct and which relatives have been affected.

   Familial combined hyperlipidaemia is associated with obesity or glucose intolerance and may be expressed as type IIa, IIb or IV hyperlipidaemia (see Table 5.3). This is also an autosomal dominant trait. Patients develop hypercholesterolaemia and often hypertriglyceridaemia in puberty. Once again, there usually is a strong family history of premature coronary artery disease. There is no doubt that an elevated triglyceride level adds to the risk of hypercholesterolaemia.

   Familial dysbetalipoproteinaemia is also associated with coronary artery disease. These patients have elevated cholesterol and triglyceride levels and are usually found to have obesity, hypothyroidism or diabetes mellitus. Find out whether there is any history of these and whether there has been atheromatous disease or vascular disease involving the internal carotid arteries and the abdominal

TABLE 5.3 Hyperlipoproteinaemias

Type	Lipoprotein elevated	Electrophoretic mobility	Mechanism	Secondary causes	Clinical features	Associations
I	Chylomicrons	Origin	Deficiency / Extrahepatic lipoprotein lipase or apo C-II deficiency	Rarely SLE	Eruptive xanthomata; lipaemia retinalis	Pancreatitis
IIa	LDL	β	Receptor defect	Cushing's; hypothyroidism	Xanthelasma; corneal arcus	CAD, PVD
IIb	LDL & VLDL	β & pre-β		Cholestasis; nephrotic syndrome	Tendon xanthomata	
III	IDL	Broad β	Oversynthesis and/or abnormal apo E	Renal and liver disease	Palmar crease and tuboeruptive xanthomata; xanthelasma	CAD, PVD
IV	VLDL	Pre-β	Oversynthesis and/or under catabolism of VLDL	Diabetes mellitus; alcoholism; chronic renal failure	Usually no xanthomata	
V	VLDL & chylomicrons	Origin and pre-β	Saturation lipoprotein lipase by VLDL	As for IV	As for I	As for I

Notes
- Apo A-1 deficiency is associated with the absence of plasma HDL and severe premature CAD.
- Apo B deficiency is the defect in abetalipoproteinaemia (autosomal recessive), which is characterised by haemolytic anaemia (acanthocytosis), fat malabsorption and neurological defects (proprioceptive loss, retinitis pigmentosa).
- LCAT deficiency results in decreased HDL, cloudy corneas and progressive renal disease.

apo = apolipoprotein; CAD = coronary artery disease; HDL = high-density lipoprotein; IDL = intermediate-density lipoprotein; LCAT = lecithin cholesterol acyltransferase; LDL = low-density lipoprotein; PVD = peripheral vascular disease; SLE = systemic lupus erythematosus; VLDL = very-low-density lipoprotein.

aorta or its branches. Ask about claudication, which occurs in about one-third of patients.

2. The patient may be able to tell you his or her cholesterol and triglyceride levels and what they have been in the past. Some patients even know their LDL and high-density lipoprotein (HDL) levels.

3. If there is no history of coronary artery disease and the patient either knows the triglyceride level to have been very high or has a history of pancreatitis, the likely diagnosis is *familial hypertriglyceridaemia*. This is also a common autosomal dominant disorder and is associated with obesity, hyperglycaemia, hyperinsulinaemia, hypertension and hyperuricaemia. Although there is a slightly increased incidence of atherosclerosis, this is probably related to diabetes mellitus, obesity and hypertension than to the hypertriglyceridaemia itself.

   Ask about the patient's alcohol consumption, any history of hypothyroidism or the ingestion of oestrogen-containing oral contraceptives. Any of these can precipitate a rapid rise in the triglyceride level, which may precipitate pancreatitis or the characteristic eruptive xanthomas. Between attacks, patients have moderate elevations of the plasma triglyceride level.

4. Next, find out about treatment. In familial hypercholesterolaemia, this will have been aimed at the cholesterol level itself and at any cardiovascular complications that have occurred. The patient should be well informed about a low saturated fat diet and may be aware of side effects from medication usage.

5. The need for drug treatment of hyperlipidaemia depends on the lipid levels and on the patient's other vascular risk factors. Ask about a family history of premature coronary disease (first-degree relatives under the age of 60), previous vascular disease (coronary, cerebral or peripheral), smoking and diabetes mellitus.

6. Ask about any history of cutaneous xanthoma. These may have resolved with treatment or been surgically removed.

The examination

1. Examine the cardiovascular system. There may be evidence of cardiac failure from previous myocardial infarcts or a sternotomy scar from previous coronary surgery. Occasionally one sees the scandalous situation of a patient with untreated hyperlipidaemia presenting with more angina after initially successful coronary surgery.

2. Look specifically for the interesting skin manifestations of these conditions.

   (a) Patients with the heterozygous or homozygous form of familial hypercholesterolaemia may have *tendon xanthomas*. These are nodular swellings that tend to involve the tendons of the knee, elbow and dorsum of the hand and the Achilles tendon. They consist of massive deposits of cholesterol, probably derived from the deposition of LDL particles. They contain both amorphous extracellular deposits and vacuoles within macrophages, and sometimes become inflamed and cause tendonitis.

   (b) Cholesterol deposits in the soft tissue of the eyelid cause *xanthelasma* and those in the cornea produce *arcus cornea* (previously insensitively called *arcus senilis*). Xanthelasma occur in about 1% of the population and arcus cornea in 30% of people over 50. When corneal arcus is seen in younger people it is more often associated with hyperlipidaemia. Surveys of people with xanthelasma indicate a slightly higher than average cholesterol level.

   Tendon xanthomas are diagnostic of familial hypercholesterolaemia, but the other signs are not as specific.

The majority of patients with the homozygous form have even more interesting signs.

- Yellow xanthomas may occur at points of trauma and in the webs of the fingers.
- Cholesterol deposits in the aortic valve may be sufficient to cause aortic stenosis; occasionally mitral stenosis and mitral regurgitation can occur for the same reason.
- Painful swollen joints may also be present. Obesity is uncommon in these patients.

These skin manifestations may or may not resolve with treatment of the cholesterol level. Surgical treatment is sometimes indicated.

Eruptive xanthomas are a sign of hypertriglyceridaemia (levels often over 20 mmol/L). This is type V hyperlipoproteinaemia. Eruptive xanthomas occur on pressure areas, such as the elbows and buttocks, and resolve rapidly with treatment. The association here is with pancreatitis. The problem is often hereditary, but exacerbated with obesity, diabetes and alcohol consumption. It is a less definite risk factor for cardiovascular disease. Palmar xanthomata are a sign of dysbetalipoproteinaemia (type III hyperlipoproteinaemia). They also resolve with treatment.

3. If the history suggests combined hyperlipidaemia or hypertriglyceridaemia, obesity is likely to be present. Look also for signs of the complications of diabetes mellitus and for signs of hypothyroidism or the nephrotic syndrome (see Table 11.2).
4. In sick patients with hypertriglyceridaemia, there may be signs of acute pancreatitis.

Investigations

1. A cholesterol level over 8 mmol/L with a normal triglyceride level suggests one of the familial hyperlipidaemias. This diagnosis can be confirmed by an assay of the number of LDL receptors on blood lymphocytes. The diagnosis is more often made from a combination of the lipid pattern, the history and the clinical examination (see Table 5.3). The other necessary investigations are those required for coronary artery disease.
2. Investigation of hypertriglyceridaemia includes tests to exclude possible underlying causes, such as hypothyroidism, diabetes mellitus and excessive alcohol intake. In familial hypertriglyceridaemia the plasma triglyceride level tends to be moderately elevated—3–6 mmol/L (type IV lipoprotein pattern). The cholesterol level is normal. The triglyceride level may rise to values in excess of 12 mmol/L during exacerbations of the condition.
3. Familial combined hyperlipidaemia produces one of three different lipoprotein patterns—hypercholesterolaemia (type IIa), hypertriglyceridaemia (type IV) or both hypercholesterolaemia and hypertriglyceridaemia (type V).
4. Familial dysbetalipoproteinaemia (type III hyperlipoproteinaemia) results in the accumulation of large lipoprotein particles containing triglycerides and cholesterol. These particles resemble the remnants and intermediate-density lipoprotein (IDL) particles normally produced from the catabolism of chylomicrons and very-low-density lipoproteins (VLDL). These patients are homozygous for the apolipoprotein E2 (apo-E2) allele, which is unable to bind to hepatic lipoprotein receptors, thus preventing the rapid hepatic uptake of IDL and chylomicrons. The condition is usually expressed only in patients with hypothyroidism or diabetes mellitus and tests for these disorders are necessary. Apo-E genotyping may sometimes be useful.

Management

1. A combination of diet and treatment of the underlying condition is usually required. Underlying diabetes mellitus and hypothyroidism must be treated.

2. Some patients with dysbetalipoproteinaemia respond dramatically to the introduction of thyroxine. Effective management of the condition tends to cause disappearance of the skin signs and improves the prognosis as far as vascular disease goes. Effective treatment of familial hyperlipidaemia from early adult life delays the onset of coronary artery disease.

3. Treatment is almost always begun with hydroxymethylglutaryl coenzyme A (HMG-CoA) reductase inhibitors (statins, e.g. pravastatin, lovastatin, artorvastatin, rosuvastatin). Except for artorvastatin, these drugs should be taken at night. They are relatively short acting and most cholesterol is manufactured at night. They work by inhibiting the synthesis of cholesterol in the liver by impeding the activity of the rate-limiting enzyme. Patients need to have their liver function checked after about a month. They are effective drugs; total cholesterol levels may be expected to fall at least 30%.

   (a) The Four-S trial in Scandinavia was the first of a number of trials to show a definite survival advantage for patients treated with these drugs for secondary prevention (i.e. those patients who have already had an ischaemic event). Secondary prevention trials for high- and intermediate-risk patients have also been positive. It is now clear that patients with existing coronary artery disease or multiple risk factors benefit most from lipid-lowering treatment. Previous concern about an apparent increase in overall mortality associated with lipid lowering seems to have been allayed.

   (b) The current indications for drug treatment of cholesterol allow a statin for patients with established symptomatic coronary artery disease at any total cholesterol level.

   (c) The most frequent problem with these drugs is the occurrence of myalgias. These are, however, uncommon. The relatively long experience with the statins suggests they are safe in quite large doses and current starting doses are two to four times those used in the past. Artorvastatin and rosuvastatin are the most potent statins and should be the drugs of choice for severe hypercholesterolaemia. All the statins favourably affect the HDL/LDL ratio.

   (d) There is controversy about the need to treat levels that are already below 4 mmol/L. There is evidence that there are pleotrophic effects of the statins that reduce coronary risk separately from their effect on cholesterol. This also implies that, for secondary prevention, the use of statins may be beneficial for patients whose total cholesterol is below 4 mmol/L before drug treatment.

4. Ezetimibe reduces cholesterol absorption from the gut and thus interrupts its enterohepatic circulation. It does not seem to interfere with the absorption of fat-soluble vitamins. Its effect on cholesterol levels is substantial, although not as great as that of the statins. It is useful for patients who are intolerant of the statins or, when used in combination with a statin, for patients whose cholesterol level is not controlled on a statin alone.

5. Gemfibrozil increases the activity of lipoprotein lipase and is useful in hyper-triglyceridaemia resulting from increased VLDL or IDL levels. Its main use is for patients with elevation of both cholesterol and triglyceride levels. Clofibrate is no longer in common use for lipid control.

6. A few patients may be taking one of the bile-sequestering resins—cholestyramine or colestipol. These are less often used as initial treatment now that the

HMG-CoA reductase inhibitors (statins) are generally available. Some patients may use a statin and a resin in combination. Resins bind bile salts in the gut so that cholesterol is withdrawn from the circulation by the liver to make more. They are not absorbed, but can cause constipation and flatulence and can block the absorption of other drugs. Patients may need to take up to two sachets (8 g) three times daily.

7. If the cholesterol cannot be brought down to normal levels with diet and a resin, nicotinic acid (which blocks VLDL synthesis) can be added. This is an effective drug and may help block the compensating increase in hepatic cholesterol synthesis that occurs with bile-sequestering resins. It is also used to try to raise HDL levels. Side effects include flushing, pruritus, abnormal liver function tests, hyperglycaemia and aggravation of peptic ulcer disease. The patient will probably have been begun on a small dose and had this gradually increased as tolerance improved. In practice it is a very difficult drug to use because of its side effects.

8. A patient with one of the combined hyperlipidaemias is likely to need to lose weight, as well as to control the cholesterol and saturated fat intake, and with dysbetalipoproteinaemia may require treatment for hypothyroidism. All these patients need to avoid alcohol and oral contraceptives. Diet is the mainstay of treatment for reducing triglyceride levels; gemfibrozil or one of the newer fibrates may be used if diet fails.

9. The indications for treatment of hyperlipidaemia with drugs on the Pharmaceutical Benefits Scheme (PBS) are complicated. Total cholesterol, HDL, LDL and triglyceride levels, as well as the presence of other risk factors, are all part of the formula. Candidates should be familiar with the latest PBS rules.

10. A patient with familial hypertriglyceridaemia will have been managed in a similar way and may have required treatment for acute pancreatitis.

11. Patients with homozygous familial hypercholesterolaemia are unlikely to live long enough to be present in clinical examinations, but treatment can sometimes involve repeated plasma exchange and even liver transplantation.

Hypertension

Many long cases are likely to provide the examiners with an opportunity to ask about the management of hypertension. Although it is an increasingly complicated subject, it is unlikely to be a patient's major problem. The examiners will want to hear sensible discussion from the candidate about a number of aspects of hypertension, including the diagnosis, appropriate investigations and approaches to treatment.

The history

1. Many patients are well informed about and very interested in their blood pressure. Find out when the diagnosis was made and what sorts of blood pressure readings were obtained before and after treatment. It is common for measurements to be made in a number of ways and in different settings. Apart from clinic measurements, the patient may have taken and continue to take his or her own blood pressure at home. There may have been ambulatory blood pressure (ABP) recordings made. It seems clear that hypertensive risk is more closely related to non-clinic and ABP results than to those obtained in the outpatient clinic. ABP should, however, be lower than clinic readings to be considered normal. Measurements of <135/85 mmHg during the day and <120/75 mmHg at night are considered normal for ABP recordings. See Table 5.4 for the current classification of clinic blood pressure levels.

TABLE 5.4 Classification of blood pressure by severity

Category	Systolic (mmHg)	Diastolic (mmHg)
Optimal	<120	<80
Normal	120–129	80–84
High normal	130–139	85–89
Mild hypertension (grade 1)	140–159	90–99
Moderate hypertension (grade 2)	160–179	100–109
Severe hypertension (grade 3)	≥180	≥110
Isolated systolic hypertension	>140	<90

Source: European Society of Cardiology adaptation of WHO/ISH classification, 1999.

2. Ask about current and past antihypertensive treatment and about problems or side effects caused by treatment. Next find out about possible complications of hypertension. These include stroke, heart failure, peripheral vascular disease and renal failure.
3. Occasionally there may be symptoms that suggest a secondary cause of hypertension: paroxysmal sweating, palpitations and headache (phaeochromocytoma) or daytime sleepiness (sleep apnoea). Rarely, the patient may be aware of a diagnosis of renal artery stenosis, coarctation of the aorta or an adrenal tumour. Primary hyperaldosteronism is now more often recognised.
4. Ask about other risk factors for vascular disease, especially type 2 diabetes, but also hyperlipidaemia, a family history of premature coronary disease or stroke. The presence of any of these conditions, or of existing heart failure, coronary or cerebrovascular disease, is a strong indication for treatment.
5. There are often a number of factors that contribute to the problem. These include obesity, excess alcohol consumption, lack of physical exercise and a high salt intake. Other factors, such as cigarette smoking, add to the patient's overall risk. Ask what the patient knows about these factors and what efforts (if any) have been made to correct them. Some racial groups have a high risk of premature vascular disease and will benefit more from early and aggressive treatment. These include Aboriginal Australians, Torres Strait Islanders and Pacific Islanders.

The examination
See page 288.

Investigations
1. **Test the urine for protein.** Measure the serum electrolyte and creatinine, blood sugar, cholesterol and haemoglobin levels.
2. **Measure the serum potassium.** The presence of hypokalaemia in patients who are not on diuretics should prompt investigations for primary aldosteronism. Measurement of plasma renin activity (PRA) and plasma aldosterone (PA) levels may be indicated. A high PA level and a low PRA level leading to a high aldosterone:renin ratio is consistent with primary hyperaldosteronism. The test is better performed off treatment. Other causes of hypokalaemia and hypertension include renovascular disease (where both aldosterone and renin are elevated), Cushing's syndrome, chronic liquorice ingestion, Liddle's syndrome and, in young patients, renin-secreting cancers (rarely).
3. **Ask about snoring.** A history of snoring and obesity should be investigated with sleep studies for sleep apnoea.

4. **Perform a CT angiogram or conventional renal angiogram for patients with intractable hypertension (especially young patients).** These are the most sensitive tests for renal artery stenosis.
5. **Ask about symptoms consistent with a phaeochromocytoma.** These need investigation with 24-hour urinary catecholamines.
6. **Investigate for Cushing's syndrome if there is any clinical suspicion.**
7. **Perform an ECG to look for evidence of ischaemic heart disease and for voltage changes that suggest left ventricular hypertrophy (LVH) (see Fig 5.6).** The presence of LVH on the ECG in hypertensives is associated with an adverse prognosis. Occasionally an echocardiogram is indicated if there is doubt about the presence of LVH.

Figure 5.6 Sinus rhythm. Left ventricular hypertrophy—the R waves are tall in the lateral leads and the S waves are deep in the septal leads. There are also lateral ST and T wave changes, called a strain pattern.

Treatment

The decision to begin drug treatment is an important one because it is likely to be lifelong. The current recommendations are that a blood pressure of >140 mmHg systolic or >90 mmHg diastolic, or both, warrants a 'treatment plan'. It is now very clear that the aggressiveness of intervention depends very much on factors other than the blood pressure level. The whole gamut of cardiovascular risk factors must be taken into account.

Tables have been published by many cardiovascular societies that show the calculated risk of vascular events and the calculated reduction in number of events over time with treatment for patients with different risk factors. The decision to use drug treatment should be based on information of this kind. Typically, calculators of risk take into account age, sex, smoking status, level of blood pressure, cholesterol, race and existing cardiovascular disease.

Except for very severe hypertension, attempts should be made to bring the blood pressure down by modifying the factors that are known to increase it. Many patients, when faced with the threat of lifelong drug treatment, are amenable to suggestions to change the way they live.

Primary hyperaldosteronism can be treated effectively with spironolactone. Renal artery stenosis may be amenable to balloon angioplasty. This usually makes blood pressure control easier, but does not cure the condition. Treatment of sleep apnoea with an appropriate continuous positive airways pressure (CPAP) mask (p 84) can also make blood pressure control easier.

Patients with only a mild risk of cardiovascular problems and blood pressure <150/95 mmHg should probably continue with conservative measures. However, at higher levels of blood pressure than this, drug treatment should be considered. Patients with very high risk (e.g. those with target organ disease or of Aboriginal race) should begin drug treatment if the blood pressure remains above 140/90 mmHg. Otherwise, drug treatment is probably indicated at levels above 150/95 mmHg. Isolated systolic hypertension in the elderly deserves therapy!

Blood pressure reduction without drugs

1. **Weight reduction.** On average, 1 kg of weight loss will reduce systolic blood pressure by 2 mmHg. The goal should be reduction to a body mass index (BMI) of 25 kg/m^2 and a waist circumference of <94 cm for men and <80 cm for women. Even lower BMIs should be recommended for some racial groups, such as Asians and Aboriginal Australians, whose cardiovascular risk increases at lower BMIs than does Europeans.
2. **Exercise.** Thirty minutes of moderately intense exercise (e.g. brisk walking) at least five days a week can lower blood pressure by about 4/2.5 mmHg.
3. **Alcohol.** Reductions of 4–5 mmHg can be achieved by alcohol restriction to two standard drinks per day for men and one per day for women.
4. **Salt.** Reduction in salt consumption to 90 mmol/day can reduce blood pressure by more than 5 mmHg. Warn patients that prepared and snack foods are usually heavily salted.

The cumulative effect of these measures can be considerable, but repeated encouragement is likely to be required for patients to achieve them.

Drug treatment

Remember that all classes of drugs (see Table 5.5) are fairly similar in their effect on blood pressure. The majority of patients will require more than one drug for effective blood pressure control.

TABLE 5.5 Classes of antihypertensive drugs
Thiazide diuretics
ACE inhibitors
Beta-blockers
Non-dihydropyridine calcium channel blockers
Dihydropyridine calcium channel blockers
Angiotensin II receptor antagonists
Others: centrally acting (methyldopa), vasodilators (prazosin, hydralazine)

There are many factors to be taken into account when a choice of antihypertensive drug is made (see Table 5.6):
- previous intolerance to a class of drugs
- known contraindications to a class of drugs (e.g. renal artery stenosis and ACE inhibitors)
- convenience of drug regimen (e.g. once-daily dosage)
- interaction with other medications (e.g. concerns about bradycardia with beta-blockers and verapamil)

TABLE 5.6 Factors affecting choice of antihypertensive drug

Condition	Drug
Contraindication or relative contraindication	
Asthma or COPD	Beta-blockers
Bradycardia or heart block	Beta-blockers, non-dihydropyridine calcium channel blockers (verapamil, diltiazem)
Cardiac failure	Calcium channel blockers
Diabetes mellitus	Thiazides, beta-blockers (relative contraindication)
Gout	Diuretics
Peripheral vascular disease	Beta-blockers
Pregnancy	Most antihypertensives, especially ACE inhibitors; methyldopa, hydralazine and labetalol are safe
Renal vascular disease	ACE inhibitors, AR antagonists
Possible indication or beneficial effect	
Angina	Beta-blockers, calcium channel blockers
Cardiac failure	ACE inhibitors, AR antagonists, diuretics, some beta-blockers
Myocardial infarction	ACE inhibitors, beta-blockers
Diabetes	ACE inhibitors, AR antagonists

COPD = chronic obstructive pulmonary disease; ACE = angiostensin-converting enzyme; AR = antiotensin receptor.

- existing medical problems that favour the use of a class of drugs (e.g. cardiac failure and ACE inhibitors)
- cost
- possible additional protective effects of some antihypertensives (e.g. ACE inhibitors and patients who have had a stroke or have diabetes).

The current Heart Foundation recommendation is that treatment begin with a small dose of a single drug. Intolerance suggests the need to try a different class. The Foundation recommends that failure to achieve control should be managed with the addition of a small dose of another class of drug. The idea is to minimise side effects. The disadvantage of this approach is that almost all patients will end up on multiple drugs, which can be a problem for compliance and cost. The other approach is to titrate up the dose of one drug to the maximum recommended unless side effects occur. Then a second drug from another class is added. Some drugs are especially effective in combination:

- beta-blocker and dihydropyridine calcium channel antagonist
- ACE inhibitor or AR antagonist and thiazide
- ACE inhibitor or AR antagonist and calcium antagonist
- beta-blocker and alpha-blocker
- beta-blocker and thiazide.

Fixed-dose combinations of some of these are available: ACE inhibitor and thiazide, beta-blocker and alpha-blocker (labetolol). These combinations should not be used to initiate treatment. Candidates should be familiar with the doses of the common antihypertensive drugs and their important side effects.

Heart transplantation

Cardiac transplantation is now an accepted form of treatment for intractable cardiac failure. Increasing numbers of patients who have either had a transplant or are on the waiting list for one are available for clinical examinations. Those awaiting transplantation are sick enough to require frequent admissions to hospital and those who have had a transplant are often readmitted for various routine investigations. Patients are usually well informed about their condition and should be able to supply a lot of useful information to the candidate.

Although this fact should not be discussed with our surgical colleagues, heart transplantation is technically not a very difficult operation. Improvements in prognosis have followed medical advances, particularly in the area of the management of rejection. The five-year survival rate is now slightly more than 75% for patients who have received a transplant since 1981 and the one-year survival rate is currently about 90%.

As in all transplantation long cases, the examiners will expect the candidate to be familiar with the indications for and contraindications to the procedure. It is also important to know what investigations are required before a patient can be accepted for surgery and to understand the management problems that can occur in patients who have had the operation (see Table 5.7).

TABLE 5.7 Evaluation for heart transplantation

1. History and examination

2. Body weight

3. Cardiac assessment

    (a) Ejection fraction: estimated by resting gated blood pool scan

    (b) Echocardiogram: with measurement of left ventricular dimensions and assessment of the cardiac valves; examination for left ventricular thrombus

    (c) Coronary angiography in patients with suspected ischaemic heart disease

    (d) 24-hour Holter monitoring to evaluate for ventricular arrhythmias

    (e) Right heart catheterisation to measure pulmonary vascular resistance and its response to vasodilators; fixed pulmonary hypertension is a contraindication to cardiac transplantation

4. HLA tissue typing

5. Chest X-ray and respiratory function tests, if indicated

6. Full blood count, ESR and coagulation studies

7. Biochemical profile, including liver function tests, electrolyte levels and estimation of creatinine clearance, serum cholesterol, triglycerides and blood sugar levels

8. Serology for antinuclear antibodies and immunoelectrophoresis

9. Bacteriology: swabs for methicillin-resistant *Staphylococcus aureus* and a Mantoux test if indicated; hepatitis A and B, toxoplasma, CMV, EBV, HIV and herpes simplex serology

10. Psychiatric, renal and dental consultations, if required

11. Social work report

If the cause of the cardiomyopathy is unknown, a myocardial biopsy, viral titres (including coxsackie A virus, echovirus, adenovirus and influenza titres) and iron studies (for haemochromatosis) are required.

Contraindications for heart transplantation: alcoholism, chronic renal disease, pulmonary parenchymal disease, continued tobacco use, advanced liver disease and advanced age. Diabetes mellitus is a relative contraindication.

CMV = cytomegalovirus; EBV = Epstein-Barr virus; ESR = erythrocyte sedimentation rate; HIV = human immunodeficiency virus; HLA = human leucocyte antigen.

The history

1. Try to establish the cause of the patient's cardiac failure. In younger patients cardiomyopathy is more likely to be the problem, but nearly half the patients currently undergoing heart transplantation have ischaemic heart disease. Rheumatic valvular heart disease can also affect younger patients. Combined heart and lung transplantation is occasionally carried out for patients with primary pulmonary hypertension or cystic fibrosis. It may also be the treatment of choice for some forms of congenital heart disease either in childhood or adult life; if pulmonary hypertension is present, these patients have to be considered for combined heart and lung transplantation.

    Ask about previous myocardial infarction or angina and whether the patient knows the results of cardiac catheterisation. All patients undergoing a transplant are required to have cardiac catheterisation. There may have been a preoperative cardiac biopsy performed and the patient may be aware of the results of this test. Also ask about previous thoracotomies.

2. Ask about the patient's symptoms before surgery. Obtain an idea of the exercise tolerance and the severity of angina, if present. The patient may know the results of investigations of cardiac function, such as exercise tests and gated blood pool scans, before and after surgery.

3. Ask what treatment the patient was receiving before transplantation—particularly the doses of diuretics, ACE inhibitors and beta-blockers (e.g. carvedilol). Find out whether frequent admissions to hospital have been necessary and whether intravenous inotropes were required. There may have been recurrent ventricular arrhythmias before surgery. Treatment may have been with drugs, especially amiodarone or an implanted defibrillator and antitachycardia pacemaker. Some patients have undergone previous surgery for arrhythmias. This may include resection of an aneurysm or myocardial resection following ventricular mapping. Occasionally, transplantation is used to treat intractable ventricular arrhythmias.

4. Find out how long it is since the transplant was performed. Ask whether there were any problems with the surgery—either technical or involving acute rejection. Find out how long the patient was in hospital and what further admissions to hospital have occurred since the operation. Ask whether a permanent pacemaker was inserted. Some patients awaiting transplant may have been given a ventricular assist device as a bridge to transplant: ask whether that was necessary.

5. Endomyocardial biopsies are fairly memorable events and the patient should be able to tell you how often these have been performed and when the last one was obtained. It is now routine to perform them at weekly intervals for the first three weeks after operation, every two weeks for the following month and every six months after that for patients whose condition is stable.

6. Find out what drugs the patient is taking currently. Transplant patients should not require antifailure treatment but will, of course, be taking immunosuppressive drugs. Almost all patients are now maintained on cyclosporin; the dose is determined by its serum level. Cyclosporin and tacrolimus are nephrotoxic and cause hypertension and hyperlipidaemia. Newer immunosuppressive drugs include mycophenolate and rapamycin. Diltiazem is often used as a cyclosporin-sparing agent. It dramatically reduces cyclosporin metabolism and therefore the cost of treating patients. Often azathioprine is also prescribed and the dose is adjusted according to the white cell count.

7. Patients are often well informed about symptoms suggesting rejection—often these resemble an attack of pericarditis. The patient may know of boosts of prednisone that have been given for rejection episodes. Early episodes of

rejection are often treated with 1 g of methylprednisolone IV for three days. Later rejection tends to be milder and may respond to an increase in oral steroids. Severe rejection is often treated with antithymocyte globulin or the murine monoclonal muromonab-CD3. Repetitive rejection may be treated with total lymphoid irradiation or methotrexate.

8. Enquire about complications of immunosuppression (see Table 5.8). Many patients are also taking regular antibiotics to prevent *Pneumocystis jirovecii* (formerly *carinii*) infection. Cotrimoxazole twice daily three days a week is a common regimen.

TABLE 5.8 Commonly used immunosuppressants for heart transplant patients

Drug	Side effects	Monitoring/avoidance
Steroids	Cushingoid, diabetes, osteoporosis	Minimal dose
Cyclosporin	Renal impairment, hypertension, neurotoxicity	Blood levels, drug interactions
Mycophenolate	Mild marrow suppression, gastrointestinal upset	Reduce dose, check FBC
Methotrexate	Hepato- and marrow toxicity	FBC
Azathioprine	Hepato- and marrow toxicity, pancreatitis	FBC, liver function tests
FBC = full blood count.		

9. Some general questions about the transplant patient's current life are very relevant. Find out how much difference has occurred in the patient's exercise tolerance and whether he or she has been able to go back to work. If the patient is currently an inpatient, find out why he or she has been admitted to hospital on this occasion. Ask about the patient's family and how they have coped with the illness and the transplant itself. Make some discreet enquiries about the patient's finances and whether there have been any problems returning to the transplant hospital for the various investigations required.

10. Ask about routine cardiac catheterisation. This is typically performed biannually in patients who have had transplants. Coronary artery intimal proliferation can cause ischaemic heart disease in the transplanted heart. Because the heart has been denervated there is not usually any pain. However, there are now patients in whom re-innervation seems to have occurred and led to symptoms of angina. This allograft arteriopathy is one of the most important problems after transplant. It represents a rejection phenomenon. The condition is usually diffuse, but once lesions causing 40% coronary stenosis have occurred, the prognosis is quite poor: the two-year survival rate is only about 50%. The condition is present in 10% of recipients at one year post-transplant and in 50% at five years. Once myocardial infarction has occurred, the two-year survival rate is only 10–20%. Although the disease is a form of rejection, it is still considered important that the patient's cholesterol level be kept as low as possible. Find out whether the patient knows what his or her cholesterol level is and what treatment is being used to keep it low. Intravascular ultrasound is used increasingly to detect subclinical vasculopathy and to study the benefits of various antirejection regimens.

11. Hypertension is another important post-transplant problem. It is associated with the use of cyclosporin. Ask about blood pressure control and treatment.

12. Transplant patients have an increased risk of malignancy. Skin cancers (basal cell and squamous cell carcinomas) are common. There is also a higher incidence of lymphoproliferative disorders. Post-transplant lymphoproliferative disease (PTLD) is an increasingly recognised complication of the immunosuppression required for organ transplants. The incidence in heart transplant patients is less than that for those with liver transplants but more than that for those with renal transplants. Primary or reactivated Ebstein-Barr virus infection is thought to be the cause. The lesions tend to occur in unusual extranodal sites. Reduction in the amount of immunosuppression will sometimes help, but antiviral treatment with acyclovir or interferon may be necessary.

The examination
1. If the transplant has been successful, there should not be many signs. A median sternotomy scar will be present.
2. Look for signs of cardiac failure and pericarditis. Pericarditis can be an indication of rejection.
3. Note the small scars in the neck at the point of introduction of the endomyocardial biopsy forceps.
4. Look for any evidence of Cushing's syndrome from steroid therapy.
5. Examine the chest carefully for signs of infection, examine the mouth for candidiasis, look for infection at intravenous access sites and look at the temperature chart.

Investigations
These depend somewhat on the reason the patient has been admitted to hospital on this occasion.
1. Endomyocardial biopsies are performed routinely and at any suggestion of rejection. Ask about the results of these biopsies.
2. A full blood count (FBC) may be indicated because of possible infection and to monitor the azathioprine dose.
3. Chest X-ray may show signs of cardiac enlargement, although this is a late sign of rejection. Changes of rejection on the ECG include a reduction in voltage caused by myocardial oedema or atrial arrhythmias. Sometimes the patient's ECG shows two sets of P waves: one comes from the transplanted heart and one arises from the residual atrium.
4. Recent assessments of myocardial function, including gated blood pool scans and resting or stress echocardiograms, may be available.
5. Routine coronary angiography may have been performed.
6. If there have been problems with possible infection, results of blood, urine and other cultures should be sought.

Management
The discussion should revolve around the patient's current problem or reason for admission. However, there is likely to be time to discuss the management of rejection, infection, cardiac failure or social problems.
1. Rejection may have been suspected because of pleuritic chest pain, deterioration in left ventricular function or ECG changes. It is diagnosed on the basis of a routine biopsy. The usual approach is to give the patient a boost of methylprednisolone—usually 1 g intravenously daily for three days followed by a repeat biopsy.
2. Infections occurring as a result of immunosuppression are a major cause of death. Possible episodes of infection should be investigated thoroughly and treated aggressively with appropriate therapy. Opportunistic infections are relatively

common as a late complication. Cytomegalovirus, herpes, *Pneumocystis jirovecii*, fungal infection, and *Nocardia* and *Toxoplasma* are all more common than in non-immunosuppressed people.

3. Further cardiac failure may be an indication of rejection, which should be treated. Cardiac failure may also be an indication of silent myocardial infarction.

4. Hyperlipidaemia should be sought routinely and treated most vigorously with drugs and diet.

There may be discussion about the patient's prognosis. The one-year survival rate after transplant is about 90% and the five-year survival rate is about 75%. The 10-year survival rate approaches 50%.

The discussion of a patient awaiting cardiac transplantation will probably run along similar lines. However, it is important to know how well informed the patient is about what is likely to happen, whether he or she appears to fulfil the criteria for transplantation (see Table 5.7) and whether there appear to be any contraindications. Some patients awaiting transplantation are sick enough to require intravenous inotropes. There may even have been talk about the use of external circulatory assistance devices for use as a bridge to transplant.

Cardiac arrhythmias

The management of some cardiac rhythm disturbances is complicated. These patients may be in hospital while waiting for diagnostic tests or, in cases of serious arrhythmias, for treatment to become effective.

They sometimes represent diagnostic, but more often management, problems. Ventricular arrhythmias are a more common reason for admission than supraventricular arrhythmias, but patients with the latter may be awaiting diagnostic or therapeutic procedures. Atrial fibrillation, the most common of the significant cardiac arrhythmias, is unlikely to be the patient's only problem if it appears in a long case.

The history

Ask why the patient is in hospital—all may be revealed without much further effort. Otherwise, the patient may know the name of the arrhythmia or be able to describe symptoms that make the diagnosis likely. If the rhythm problem is a serious and continuing one, the candidate may be fortunate enough to find the patient on an ECG monitor.

Possible presenting symptoms include:

1. rapid and irregular palpitations—suggest atrial fibrillation (AF) (see Fig 5.7)

2. rapid and regular palpitations, with or without dizziness and perhaps terminated by Valsalva manoeuvres—suggest supraventricular tachycardia (SVT) (see Fig 5.8)

3. rapid and regular palpitations with dizziness, syncope or near syncope—suggest ventricular tachycardia (VT), *particularly if there is a history of ischaemic heart disease*

4. syncope with bradycardia or no palpitations—suggests heart block (see Fig 5.9)

5. symptoms of AF and episodes of syncope—suggest sick sinus syndrome

6. a family history of sudden death—suggests the possibility of congenital long QT interval (see Fig 5.10), Brugada syndrome (ionopathy) or a structural cardiac problem such as hypertrophic cardiomyopathy

7. the occurrence of syncope in association with antiarrhythmic drug treatment— suggests the possibility of proarrhythmia; ask about class 1C drugs and sotalol, perhaps prescribed because of paroxysmal AF, as these drugs may also worsen bradyarrhythmias in patients with sick sinus syndrome.

Figure 5.7 **Atrial fibrillation. The ventricular response rate is rapid—between 95 and 160 beats/minute.**

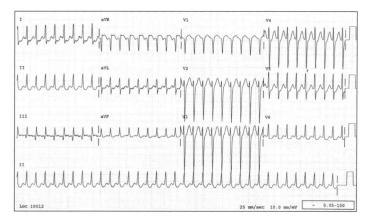

Figure 5.8 **Supraventricular tachycardia. The complexes are narrow. The heart rate is about 200 beats/minute and the rhythm is regular.**

Figure 5.9 **Sinus rhythm. First-degree heart block. Right bundle branch block (RBBB) and left anterior hemi-block (LAHB). This combination of abnormalities is called *trifascicular block*. It is a sign of significant conduction system disease and, in a patient with recurrent syncope, suggests that intermittent complete heart block may be the cause of the symptoms.**

Figure 5.10 (a) Sinus rhythm. The QT interval is prolonged (423 ms) and the corrected QT (QTc) is 460 ms (normal <440 ms). These patients are at risk of syncope or sudden death as a result of the development of polymorphic VT. (b) Polymorphic VT or *torsade de pointes*. This apparent twisting of the QRS complexes is named after the gold braid on French military uniforms.

Ask about previous known heart disease (e.g. ischaemic heart disease and VT, aortic stenosis and heart block) and recent cardiac, thoracic or abdominal surgery.
- Cardiac surgery may be complicated by heart block and all of the above may precipitate AF.
- The 'grown-up' congenital heart disease patient may have persisting problems with atrial or ventricular arrhythmias following cardiac surgery in childhood.
- Atrial septal defects are often complicated by atrial arrhythmias.
  Consider the common causes and associations of AF:
  1. advancing age (3% of 65-year-olds, >6% of people in their 80s)
  2. ischaemic heart disease and myocardial infarction
  3. mitral valve disease
  4. thyrotoxicosis
  5. recent thoracic or abdominal surgery
  6. atrial septal defect
  7. Wolff-Parkinson-White (WPW) syndrome (see Figs 5.11 and 5.12)
  8. recent alcoholic binge
  9. pulmonary embolism
  10. hypertension.

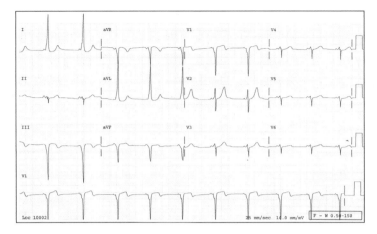

Figure 5.11 Sinus rhythm. Wolff-Parkinson-White conduction. The PR interval is short and delta waves are visible. There are positive delta waves in lead I—seen as a slurred upstroke at the start of the R wave—and negative delta waves in lead III—seen as a slurred Q wave. These patients' ECGs are usually abnormal between their attacks of tachycardia but the *pre-excitation* **(delta wave) may occur only intermittently. They are at risk of sudden death or syncope if atrial fibrillation or flutter occurs (they are often at increased risk of this arrhythmia) because very rapid ventricular rates may occur if the accessory pathway can conduct at high rates. Treat acute atrial fibrillation or flutter in this setting if unstable using electrical cardoversion (never use verapamil, adenosine or digoxin).**

Ask whether the rhythm has been paroxysmal and self-limiting, persistent and requiring cardioversion, or permanent.

Find out about treatment.

1. Has the patient required intravenous drugs to control the heart? Have these been by infusion or bolus injection? Intravenous adenosine is now the drug treatment of first choice for SVT. Patients may well remember its use. It causes a brief but distressing sensation of impending death.
2. Have physical manoeuvres been tried?
3. What oral drugs have been used in the past and during this admission? Make enquiries about the known side effects of these drugs.
4. The investigations the patient has undergone or may be about to undergo can help sort out the diagnosis.
   (a) Certain tests, such as electrophysiological studies (EPS), are more memorable than others. An EPS with induction of VT may mean that direct current (DC) cardioversion was required; despite sedation and reduced cardiac output, some memory of this may remain.
   (b) A cardiac biopsy may have been performed to look for right ventricular cardiomyopathy (RV dyplasia), a cause of VT.
   (c) Cardiac MRI and CT scans are commonly used to look for the patchy changes of cardiac sarcoid or right ventricular (RV) cardiomyopathy (RV dysplasia)
   (d) Other procedures may have been entirely therapeutic: for example, DC cardioversion performed electively under general anaesthesia suggests AF or atrial flutter; catheter ablation, often a fairly prolonged procedure, suggests SVT or VT; pacemaker insertion suggests bradycardia; antiarrhythmia surgery suggests VT or, less often now, SVT.
5. Catheter ablation is now a routine treatment for SVT that does not respond to

simple drug treatment. Rarely there may be failure to suppress the arrhythmia, or a complication such as complete heart block or cardiac rupture can occur. Ablation is also very effective for some forms of VT. These include right, and the less common left, ventricular outflow tract tachycardias. These benign forms of VT can cause frequent recurrent episodes of self-limiting VT with a left or right bundle branch block morphology, respectively. They may respond to treatment with verapamil but are otherwise managed with catheter ablation.

6. Patients with automatic implantable cardioverter-defibrillators (AICDs) can often provide vast amounts of useful information about their devices and about their arrhythmia.

The examination

Examine the cardiovascular system. Is the patient in sinus rhythm clinically? Look for thoracotomy scars, pacemakers and implanted defibrillators. Look for signs of cardiac failure, valvular heart disease and evidence of recent abdominal surgery or thyrotoxicosis.

Investigations

These depend on the actual rhythm problem.

1. **Resting ECG.** Look for:
   (a) the current rhythm
   (b) evidence of pre-excitation (Wolff-Parkinson-White conduction [see Fig 5.12], Lown-Ganong-Levine syndrome)
   (c) heart block
   (d) old infarct
   (e) paced rhythm (ventricular-ventricular inhibited [VVI] or dual chamber—atrial sensing and ventricular pacing or dual-chamber pacing)
   (f) long QT interval (increased risk of polymorphic VT—*torsade de pointes*).

Figure 5.12 **Sinus rhythm in WPW conduction. The delta waves and overall QRS are directed anteriorly in V1, superficially resembling RBBB. This is type A WPW where the bundle of Kent inserts into the left ventricular myocardium. Where the delta wave is initially isoelectric, the PR interval appears normal. Note also the close resemblance to an inferoposterior infarction.**

2. **The examiners may produce previous ECGs or parts of 24-hour Holter monitors.** Remember that a broad complex tachycardia should be considered VT unless there is good reason to consider otherwise. There are a number of ECG criteria for distinguishing VT from SVT with aberrant conduction.

Findings suggestive of VT include:

(a) a QRS >0.14 seconds (if a RBBB pattern) or >0.16 seconds (if a LBBB pattern)

(b) left-axis deviation (between −90° and −180°)

(c) atrioventricular (AV) dissociation (with P waves 'marching through' the QRS complexes)

(d) changes from the pre-existing QRS morphology in pre-existing bundle branch block (but note, these rules do not apply in SVT with aberration caused by WPW conduction).

The presence of known ischaemic heart disease, or cardiac failure, is particularly useful. *Broad complex tachycardia in a patient with ischaemic heart disease is usually VT (95%).*

3. **EPS** may be used to assess inducibility of atrial and ventricular arrhythmias before and after treatment. It is now used in conjunction with catheter ablation as curative treatment for SVT caused by accessory pathways and for some types of VT. It can also be performed to ablate the AV node or the regions around the four pulmonary veins for patients with intractable and disabling AF.

4. **Routine investigations for patients with AF** include echocardiography, thyroid function testing and sometimes exercise testing. Echocardiography may reveal an underlying pathology that is responsible for the AF (e.g. mitral stenosis). It is important in helping quantify embolic risk. Look for:

(a) valve abnormalities

(b) cardiomyopathy

(c) diastolic dysfunction of the left ventricle (especially important in hypertensive patients)

(d) left ventricular hypertrophy

(e) atrial size (consider atrial septal defect)

(f) mitral valve disease

(g) segmental wall abnormalities consistent with ischaemic heart disease.

5. Tests may be needed because of actual or potential drug side effects (e.g. liver function or thyroid function tests for patients on amiodarone).

6. **Cardiac catheterisation** is often indicated for patients with ventricular arrhythmias, as they may have an ischaemic substrate.

Management

Much depends on the rhythm abnormality.

1. Arrhythmias that are not life-threatening are usually managed, at least at first, with drugs. Candidates will be expected to have a thorough working knowledge of the common antiarrhythmic drugs, their methods of action, indications and side effects. Remember that many antiarrhythmic drugs have a potentially dangerous proarrhythmic effect.

2. The indications for permanent pacing (see Table 5.9) and different uses for VVI, VVIR (rate-responsive) and DDD (dual-chamber) pacers (see Figs 5.13 and 5.14) should be well understood. A basic understanding of antitachycardia devices and indications for their use (see Table 5.10) is also important.

3. Automatic implanted cardioverter-defibrillators (AICDs) are increasingly used to manage recurrent VT:

• They are often used in combination with antiarrhythmic drugs of some sort. They are becoming smaller, cheaper (between $25,000 and $50,000) and more complicated. It is now established that they improve mortality rates in selected patients.

• They are usually the treatment of choice for hypotensive VT or missed sudden death from VF. Drug treatment of these conditions is not very effective.

- The current models have leads that can be placed intravenously into the vena cava and for pacing purposes into the right ventricle.
- They are small enough to be implanted like pacemakers in the chest wall, but are still noticeably larger than pacemakers (see Fig 5.15). Implantation takes place under local anaesthetic in the electrophysiology laboratory.
- The periprocedural mortality rate is less than 1%, compared with over 5% when surgical implantation was required.

TABLE 5.9 Indications for permanent pacemaker insertion in adults

Generally agreed indications

1. Intermittent or permanent complete heart block, with:
   (a) symptomatic bradycardia
   (b) cardiac failure
   (c) arrhythmias that require treatment with drugs that slow conduction
   (d) documented asystole of more than 3 seconds or escape rhythm with a rate <40 beats/minute
   (e) confusional states that improve with temporary pacing
2. Intermittent permanent second-degree AV block with symptomatic bradycardia
3. Sinus node dysfunction with symptomatic bradycardia

Less certain indications

1. Asymptomatic complete heart block; heart rate ≥40 beats/minute
2. Symptomatic type 2 second-degree heart block
3. Bifascicular or trifascicular block with syncope of unknown aetiology

Not indicated

1. First-degree heart block
2. Asymptomatic type 1 second-degree heart block

Figure 5.13 Atrial sensing and ventricular pacing. This is the ECG of a patient with a dual-chamber pacemaker. Normal P waves are followed by an atrioventricular (PR) interval and then a pacing spike, which precedes a wide QRS complex with a LBBB pattern (pacing is from the right ventricular apex).

Figure 5.14 Dual-chamber pacing. Pacing spikes precede both atrial and ventricular complexes.

TABLE 5.10 Indications for implanted cardioverter-defibrillators (ICDs)
Generally agreed indications
1. Confirmed VF or hypotensive VT not related to acute infarct or severe electrolyte abnormality, but VF/VT not inducible at EPS—this means drug treatment cannot be tested by EPS
2. VF/VT with contraindications to drug treatment (intolerance)
3. Persistently inducible VT/VF despite drug treatment, ablation or surgery
4. Persistent spontaneous VT/VF despite drug treatment
5. Symptomatic long QT syndrome despite drug treatment
Less certain indications
1. Inducible but not spontaneous VT despite other treatment in high-risk patients
2. VT/VF apparently controlled but in a high-risk patient
3. Serial drug testing possible but defibrillator preferred
Not generally indicated
1. Very frequent or incessant VT
2. Reversible cause
3. Recurrent syncope, VT/VF not inducible
4. Poor life expectancy (e.g. class IV cardiac failure but not a transplant candidate)
Note: Increasingly proven VT or VF in a patient with poor LV function is considered an indication regardless of EPS findings.
VF = ventricular fibrillation; VT = ventricular tachycardia; EPS = electrophysical study.

The programming of these machines is complicated, but candidates should know that they are usually set to attempt reversion of VT by overdrive pacing (antitachycardia pacing, ATP) before administering a DC shock. Patients are usually, but not always, aware of the onset of ATP and almost always aware of DC shock administration. Ask how the device has affected the patient's life and confidence, including how often it goes off and whether the box itself causes problems because of its size. Although AICDs can prevent sudden death, their presence is often associated with a feeling of insecurity. Patients may have clear memories of events leading up to activation of the device. They may avoid places where arrhythmias and activations have occurred. They often require repeated explanation and reassurance.

Figure 5.15 (a) PA chest X-ray showing implanted cardioverter defibrillator and biventricular pacemaker. (b) Lateral view: the large defibrillation electrode (which also serves as an RV pacing electrode) (arrow) and the right atrial and left ventricular pacing leads are visible.

Figures reproduced courtesy of The Canberra Hospital.

The particular management problems of atrial fibrillation

Examiners require candidates to have a sensible approach to the management of AF and the opportunity for examiners to ask about this common condition will often arise. The principles of management are to:

- maintain sinus rhythm
- control the heart rate (if maintaining sinus rhythm proves difficult)
- protect from embolic events.

1. There is good evidence from recent trials that control of heart rate is at least as satisfactory an approach as that of trying aggressively to maintain sinus rhythm. Nevertheless, patients with paroxysmal AF often find the arrhythmia very disturbing. They should be told at the outset that it may not be possible to keep them in sinus rhythm, but that rate control and freedom from embolic episodes can be almost guaranteed. The prophylactic drug treatment of paroxysmal AF involves the use of a class III drug (sotalol or amiodarone) in most cases, but occasionally the class 1C drug flecainide can be used if the heart is known to be structurally normal.

2. Rate control of persistent or paroxysmal AF can be achieved with less-toxic drugs. Digoxin is a common first-line treatment and is usually well tolerated. It is not very effective on its own at controlling the heart rate during exercise. Many patients with chronic AF have persistent dyspnoea during exercise because of inadequate rate control. They benefit from the use of a beta-blocker or one of the non-dihydropyridine calcium channel blockers (diltiazem or verapamil). These can be used with or without digoxin. Control of the heart rate can prevent or reverse the impairment of left ventricular function that is associated with tachycardias (tachycardia-induced cardiomyopathy).

3. When patients remain unhappy with their symptoms despite rate control, further intervention should be considered. AV nodal ablation is a relatively simple procedure that prevents fibrillation waves reaching the ventricles. The patient then requires an artificial pacemaker. Although atrial systole is lost, the regularisation of the heart rate is usually enough to improve symptoms dramatically. If the patient's AF has been paroxysmal, a dual-chamber pacemaker with a 'mode switch' may be used. When the patient is in sinus rhythm, atrial sensing occurs and the ventricles are paced after an appropriate AV interval. When episodes of AF occur, the pacemaker mode switches and paces the ventricle at a steady rate.

4. DC cardioversion of AF can be a reasonable treatment for the first episode or for patients with infrequent episodes. DC cardioversion is safe in the absence of digoxin toxicity or hypokalaemia but is associated with a risk of embolism if the patient's AF has been present for more than 48 hours. In this case, one month's therapeutic anticoagulation with warfarin should be instituted before the procedure and continued for four weeks afterwards. An alternative is to perform a transoesophageal echocardiogram to look for left atrial appendage thrombus or spontaneous echocardiograph contrast (a sign of slow blood flow). The absence of these means that DC cardioversion is safe, but that warfarin must be given for four weeks afterwards because there is a persisting risk over this period.

5. Reversion of AF with drug treatment is difficult. Many episodes terminate spontaneously but drug treatment is given the credit. It is known that digoxin does not increase the reversion rate, but the class III drugs and flecainide do improve the chances somewhat. Sometimes control of the heart rate and awaiting spontaneous reversion can be an option. A decision to go on to DC cardioversion, however, should be made before 48 hours has passed.

6. Over many years attempts have been made to prevent AF by surgical or catheter

ablation techniques. Pulmonary vein isolation is now commonly performed for intractable symptomatic AF. Radiofrequency energy is used to isolate the two pairs of pulmonary veins in the left atrium. The rationale for this approach is that almost all AF seems to be initiated by electrical activity arising from this part of the heart. Isolation of this area from the rest of the heart prevents the initiation of AF. The procedure is complicated and time-consuming (4–6 hours per case). It is not a practical solution for most cases of AF. Success rates of about 60% are usually quoted. Until recently, an uncommon but severe complication involved the late occurrence of pulmonary vein stenosis. Newer techniques have made this a rare problem. Other complications include heart block and cardiac perforation. Successful treatment spares a patient the need for anticoagulation.

7. Protecting patients from embolic events is perhaps the most important aspect of the management of AF. Cerebral embolus is the most feared complication, but life-threatening peripheral embolisation (e.g. to the mesenteric bed) can occur. Patients should have this aspect of AF explained to them early on. The risk of embolism is low in people under the age of 60 and without any risk factors (see Table 5.11): <0.5% a year. It can be as high as 30% for patients with mitral stenosis.

   Use the **CHADS2** scoring system to help you decide who to anticoagulate with persistent AF:
   Congestive heart failure: 1 point
   Hypertension: 1 point
   Age 75 and over: 1 point
   Diabetes mellitus: 1 point
   Stroke or TIA: 2 points

CHADS2 scoring system	
CHADS2 score = 0	aspirin alone
CHADS2 score = 1 or 2	warfarin or aspirin considered acceptable
CHADS2 score = 3 or more	warfarin

TABLE 5.11 Risk factors for embolic events for patients with AF

1. Age >65 years

2. Previous embolic event

3. Mitral valve disease, especially mitral stenosis or a mechanical valve

4. Cardiac failure

5. Hypertension or left ventricular hypertrophy on echocardiography

6. Diabetes mellitus

7. Thyrotoxicosis

8. Thrombus or spontaneous echocardiographic contrast on transoesophageal echocardiography

8. Patients with risk factors remain at risk of stroke even if sinus rhythm has been restored. Those with self-limiting paroxysmal AF are also at risk if episodes are more than a rare event. Aspirin gives some protection to those unwilling or unable to take warfarin. There is evidence that combination anti-platelet

treatment (e.g. with aspirin and clopidogrel) is somewhat more effective than aspirin alone.

9. An assessment of the patient's ability to manage regular blood tests and dosage adjustments is necessary before treatment can begin. Patients are often reluctant to undertake the complexities of treatment but should not be allowed to decline treatment until all the risks of this approach have been carefully explained.

10. The availability of home international normalised ratio (INR) testing machines that use a capillary blood sample has made the use of warfarin more acceptable to some patients (e.g. those who travel frequently). A number of studies have shown that this approach is safe for selected patients. The safe therapeutic range is an INR of between 2 and 2.5.

11. Find out from the patient how the warfarin is managed and whether he or she knows the last few readings and dosage. Patients should be encouraged to keep a record of their INR results and warfarin doses. The examiners will expect considerable detail about the patient's warfarin management.

Chapter 6

The respiratory long case

I here present the reader with a new sign, which
I have discovered for detecting diseases of the
chest. This consists in percussion ...
Leopold Auenbrugger (1760)

Bronchiectasis

Bronchiectasis is a reasonably common subject for a long case and usually poses a management problem. It is defined as pathological and permanent dilatation of the bronchi. There are associated destructive and inflammatory changes in the walls of the segmental and subsegmental bronchi.

The history

1. Find out when the patient's respiratory problems began. Classically the cough and sputum begin in childhood, although adult onset is becoming more common. Ask about childhood whooping cough or measles. Lower respiratory tract infection with influenza and adenoviruses is an increasingly common cause of the disease. Potentially necrotising bacteria are also a cause if antibiotic treatment is inadequate—these include *Staphylococcus aureus* and *Klebsiella* organisms. The abnormal pulmonary defence mechanisms, or mucus clearance, associated with cystic fibrosis, tuberculosis, immunoglobulin deficiency, HIV infection and primary ciliary dyskinesia (immotile cilia syndrome) make these important causes of the condition. Localised bronchiectasis can occur in association with a space-occupying lesion, which can be endobronchial or external.

    Symptoms include:
    (a) recurrent haemoptysis
    (b) dyspnoea and wheeze
    (c) chronic sinusitis (70%)
    (d) recurrent pneumonia and pleurisy
    (e) systemic symptoms of weight loss, fever and anorexia
    (f) symptoms of right heart failure—a late event.
2. Ask about recent precipitating causes of admissions to hospital (e.g. infection, haemoptysis).
3. Enquire about treatment—physiotherapy, postural drainage, antibiotics (as prophylaxis or treatment), bronchodilators, lung resection.
4. Determine whether the patient had childhood immunisations (e.g. MMR).
5. Ask about investigations in the past (e.g. CT scanning, ciliary function studies, sweat test, bronchograms [memorable!]).

6. Establish aetiology such as childhood or early adult infections (e.g. pneumonia, measles, whooping cough) (see Table 6.1).
7. Ask how the disease interferes with the patient's life (e.g. work). Infertility is usual in men with primary ciliary dyskinesia and is variable in affected women.

TABLE 6.1 Causes of bronchiectasis
1. Congenital
(a) Cystic fibrosis
(b) Primary ciliary dyskinesia, including the immotile cilia syndrome
(c) Congenital hypogammaglobulinaemia (especially IgA and IgG subclasses)
2. Acquired
(a) Infections in childhood (e.g. pneumonia, measles, whooping cough)
(b) Localised disease (e.g. bronchial adenoma, tuberculosis, foreign body)
(c) Allergic bronchopulmonary aspergillosis (proximal bronchiectasis)
(d) Rheumatoid arthritis, Sjögren's syndrome
(e) Idiopathic (up to 50%)
Note: Lung carcinoma rarely causes bronchiectasis, as death tends to intervene first.

The examination
Examine the respiratory system carefully (see p 291).
1. Particularly note the unpleasant purulent sputum.
2. Examine carefully for clubbing and localised crackles and wheezes.
3. Look for the position of the apex beat (don't miss dextrocardia—Kartagener's syndrome) and for the signs of right heart failure.
4. Consider the complications and look for them. These include:
   (a) pneumonia
   (b) pleurisy
   (c) empyema
   (d) lung abscess
   (e) cor pulmonale
   (f) cerebral abscess (very rare)
   (g) amyloid (rare, but an important topic in the examination).

Investigations
Investigations should include:
- **chest X-ray film** (see Fig 15.15(a)), which may be normal, or it may show 1–2 cm cystic lesions or, more often, streaky infiltration and thickened bronchial walls (tram tracking), especially in the lower lobes
- **sputum microscopy**; the common organisms are *Haemophilus influenzae, Pseudomonas, Escherichia coli*, pneumococcus and *Staphylococcus aureus*
- **immunoglobulin (IgG, IgM, IgA) levels** (hypogammaglobulinaemia)
- **blood film for eosinophilia**, which may indicate allergic bronchopulmonary aspergillosis or asthma
- **ventilatory function tests**, which may show a restrictive defect or an obstructive pattern
- **arterial blood gas estimations**, which may show mild or moderate hypoxia and, later, respiratory failure—defined as an arterial oxygen tension (PaO_2) <60 mmHg or an arterial carbon dioxide tension ($PacO_2$) >50 mmHg
- **high-resolution CT scanning of the chest** (see Fig 15.15(b)), which has replaced bronchography and is indicated in most patients to confirm the diagnosis.

The extent of the disease is usually generalised. If the bronchiectasis is localised, resection may be indicated as long as the underlying cause is not systemic.

Treatment

The principles of treatment are as follows:

1. The facilitation (or maximisation) of clearance of sputum and the treatment of infection with antibiotics and of bronchoconstriction with bronchodilators.
2. Inhaled steroids may be of value if there is bronchial reactivity.
3. Twice-daily postural drainage (20 minutes morning and night) or newer physiotherapy techniques should be recommended.
4. The use of antibiotics during exacerbations is routine and prednisone in tapered doses may be useful. Prophylactic oral or nebulised antibiotics are controversial treatments. Problem pathogens include *Mycobacterium avium* complex (MAC), *Pseudomonas* and *Aspergillus*.
5. Influenza and pneumococcal vaccines are advisable for all patients.
6. Treatment of heart failure should go *pari passu* with that of the lung disease.
7. Immunoglobulin deficiency can be treated with monthly IV injections of immunoglobulin, which decrease the incidence of infection and the need for hospitalisation.
8. Massive haemoptysis may occur as a result of bronchial wall erosion and the increased vascularity of the bronchial walls. It may respond to bronchial artery embolisation.
9. Smoking (including of marijuana) cessation is always essential.
10. Surgery should be considered for localised disease to prevent progression or as treatment of intractable haemorrhage.
11. Transplant is occasionally appropriate for end-stage disease.

Lung carcinoma

Lung carcinoma is a common disease that candidates often encounter in the examination. It can pose a diagnostic and management problem, and remains a leading cause of cancer death in men and women. At diagnosis only 20% of patients will have local disease and half will have disseminated disease. The overall five-year survival rate is less than 15%. The major cell types are set out in Table 6.2. Over the last 20 years, adenocarcinoma has become more common than squamous cell carcinoma.

TABLE 6.2 Carcinoma of the lung—cell types		
Type	Frequency	Overall five-year survival rate
Adenocarcinoma	32%	17%
Squamous cell	29%	15%
Small (oat) cell	18%	5%
Large cell	9%	11%
Bronchioalveolar	3%	42%

The history

1. Find out how the diagnosis was made or suspected—a proportion of patients are asymptomatic and were diagnosed after a routine chest X-ray or scan.
2. Ask about the duration of illness and respiratory symptoms (e.g. haemoptysis, dyspnoea, increasing cough, chest pain).
3. Enquire about a history of unresolved pneumonia, pleural effusion or lung abscess.

4. Ask about systemic symptoms (e.g. weight loss).
5. Determine metastatic and non-metastatic symptoms (see Table 6.3).
6. Ask about aetiology:
   (a) smoking and exposure to the cigarette smoke of others (a dose–response relationship—long-term smokers have a 10- to 30-fold risk; discontinuation of smoking reduces the risk over 10–15 years, but the relative risk does not return to 1.0); women have a higher risk for a given level of exposure to cigarette smoke than men (1.5:1); there is a familial association for first-degree relatives
   (b) occupational history (e.g. asbestos exposure, uranium miners); remember, the effect of asbestos plus smoking is synergistic, *not* additive
   (c) chronic scarring (e.g. tuberculosis, scleroderma, interstitial lung disease [ILD] may be associated with adenocarcinoma).
7. Ask about investigations performed, such as chest X-ray changes (the only abnormal finding in 5% of cases), CT scans, bronchoscopy, sputum cytology, needle biopsy and thoracotomy.
8. Enquire about the patient's work and home environments, including the number of dependants and the patient's ability to work.
9. Ask about treatment offered and begun.
10. Find out the patient's understanding of the condition and the likely prognosis.

TABLE 6.3 Metastatic and non-metastatic manifestations of lung carcinoma
Local extension
1. Pleural effusion
2. Rib involvement
3. Nerve involvement (e.g. Pancoast's tumour, Horner's syndrome, recurrent laryngeal nerve palsy, diaphragmatic paralysis)
4. Superior vena caval obstruction
5. Pericardial effusion
6. Oesophageal obstruction
7. Tracheal obstruction
8. Lymphangitis
Distant metastases
1. Cervical adenopathy
2. Cerebral, liver or bone metastases
Non-metastatic features
1. Anorexia, weight loss, cachexia, fever
2. Endocrine:
(a) hypercalcaemia (increased parathyroid hormone occurs usually in squamous cell carcinoma)
(b) hyponatraemia (antidiuretic hormone—small cell carcinoma)
(c) ectopic adrenocorticotrophic hormone (ACTH) syndrome (usually small cell carcinoma)
(d) gynaecomastia (all types—caused by ectopic gonadotrophin secretion)

TABLE 6.3 Metastatic and non-metastatic manifestations of lung carcinoma (Continued)

Non-metastatic features (continued)

   (e)   carcinoid syndrome (small cell carcinoma)

   (f)   insulin-like activity (squamous cell carcinoma)

3. Skeletal (very rare with small cell carcinoma):

   (a)   clubbing

   (b)   hypertrophic pulmonary osteoarthropathy (may be more common with adenocarcinoma)

4. Neurological:

   (a)   Eaton Lambert's syndrome (small cell carcinoma)

   (b)   peripheral neuropathy or autonomic neuropathy

   (c)   subacute cerebellar degeneration

   (d)   polymyositis/dermatomyositis

   (e)   cortical degeneration with dementia

   (f)   acute transverse myelopathy

5. Haematological:

   (a)   migrating venous thrombophlebitis, arterial thrombosis

   (b)   diffuse intravascular coagulation

   (c)   anaemia, leucoerythroblastosis, red cell aplasia, polycythaemia, eosinophilia

6. Skin: e.g. acanthosis nigricans, fibrinolytic purpura, scleroderma (alveolar cell carcinoma)

7. Renal: e.g. nephrotic syndrome (owing to membranous glomerulonephritis)

8. Opportunistic infections (most often in those treated with chemotherapy)

The examination

1. Finger clubbing is a most important sign (see Table 15.11). This is very rare in small cell carcinoma.
2. Chest signs will vary—listen carefully for a fixed inspiratory wheeze over a large bronchus.
3. Recurrent laryngeal nerve palsy may have caused hoarseness, and phrenic nerve paralysis may have caused an elevation of a hemidiaphragm.
4. An apical tumour may be responsible for Pancoast's syndrome (C8, T1 thoracic nerve destruction or compression, or Horner's syndrome, or both).
5. Look for metastatic (e.g. supraclavicular lymphadenopathy and hepatomegaly) and non-metastatic manifestations, especially the neurological and endocrinological changes (see Table 6.3).

Investigations

Screening of high-risk patients with chest X-ray or CT scanning may lead to an early diagnosis but has not been shown to affect survival. The diagnosis may be difficult, even when suspected.

1. Sputum cytology may be helpful in centrally located lesions, but fibre-optic bronchoscopy is now more often done first.
2. The chest X-ray or CT may suggest the cell type: for example, peripheral nodule—adenocarcinoma; central lesion with obstructive pneumonitis—squamous;

mediastinal or hilar mass—small cell; or alveolar infiltrate—bronchoalveolar cell.

3. A suspect shadow on the chest X-ray film should be investigated by fibre-optic bronchoscopy and biopsy or fine-needle aspiration (see Fig 6.1). Bronchial brushings and washings, taken at bronchoscopy, should also be sent for cytological examination but have a lower yield than biopsy.

4. For peripheral lesions, especially those less than 2 cm in size, transthoracic fine-needle biopsy with CT guidance is very useful, but complications (e.g. pneumothorax, significant bleeding) can occur.

5. In patients with a malignant pleural effusion, thoracocentesis and pleural biopsy provide a high diagnostic yield (see Table 15.12).

6. Other investigations may include bone marrow biopsy, mediastinoscopy and thoracotomy. Video-assisted thoracoscopy has replaced open biopsy in many centres.

7. Other possible causes (e.g. of a coin lesion) must be excluded. For this purpose CT is helpful; demonstration of central or lamellar calcification usually indicates that a coin lesion is benign. Follow-up scans to confirm a lesion is unchanged are helpful. Positron emission tomography (PET) scans may be of value in these cases.

8. Once the diagnosis is made and the cell type identified, further investigations may be indicated to stage the disease.
   - Symptoms and signs that suggest central nervous system, liver, bone, chest wall or mediastinal involvement need to be sought carefully.
   - Full blood count (see Table 6.4), serum calcium and liver function tests may suggest tumour spread.

Figure 6.1 (a) PA film. A round opacity is visible in the right middle lobe (arrow).
Figure reproduced courtesy of The Canberra Hospital.

Figure 6.1 Continued (b) Lateral film. A round opacity is visible in the right middle lobe (arrow).
Figure reproduced courtesy of The Canberra Hospital.

- CT scanning of the chest and abdomen with contrast is an important aid in determining whether disease is localised.
- In small cell carcinoma, stage the disease into limited disease (lung primary, ipsilateral and contralateral hilar, mediastinal and supraclavicular nodes) or extensive disease—70% of patients (contralateral lung, distant metastases).
- Non-small cell carcinoma is staged according to the tumour node metastases (TNM) international staging system (see Table 6.5).

9. Assessment for resectability should include respiratory function tests. If the forced expiratory volume (FEV_1) is 1.5 L or more, this indicates that the patient could tolerate a pneumonectomy (a postoperative FEV_1 of 1 L or more is usually considered the minimum that will be tolerated). Otherwise, a patient who can climb three flights of stairs is usually considered well enough to tolerate surgery.

Treatment
The average five-year survival rate for all types of carcinoma of the lung is about 15%.

Small cell carcinomas
1. These are only occasionally resected as they have usually metastasised at the time of diagnosis.

TABLE 6.4 Full blood count and liver function tests from a female patient with carcinoma of the lung

Parameter	Value	Normal value
Haemoglobin	84 g/L	115–165 g/L (female)
Mean corpuscular volume (MCV)	95 fL	80–100 fL
White cell count (WCC)	4.0×10^9/L	$4.5–13.5 \times 10^9$/L
Platelets	95×10^9/L	$150–400 \times 10^9$/L
Erythrocyte sedimentation rate (ESR)	70 mm/h	3–19 mm/h (female <50 years)
Bilirubin	84 mmol/L	<20 mmol/L (total)
Aspartate aminotransferase (AST)	57 U/L	<40 U/L
Alanine aminotransferase (ALT)	50 U/L	<35 U/L
Lactate dehydrogenase (LDH)	780 U/L	110–230 U/L
Protein	60 g/L	62–80 g/L (total)
Albumin	33 g/L	32–45 g/L

Blood film: normochromic red cells, poikilocytosis, tear drop cells. Some nucleated red cells (normoblasts) and myeloid cells (metamyelocytes and myelocytes). Some rouleaux formation. *Comment:* The combination of normochromic anaemia and the presence of marrow precursors in the peripheral blood is called a leucoerythroblastic reaction. It is typical of bone marrow infiltration by carcinoma or fibrosis. The abnormal liver function tests are non-specific, but suggest liver involvement in this setting. The elevated LDH level probably indicates liver damage, but can also occur when there is haemolysis.

TABLE 6.5 TNM international staging system for carcinoma of the lung (non-small cell)

Stage	TNM			5-year survival rate	Management
IA	T1	N0	M0	61%	Surgery
IB	T2	N0	M0	38%	Surgery
IIA	T1	N1	M0	34%	Surgery ± radiotherapy or chemotherapy
IIB	T2	N2	M0	24%	Surgery ± radiotherapy or chemotherapy
IIIA	T3	N1	M0	9%	Surgery + chemotherapy
	T1–3	N2	M0	13%	
IIIB	T4	N0–2	M0	9%	
	T1–4	N3	M0	3%	Chemotherapy or palliation
IV			M1	1%	Chemotherapy or palliation

T1–T4 = ascending degrees of increase in tumour size and involvement; N0 = no lymph nodes; N1–4 = ascending degrees of nodal involvement; M0 = no metastases; M1–4 = ascending degrees of metastatic involvement.

2. In patients with limited disease, chemotherapy and concurrent radiotherapy improve the prognosis. Untreated, the median survival is only about four months. Treatment often includes etoposide and cisplatin or carboplatin.

3. Prophylactic cranial irradiation may be given to patients with complete responses. There is a risk of leukaemia, central nervous system metastases, dementia and second primary malignancies with treatment.

Limited small cell carcinoma has a median survival with treatment of 11–18 months; 10–20% are disease-free at two years. Extensive small cell carcinoma has a median survival of 6–12 months with therapy.

Non-small cell carcinomas

1. These may be resectable—unless tumour has spread to the contralateral lung or outside the thorax or there is significant cardiopulmonary disease.
2. The most important prognostic factor is the stage of disease. Staging usually involves bronchoscopy and CT scanning of the chest, abdomen and brain, as well as a physiological assessment of the patient's fitness for surgery, from the point of view of both lung function and general health. One-third of patients have disease sufficiently localised for an attempt at resection.
3. Radiotherapy with 'curative intent' may be offered to patients if they refuse surgery or are unfit for surgery for other reasons. About 6% are alive after five years.
4. Adjuvant chemotherapy is not routine for surgical patients, but regimens including cisplatin may provide a small survival advantage. Median survival is only a few months in patients with intracranial metastases or bone involvement.
5. Airway obstruction as a result of carcinoma may be relieved by using Nd-YAG laser or brachytherapy for palliation.
6. Combination chemotherapy is sometimes appropriate. Survival benefit is only one or two months.

Chronic obstructive pulmonary disease

This general term is usually applied to patients with chronic bronchitis and emphysema. Although these two conditions are different, they usually occur together. Chronic obstructive pulmonary disease (COPD) is common and presents major management problems. However, in the examination it is unusual for it to be the patient's only medical problem. The vast majority of patients with COPD (more than 95%) are or have been smokers. However, only about one-fifth of smokers experience a rapid enough decline in FEV_1 ever to develop COPD.

The history

1. Find out about symptoms, such as cough and sputum, dyspnoea, wheeze, impaired exercise tolerance, ankle oedema and weight loss. Remember that the diagnosis of chronic bronchitis is made largely from the history.
2. Ask about precipitating causes of disease exacerbation, such as an upper respiratory tract infection, pneumonia, omission of drugs, symptoms of right ventricular failure, resumption of smoking, pneumothorax, sleep apnoea, oropharyngeal aspiration and gastro-oesophageal reflux disease.
3. Enquire about smoking habits. Ask about the number of cigarettes smoked per day and the length of use (10 packet years of smoking is usually a prerequisite), as well as exposure to other people's cigarette smoke—passive smoking. Absence of a smoking history weighs heavily against the diagnosis unless chronic asthma or alpha1-antitrypsin deficiency is present. Find out at what age the patient began to smoke. Commencement in adolescence when lung development is incomplete may lead to a more rapid decline in lung function.
4. Ask about occupational history. This may be important, particularly as an additive feature if the patient has pneumoconiosis or has been exposed to

toluene in plastics factories. Exposure to the fumes of solid fuel fires and to air pollution is also a risk factor.
5. Ask about medications, especially steroids, home oxygen and bronchodilators.
6. Enquire about management at home and work and the social effects of the disease. Find out in detail how limited the patient is physically and whether ADLs are managed. Ask about financial problems associated with chronic illness and symptoms of depression caused by chronic disability and loss of self-esteem.
7. Ask about family history, such as alpha$_1$-antitrypsin deficiency causing emphysema (autosomal codominant inheritance; the most common variant associated with severe deficiency of alpha$_1$-antitrypsin (<11 mmol/L) is the *ZZ* allele, responsible for 2% of cases of emphysema in smokers).

The examination
Examine the respiratory system carefully (see p 291). The examination may be normal until airways obstruction is moderately severe. Look particularly for:
1. pursed-lip breathing (prolongs the expiratory time and may limit over-inflation) and use of accessory muscles
2. cyanosis and polycythaemia (*note:* clubbing does not occur unless another disease such as carcinoma has supervened)
3. intercostal recession
4. prolonged forced expiratory time (reduced in both obstructive and restrictive lung disease)
5. tracheal tug
6. reduced diaphragmatic movements, over-inflation, reduced chest wall movement and expansion, Hoover's sign (paradoxical inward movement of the lower costal margin during inspiration)
7. reduced breath sounds with or without wheezes (rhonchi) and coarse inspiratory crackles
8. sputum
9. signs of right heart failure
10. signs of cachexia in patients with advanced disease (this is probably related to the increase in tumour necrosis factor alpha associated with chronic hypoxia rather than to the increased work of breathing)
11. side effects of treatment (e.g. tremor as a result of the use of beta-agonists, or the various changes caused by steroids).

Investigations
1. **Chest X-ray film (see Fig 6.2)**—look for signs of hyperinflation (flat diaphragms and a vertical heart shadow) and cor pulmonale and exclude pneumonia. Radiolucent bullae may be visible; they are very specific for emphysema. The X-ray may be normal if the patient has mild disease. High resolution CT of the chest is more often performed and is more specific for emphysema.
2. **Ventilatory function tests**—look for a considerable reduction of the FEV$_1$/FVC (forced vital capacity) ratio. A normal FEV$_1$ excludes the condition. The amount of reversibility should be tested with bronchodilators. An increase in FEV$_1$ or FVC of more than 15% and of at least 200 mL is considered significant. Complete or almost complete reversibility means that the diagnosis is asthma rather than COPD. Some asthmatics smoke and have both conditions; many smokers claim to have asthma but have only COPD. Vital capacity or total lung capacity may be falsely decreased if measured by gas dilution techniques because of the non-homogeneity of ventilation in COPD. The diffusing capacity for carbon monoxide is reduced in emphysema—a value of <50% is associated with exertion-induced hypoxia.

Figure 6.2 COPD. Note the overinflated lungs, flat diaphragms and prominent pulmonary arteries (arrows), a sign of pulmonary hypertension.
Figure reproduced courtesy of The Canberra Hospital.

3. **Arterial blood gas levels**—look for respiratory failure at rest. The demonstration of significant hypoxia (usually a PaO_2 of <55 mmHg, or <59 mmHg if the patient has cor pulmonale) is required for the prescription of home oxygen treatment. Ventilatory failure is defined as $PaCO_2$ of >45 mmHg.
4. **Haemoglobin value**—look for polycythaemia.
5. **Sputum culture**—will usually grow *Haemophilus influenzae*, *Streptococcus pneumoniae* or *Moraxella catarrhalis* during exacerbations *and* remissions.
6. **Electrocardiogram (ECG)**—look for signs of right ventricular hypertrophy and multifocal atrial tachycardia, which can complicate chronic lung disease (see Figs 6.3 and 6.4).
7. **Alpha₁-antitrypsin measurement**—this is now generally recommended. It should particularly be considered if the patient has never smoked or has associated bronchiectasis, cirrhosis or basilar emphysema.

Figure 6.3 COPD. There is atrial fibrillation with a moderately rapid ventricular response rate. There are prominent R waves in V1 and there is marked RAD (right-axis deviation) (+110°). The right precordial T wave inversion suggests right ventricular 'strain'.

Figure 6.4 **Multifocal atrial tachycardia L2 strip.**

8. **Assessment of nutrition**—body mass index (BMI = weight in kg/height in cm²), grip strength, serum albumin, calcium and phosphate levels.
9. **Exercise testing**—to assess the need for ambulatory oxygen therapy and the degree of disability if there are discrepancies.

Differential diagnosis
1. **Asthma**—features suggesting asthma:
   (a) non-smoker
   (b) onset in childhood
   (c) family history of allergy
   (d) episodic attacks and also nocturnal symptoms
   (e) a rapid response to treatment, especially steroids
   (f) eosinophilia in the sputum
   (g) atopic diathesis
   (h) reversibility of obstruction.
2. **Bronchiectasis**—features suggesting bronchiectasis:
   (a) daily sputum production with or without haemoptysis
   (b) onset in childhood
   (c) recurrent chest infection
   (d) clubbing.

Treatment
1. The patient should stop smoking, as this decreases sputum production and bronchospasm and may reduce the rate of decline in lung function to that of a non-smoker (smoking cessation has been shown to prolong life). The candidate should have an approach to the treatment of nicotine addiction. This may involve the temporary use of nicotine substitutes, psychological counselling and encouragement, or the use of drugs such as bupropion.
2. Antibiotics can be used to shorten exacerbations (long-term chemoprophylaxis is indicated if there are four or more episodes a year), such as amoxycillin or doxycycline given as a course at home at the first sign of purulent sputum. Remember that 25% of *H. influenzae* and 75% of *M. catarrhalis* infections are ampicillin-resistant.
3. Regular bronchodilators are of value:
   - Beta$_2$-agonists from metered-dose inhalers form the basis of treatment. A small change in FEV$_1$ and FVC may produce considerable subjective improvement. Some patients find the inhaler devices difficult to use.
   - Inhaled long-acting anticholinergic drugs such as tiotropium bromide provide symptomatic improvement and reduce exacerbations, but do not prolong life.
   - Inhaled steroids in high doses (e.g. 400 µg beclomethasone) reduce the rate of episodes of exacerbation, but should be discontinued if after a trial of 4–8 weeks of treatment there is no clinical or spirometric improvement.

Candidates should have a strategy to ensure effective use of the best device for a particular patient. Long-acting drugs, such as salmeterol, provide longer acting bronchodilatation and are at least more convenient. Oral theophylline derivatives may have an additive effect with beta$_2$-agonists, perhaps because they improve respiratory muscle function. They are prescribed much less often now, partly because they cause oesophageal reflux, cardiac arrhythmias, nausea and insomnia, and partly because they are not very effective. Antitussives and mucolytics are controversial, but may be useful to prevent exacerbations.

When patients do not improve, consider problems with compliance or technique.

4. Pursed lip breathing and postural changes may be of value. Maintain adequate hydration.

5. Steroid use may be effective in an acute exacerbation and as a way of excluding asthma if there is persisting doubt. A trial of high doses for two weeks may be beneficial when bronchodilators are insufficient. Maintenance steroid treatment should be given only if a short course has been shown objectively to be effective (i.e. improved respiratory function test results). Use the lowest dose possible. The associated weight gain, loss of muscle strength and osteoporosis may make things worse.

6. Annual influenza vaccine and five-yearly pneumococcal vaccine are useful.

7. Pulmonary rehabilitation programs have been demonstrated in randomised controlled trials to improve symptoms and quality of life, but not to prolong life. Exercise and weight reduction increase patients' wellbeing, but not their lung function.

8. Domiciliary oxygen is indicated for patients with a PaO_2 of <55 mmHg or cor pulmonale and a PaO_2 of <59 mmHg. There is evidence that mortality rates are decreased by the use of domiciliary low-flow oxygen given for 19 hours per day (especially during sleep). This may work by reducing the progression of pulmonary hypertension. Find out what type of oxygen supplementation the patient uses (e.g. concentrator, cylinders) and how this is managed with regard to convenience and cost.

9. Consider treatment of cor pulmonale. Heart failure is likely to improve with successful treatment of the lung disease. Spironolactone and diuretics may be useful.

10. Alpha$_1$-antitrypsin deficiency can be treated by replenishing the missing antiprotease, which re-establishes antineutrophil elastase protection for the lower lung zones. An IV preparation can be administered weekly or monthly. This expensive treatment is indicated only if alpha1-antitrypsin levels are below 11 μmol/L. Only a small proportion of people with alpha$_1$-antitrypsin deficiency develop COPD and the treatment is not recommended unless there is demonstrated disease.

11. Lung transplantation is an option for younger (<65 years) patients with end-stage disease and without serious co-morbidity who have not had previous thoracic surgery. The one-year survival rate is more than 80% for this group.

12. Lung reduction surgery was once used as an option for some severely symptomatic patients who had stopped smoking. Those with predominately upper lobe emphysema were thought more likely to benefit. Thorascopic removal of the worst lung segments did seem to give symptomatic improvement to many patients. However, the procedure has lost favour and is now rarely performed. This is partly because lung function continues to decline. Symptomatic benefit may be lost within a year and accelerated decline in lung function may occur. Pulmonary hypertension is a contraindication and air leaks from the stapled lung are the most important postoperative problem. This operation

was combined with an intensive rehabilitation and exercise program, which may in itself account for some of the postoperative improvement.

13. The use of positive pressure ventilation (CPAP) is a possible option for long-term management.

14. The management of severe exacerbations is difficult, particularly when these are associated with severe carbon dioxide retention and a reduced level of consciousness. Steroids and theophylline are both used commonly for these patients. Evidence for their effectiveness is not strong. Non-invasive ventilation (BiPAP) via a mask may improve symptoms and avoid the need for intubation. Intensive care units usually require some evidence of a potentially reversible problem before allowing intubation and mechanical ventilation. The patient's own wishes are important and should be obtained before he or she is too sick to make a decision.

Sleep apnoea

Sleep apnoea is an increasingly recognised clinical syndrome that should be suspected in patients who have obesity, hypertension, fatigue, excessive snoring or unexplained respiratory failure. Obstructive sleep apnoea is a common cause of sleep disturbance but by no means the only explanation for it. Sleep apnoea patients commonly have some combination of these symptoms.

The history

1. Classically, in obstructive sleep apnoea, anyone else in the house will describe a history of loud snoring at night, associated with multiple periods of cessation of respiratory movement and waking and gasping for breath. Apnoeas of more than 10 seconds are considered significant, but for patients with this condition pauses of up to 2 or 3 minutes can occur and pauses of 30 seconds are common. Remember, though, that the majority of people who snore (40% of middle-aged men and 20% of middle-aged women) do not have sleep apnoea and brief apnoeas not associated with signs of arousal are normal for many people.

2. Ask the patient whether there have been problems with excessive daytime sleepiness and with working during the day.

3. Enquire whether the patient drinks alcohol and, if so, how much. Alcohol consumption is a common exacerbating factor.

4. Calculate the patient's Epworth sleepiness score (see Table 6.6).

5. Ask whether there is a history of hypertension and whether this has been treated (50% of these patients have hypertension). Find out whether the patient has had angina or arrhythmias at night; both of these may be precipitated by the hypoxia associated with apnoea. Heartburn and non-cardiac chest pain caused by gastro-oesophageal reflux are also common.

6. Enquire about medications, such as hypnotics, that may have been prescribed for poor sleeping, but actually aggravate sleep apnoea.

7. Ask about a previous diagnosis of COPD or symptoms of heart failure. The recurrent increase in afterload that occurs during apnoeic episodes can precipitate or exacerbate left ventricular failure. Fewer than 10% of patients develop right heart failure and significant pulmonary hypertension.

8. Ask about a history of tonsillar enlargement or throat surgery. In a few sleep apnoea patients there is a clear anatomical cause for the obstruction.

9. In the absence of excessive snoring, central sleep apnoea needs to be considered for a patient with the other symptoms.

TABLE 6.6 The Epworth sleepiness scale
'How easily would you fall asleep in the following circumstances?'
0 = never, 1 = slight chance, 2 = moderate chance, 3 = high chance
• Sitting reading
• Watching television
• At a meeting or at the theatre
• As a passenger in a car on a drive of more than an hour
• Lying down in the afternoon to rest
• Sitting talking to someone
• Sitting quietly after lunch (no alcohol)
• When driving and stopped at traffic lights
A normal score is between 3 and 8; a score of 11 to 20 indicates severe sleep apnoea.

10. Ask about symptoms suggestive of narcolepsy rather than sleep apnoea (see Table 6.7). The sudden sleep attacks of narcolepsy can occur at any time, including during meals, conversation or driving. Patients may also report sudden loss of muscle tone from emotion (e.g. laughter). The result is an unexpected dropping of an object or a sudden buckling at the knees and falling down; cataplexy should be considered. Cataplexy is usually associated with narcolepsy, although it may precede narcolepsy by several years.

11. Ask about symptoms of the restless legs syndrome (RLS), which may also lead to daytime sleepiness (remember, RLS is associated with iron deficiency).

12. The use of diuretics or insulin may predispose patients to inadequate sleep and should not be confused with sleep apnoea.

13. Ask whether the patient drives a motor car and whether the risks of driving have been discussed. Also ask whether it has been recommended that the anaesthetist be informed of the patient's sleep apnoea before the administration of an anaesthetic.

14. Find out whether a CPAP mask has been prescribed and whether the patient finds it comfortable enough to use. Up to 50% of patients are unable to tolerate the device. If the treatment is tolerated, find out whether it has made a difference—many patients report a dramatic reduction in daytime sleepiness and improvement in wellbeing.

15. Find out how this chronic condition has affected the patient's family and work.

TABLE 6.7 Differential diagnosis of daytime sleepiness
1. Not enough sleep (now sometimes considered related to 'poor sleep hygiene')
2. Poor adjustment to shift work
3. Use of sedative and stimulant drugs (e.g. sedatives, caffeine, narcotics)
4. Depression with or without early morning waking
5. Idiopathic hypersomnolence (sleepiness despite plenty of sleep without snoring)
6. Narcolepsy (uncommon, sudden, unexpected falling asleep)

The examination

1. Assess the BMI, but remember that up to 50% of patients with obstructive sleep apnoea and most patients with central sleep apnoea are not obese.
2. Respiratory examination is usually normal.
3. Measure the blood pressure and look in the fundi for signs of hypertension.
4. The cardiovascular system should be examined carefully for evidence of pulmonary hypertension.
5. Inspect the head, neck and mouth for signs of uvular enlargement and macroglossia or tonsillar hypertrophy—'pharyngeal crowding'. Look at and measure the neck circumference.
6. Perform a neurological examination to look for signs of autonomic neuropathy (e.g. diabetes mellitus, Shy-Drager syndrome), brain stem lesions or spinal cord disease (e.g. tumour, demyelination), which can cause central sleep apnoea.
7. Examine for neurological causes of obstructive sleep apnoea, such as myasthenia gravis or muscular dystrophy.
8. Look for signs of hypothyroidism or acromegaly.

Investigations

1. Consider sleep study monitoring (polysomnography) with the electroencephalogram, chin electromyogram, electro-ocular monitoring (to detect rapid eye movement [REM] sleep), oximetry, $PaCO_2$ monitoring and, if indicated, ECG monitoring (for arrhythmias).
2. For a definitive diagnosis, the apnoeic spells must be 10 seconds or longer in duration and at least five per hour must be recorded over several hours. The apnoea hypopnoea index (AHI) is the total number of episodes of apnoea or hypopnoea per night divided by the number of hours of sleep (mild 5–15; moderate 6–30; severe >30). A value of 5 or greater is considered abnormal, but is probably not diagnostic in the absence of symptoms.
3. For patients with typical features of the condition, home PaO_2 monitoring overnight may be an option. A positive test (several significant desaturation episodes per hour) is enough evidence to justify treatment. A negative test, however, does not exclude the diagnosis.
4. Narcolepsy can also be diagnosed by a sleep study.
5. Hypothyroidism should be excluded with thyroid function tests if there is any clinical suspicion.
6. Echocardiography may be indicated to enable estimation of pulmonary artery pressures and to assess right ventricular function.

Treatment

1. If the patient has hypothyroidism, thyroid hormone replacement may reverse sleep apnoea.
2. Concomitant diseases such as cardiac failure, hypertension and asthma need to be treated vigorously. Nasal decongestants may be helpful. Weight loss is of value but may be difficult to achieve. Respiratory depressants, such as tranquillisers, should be withdrawn.
3. CPAP is of value for long-term treatment of irreversible obstructive sleep apnoea (see Table 6.8). CPAP devices are not always well tolerated, but the devices are improving steadily in comfort and portability. Nasal CPAP is effective in the majority of patients who can adjust to it. If there is residual sleepiness despite regular use of CPAP, modafinil may be a useful adjunct.
4. Surgical correction of upper airways narrowing caused by polyps, enlarged tonsils or macroglossia can lead to significant improvement but may not fully

TABLE 6.8 The effects of treatment for sleep apnoea from randomised clinical trials

Epworth score >11 and >15 apnoeas/hour

- Reduced sleepiness
- Improved blood pressure
- Improved cognition
- Safer driving
- Improved mood and quality of life

Epworth score >11 and 5–15 apnoeas/hour

- Improved symptoms
- Improved daytime sleepiness
- Less evidence of quality of life or cognitive improvement
- No evidence of improved blood pressure

Normal Epworth score with apnoea

- No evidence of benefit of treatment

reverse the problem. Excision of soft tissue in the oropharynx is of value for well-selected patients.

5. If there has been a recent stroke, observation may be all that is required, since respiratory function may improve with time. Patients with central sleep apnoea can often be successfully treated with bilevel positive airways pressure (BiPAP) ventilation.

Interstitial lung disease, including idiopathic pulmonary fibrosis

Interstitial lung disease (ILD) may have a prolonged course, so patients are often available for the examinations. Discovering the aetiology may be difficult.

The history

The diagnosis may not be obvious until you examine the patient, at which stage you may have to ask further questions about the following:

1. presenting respiratory symptoms (e.g. dry cough, dyspnoea, lethargy, malaise)
2. whether the patient knows the cause of the respiratory symptoms
3. the onset and duration of symptoms (these are clues)—pulmonary fibrosis has a very slow onset and patients are not acutely ill; if there is the insidious onset of cough, fever, malaise and myalgias over weeks to months, think about cryptogenic organising pneumonia (COP), which has a better prognosis and responds to steroids!
4. the patient's gender and age (also clues)—for example, lymphangioleiomyomatosis (LAM) occurs essentially only in premenopausal women who often have a history of recurrent pneumothorax
5. systemic symptoms—for example, weight loss, fatigue, fever, rash and arthralgia, which may indicate a systemic disease, particularly a connective tissue disease (scleroderma, systemic lupus, Sjögren's syndrome or rheumatoid arthritis) or sarcoidosis (see Table 6.9)
6. pre-existing asthma—which may suggest Churg Strauss syndrome (ask about renal disease)
7. whether there is a history of haemoptysis and renal disease—which may indicate Goodpasture's syndrome or SLE

8. drug use—cardiac (e.g. amiodarone, hydralazine, procainamide), rheumatological (e.g. methotrexate, d-penicillamine), chemotherapeutic (e.g. busulphan, bleomycin, cyclophosphamide) and others (e.g. nitrofurantoin, bromocriptine)
9. any history of radiotherapy
10. a detailed lifetime occupational history, such as exposure to mineral dust (silicosis, asbestosis, coal worker's pneumoconiosis), chemical fumes (nitrogen dioxide, chlorine, ammonia) or organic dusts (see Table 6.10)
11. occupational history consistent with hypersensitivity pneumonitis (e.g. bird fancier's lung, farmer's lung from mouldy hay or grain dust in grain elevators); ask about recurrent Monday chest tightness (e.g. byssinosis from cotton, flax or hemp dust)
12. infections (e.g. aspiration pneumonia, miliary tuberculosis)
13. investigations (e.g. high-resolution CT of the thorax, lung biopsy or bronchial lavage)
14. treatment, if any
15. social problems as a result of the chronic disability.

TABLE 6.9 Fibrotic and granulomatous lung disease

Connective tissue diseases causing fibrosis (ILD)
1. Rheumatoid arthritis
2. Systemic lupus erythematosus
3. Scleroderma
4. Polymyositis and dermatomyositis
5. Sjögren's syndrome
6. Polyarteritis nodosa (rare)
Causes of granulomatous lung disease on lung biopsy
1. Sarcoidosis
2. Tuberculosis
3. Chronic berylliosis
4. Extrinsic allergic alveolitis

TABLE 6.10 Asbestos and the lung

Heavy exposure associated with:
1. Asbestosis
2. Bronchial carcinoma
Trivial exposure associated with:
1. Pleural fibrosis and plaques
2. Mesothelioma after a latent period of 30–40 years

The examination

1. Clubbing (consider idiopathic pulmonary fibrosis but also asbestosis); cyanosis and lower lobe crackles (fine, late, inspiratory) make the diagnosis of idiopathic pulmonary fibrosis (IPF) likely.
2. If the signs suggest upper lobe pulmonary fibrosis, consider in your differential

diagnosis silicosis, sarcoidosis, beryllium, cystic fibrosis, coal worker's pneumo-coniosis, eosinophilic granuloma, ankylosing spondytitis and tuberculosis. Lower lobe pulmonary fibrosis may be due to IPF, scleroderma, asbestosis, aspiration or drugs.

3. Look for signs of associated systemic disease, as well as sarcoidosis and connective tissue disease that would rule out IPF. For example, erythema nodosum and anterior uveitis would suggest looking for evidence of sarcoidosis.

4. Assess the severity of the disease (signs of pulmonary hypertension).

5. Look for signs of drug side effects (especially steroids).

Investigations

The goals of investigations are to find the aetiology, establish the severity of the disease and look for signs of active inflammation. If active inflammation is present, the condition may respond to immunotherapy (steroids or cyclophosphamide). If established fibrosis is present, such treatment is unlikely to help.

1. Chest radiography is the initial investigation but may be normal (see Fig 15.14).

2. High-resolution CT of the thorax is the investigation of choice (see Fig 6.5). It is the most sensitive non-invasive test. The changes of ILD are characteristic. Note whether there is a localised or diffuse abnormality or progressive massive fibrosis (caused by silicosis and coal worker's pneumoconiosis).

3. Pulmonary function tests usually reveal a restrictive pattern, with reduction of lung volumes and reduced transfer factor. An obstructive pattern may be seen in sarcoidosis, histiocytosis X (typically found in men who smoke and have a history of pneumothorax) and LAM.

Figure 6.5 CT scan of the thorax. There are increased lung markings posteriorly, more prominent on the right than on the left (arrows).

Figure reproduced courtesy of The Canberra Hospital.

4. Blood gas levels will show hypoxia with a normal or low $PaCO_2$.
5. The erythrocyte sedimentation rate is often raised.
6. There may be hypergammaglobulinaemia and a raised lactate dehydrogenase (LDH) level. Eosinophilia may be a useful clue (see Table 6.11). Serological testing for connective tissue diseases is routine.
7. A positive gallium-67 lung scan may indicate disease activity. Lung clearance studies using pertechnate may also be helpful (rapid clearance suggests active alveolitis).
8. Bronchoalveolar lavage can be performed. It is suggested that fibrosis on a transbronchial biopsy associated with a lavage showing a predominance of polymorphonuclear cells is less responsive to treatment. Lymphocytosis on lavage suggests drug-induced or granulomatous disease.
9. Diagnoses likely to be made by transbronchial lung biopsy include sarcoidosis and lymphangitic spread of carcinoma; infection can be ruled out. Other specific diagnoses are not usually apparent.
10. Open lung biopsy or video-assisted thoracoscopic biopsy may be required to confirm the presence of idiopathic ILD but only if there is clinical uncertainty and the test result could change treatment.

TABLE 6.11 Causes of pulmonary infiltrate and eosinophilia (PIE)

Prolonged pulmonary eosinophilia—this may be caused by: drugs (e.g. sulfonamides, sulfasalazine, salicylates, nitrofurantoin, penicillin, isoniazid, methotrexate, carbamazepine, imipramine, L-tryptophan); parasites (e.g. *Ascaris*); idiopathic

Loeffler's syndrome (benign and acute)

Allergic bronchopulmonary aspergillosis (always associated with asthma)

Tropical (e.g. microfilaria)

Eosinophilic pneumonia and vasculitis (e.g. polyarteritis nodosa, Wegener's granulomatosis)

Treatment

This depends on the cause (see Table 6.12).
1. Remove exposure, if appropriate.
2. Treatment will not reverse established fibrosis.
3. Steroids may help in COP, chemical injuries, hypersensitivity pneumonias (acute disease only), sarcoidosis (severe disease), histiocytosis X (controversial) and connective tissue disease. However, there is no evidence that steroids improve survival in these conditions and they are of no value in dust diseases. In IPF, 30% improve on steroids plus cyclophosphamide.
4. Treatment with prednisolone is usually begun at 1 mg/kg/day and reduced to half this dose after 4–12 weeks. Follow-up with measurement of spirometry, lung volumes and transfer factor is important to document response to treatment. Consider maintenance steroids in lower dose for patients who are improving or stabilised.
5. Immunosuppressive agents, and especially cyclophosphamide, may sometimes be of benefit and can be used in combination with low-dose steroids. Colchicine in doses of 0.6 mg daily has been shown to improve some patients. It inhibits macrophage production of fibroblast growth factors.
6. General measures, such as administration of pneumococcal and influenza vaccines, may be indicated.
7. Home oxygen therapy may provide symptomatic relief for hypoxaemic patients.
8. Unilateral lung transplantation may be considered for some patients in the final stage of their disease.

TABLE 6.12 Classification of interstitial lung disease (ILD)
Secondary to alveolitis (previously called fibrosing alveolitis)
1. Unknown cause
• Idiopathic interstitial pneumonia (e.g. idiopathic pulmonary fibrosis; cryptogenic organising pneumonia, lymphangioleiomyomatosis)
• Connective tissue disease (e.g. SLE, rheumatoid arthritis, ankylosing spondylitis, systemic sclerosis)
• Pulmonary haemorrhage syndromes (e.g. Goodpasture's syndrome)
• Graft versus host disease
• Gastrointestinal or liver diseases (e.g. Crohn's disease, primary biliary cirrhosis)
2. Known cause
• Asbestosis
• Radiation injury
• Aspiration pneumonia
• Drugs (e.g. amiodarone, bleomycin, busulfan, nitrofurantoin, penicillamine, cocaine)
• Exposure to gases or fumes
Secondary to granulomatous disease
1. Unknown cause
• Sarcoidosis
• Wegener's disease, Churg-Strauss disease
2. Known cause
• Hypersensitivity pneumonitis to organic or inorganic dusts (silica, beryllium)
SLE = systemic lupus erythematosus.

Pulmonary hypertension

Many patients with this chronic and often severe illness will have raised pulmonary artery pressures as a result of a cardiac or respiratory illness. The patient may or may not be aware of this complication of the underlying disease, but it is essential for the candidate to know when to look for it. Idiopathic pulmonary hypertension (IPH) is a rare but important condition, which is diagnosed when other causes of pulmonary hypertension have been excluded. By definition, pulmonary hypertension is present when the mean pulmonary artery pressure (PAP) exceeds 25 mmHg at rest or 30 mmHg during exercise.

The classification of pulmonary hypertension has been revised recently. The Venice classification was released in 2003 and the term 'primary pulmonary hypertension' has been replaced with 'idiopathic pulmonary hypertension' (see Table 6.13).

The history

1. Symptoms are usually non-specific but often severe. As usual, begin by asking whether the patient knows what is wrong and the reason for the admission, or visit, to hospital.
2. If pulmonary hypertension seems a possibility, ask about the possible causes (see Table 6.13). Remember to ask specifically about appetite-suppressing drugs. The use of fenfluramine and phenermine in combination and for long periods has been associated with the greatest risk.

TABLE 6.13 The Venice classification for pulmonary hypertension (2003)

1. Pulmonary arterial hypertension (PAH):

   1.1 Idiopathic (IPAH)

   1.2 Familial (FPAH)

   1.3 Associated with (APAH):

      1.3.1 Collagen vascular disease

      1.3.2 Congenital systemic-to-pulmonary shunts

      1.3.3 Portal hypertension

      1.3.4 HIV infection

      1.3.5 Drugs and toxins

      1.3.6 Other (thyroid disorders, glycogen storage disease, Gaucher's disease, hereditary haemorrhagic telangiectasia, haemoglobinopathies, myeloproliferative disorders, splenectomy)

   1.4 Associated with significant venous or capillary involvement:

      1.4.1 Pulmonary veno-occlusive disease (PVOD)

      1.4.2 Pulmonary capillary haemangiomatosis (PCH)

   1.5 Persistent pulmonary hypertension of the newborn

2. Pulmonary hypertension with left heart disease:

   2.1 Left-sided atrial or ventricular heart disease

   2.2 Left-sided valvular heart disease

3. Pulmonary hypertension associated with lung diseases and/or hypoxaemia:

   3.1 Chronic obstructive pulmonary disease

   3.2 Interstitial lung disease

   3.3 Sleep-disordered breathing

   3.4 Alveolar hypoventilation disorders

   3.5 Chronic exposure to high altitude

   3.6 Developmental abnormalities

4. Pulmonary hypertension as a result of chronic thrombotic and/or embolic disease:

   4.1 Thromboembolic obstruction of proximal pulmonary arteries

   4.2 Thromboembolic obstruction of distal pulmonary arteries

   4.3 Non-thrombotic pulmonary embolism (tumour, parasites, foreign material)

5. Miscellaneous—sarcoidosis, histiocytosis X, lymphangiomatosis, compression of pulmonary vessels (adenopathy, fibrosing mediastinitis)

3. If the patient has an illness that could be a cause, ask detailed questions about that condition, its severity and chronicity. There may be a family history in cases of IPH (6%; autosomal dominant condition with incomplete penetrance, 20–80%). The majority of familial cases are associated with a mutation on the *BMPR2* gene.

4. Find out how symptomatic the patient is now. Idiopathic and secondary pulmonary hypertension cause dyspnoea. Almost all patients have dyspnoea at the time of diagnosis. Other less common symptoms include fatigue, chest pain, syncope and oedema. Cough and haemoptysis can be present. Ask about symptoms of

connective tissue diseases and especially about scleroderma. Try to work out the patient's functional class (NYHA I–IV, often called the NYHA-WHO class when related to pulmonary hypertension).

5. Ask about previous or planned investigations. These may relate to the underlying condition; for example, respiratory function tests or scans, echocardiography (often transoesophageal echocardiography) or cardiac catheterisation. A patient who presents with symptoms and signs of pulmonary hypertension needs a number of investigations before IPH can be diagnosed.

6. What general treatment has been recommended? This may be for the underlying cardiac or respiratory condition or for thrombosis. There may be a history of cardiac surgery in childhood for congenital heart disease. Oxygen supplementation is often prescribed. Find out how this is administered (e.g. via nasal prongs or a mask), for how many hours a day and whether it comes from a concentrator or oxygen tanks. Oxygen is very expensive unless subsidised. Ask about the cost and inconvenience of the treatment with regard to portability and noise (oxygen concentrators are noisy and use a lot of electricity). Has the treatment been helpful?

7. What drugs is the patient taking? Heparin and then warfarin are routine for pulmonary embolism, but warfarin is also used for most patients with IPH because of the risk of in situ thrombosis in the pulmonary arteries. Bronchodilators and steroids may have been prescribed for lung disease. The possibility of a heart or lung transplant, or both, may have been raised with the patient. The patient may be on a therapeutic trial or taking an agent, such as bosentan, sildenafil or the inhaled prostacyclin analogue iloprost. Patients involved in trials or taking new drugs are often very well informed about what is going on.

8. As with any chronic and possibly debilitating condition, questions about the patient's ability to work and manage the activities of daily living need to be detailed and comprehensive.

The examination

1. Try to assess the severity of the patient's dyspnoea as he or she undresses or by asking the patient to walk around the room.

2. Perform a thorough respiratory and cardiac examination (see pp 291 and 263). Look particularly for an elevated JVP with a large v wave. Feel for a parasternal impulse (right ventricular heave). Feel for a palpable P2 (and listen for tricuspid regurgitation).

3. Look for signs of chronic lung disease, congenital heart disease and connective tissue disease. Examine for signs of a deep venous thrombosis (DVT).

Investigations

Investigations are directed at finding an underlying reason for pulmonary hypertension—IPH is a diagnosis of exclusion—and at assessing its severity and potential reversibility. These include:

1. **Chest X-ray**—this will be abnormal in 90% of IPH patients. It may show ILD or an abnormal cardiac silhouette—right ventricular dilatation. There may be large proximal pulmonary arteries that appear 'pruned' in the periphery, and the right ventricle may appear enlarged on the lateral film (see Fig 6.6).

2. **Respiratory function tests** (normal, restrictive or obstructive pattern)—moderate pulmonary hypertension itself is associated with a reduction in the diffusion capacity for carbon monoxide (DLCO) to about 50% of predicted.

3. **ECG**—signs of right heart strain or hypertrophy are present in up to 90% of patients (see Fig 6.7).

4. **Blood gases**—hypercapnia in hypoventilation syndromes, but hypocapnia is

more common in IPH because of increased alveolar ventilation. Mild hypoxia in IPH, but more severe when pulmonary hypertension is secondary to lung disease.

5. **CT pulmonary angiogram or ventilation–perfusion (V/Q) scan and Doppler venograms**—DVT and pulmonary embolism—assessment of extent of involvement of the pulmonary bed.

6. **High-resolution CT of the lungs**—looking for interstitial lung disease.

Figure 6.6 (a) and (b) Severe pulmonary hypertension. There is pruning of the pulmonary arteries and right ventricular dilatation.

Figure 6.7 ECG of a patient with idiopathic pulmonary hypertension. Note RAA (right atrial abnormality), 'P' pulmonale, right axis, right ventricular hypertrophy and strain pattern, and sinus tachycardia.

7. **Six-minute walking test**—predicts survival and correlates with NYHA-WHO class. Reduction in arterial oxygen concentration of >10% during this test predicts almost threefold mortality risk over 29 months. Patients unable to manage 332 metres in 6 minutes also have an adverse prognosis.

8. **Transthoracic or transoesophageal echocardiogram** (see Fig 6.8)—a transthoracic echocardiogram will usually enable left ventricular failure or severe mitral valve disease to be excluded. One or both will enable the assessment of known congenital heart disease, the detection of a left to right (or reversed) shunting (Eisenmenger's syndrome) and measurement, in many cases, of pulmonary artery pressures. The presence of tricuspid regurgitation (common in normal people and almost universal in the presence of raised right ventricular pressures) enables estimation of right ventricular and therefore pulmonary artery pressures in many patients. The pressure difference across the tricuspid valve can be calculated if the velocity of the regurgitant jet is measured by Doppler. Right atrial pressures are usually close to 5 mmHg; the right ventricular pressure can be estimated by adding 5 to the pressure difference across the tricuspid valve. The normal right ventricular and pulmonary artery systolic pressure is 20–25 mmHg. Assessment of pulmonary artery ejection characteristics can also be used to estimate pulmonary artery pressures. Right ventricular size and function can be assessed. Right ventricular dilatation and abnormal septal motion are useful signs of pulmonary hypertension. The right ventricle appears abnormal on echocardiograms in more than 90% of people with pulmonary hypertension.

9. **Catheterisation of the right heart**—this investigation is the gold standard and should also be performed if other tests have not been definitive. It is usually performed with a multiple-lumen flotation catheter and enables direct measurement of the right heart pressures. Left to right shunting can be detected by the collection of blood samples from the venae cavae, right atrium, right ventricle and pulmonary artery. A 'step-up' in the blood oxygen saturation indicates a shunt. The size of the shunt can be calculated if the cardiac output is measured by thermodilution. Measurement of the pulmonary artery wedge pressure enables the detection of mitral stenosis or the very rare pulmonary veno-occlusive disease. By definition, IPH means the pulmonary capillary wedge pressure is <18 mmHg (i.e. the raised pulmonary pressures are not secondary to left ventricular failure). Pulmonary vascular resistance can be calculated using the cardiac output, pulmonary artery pressure and pulmonary artery wedge pressure measurements. The formula is:

$$\text{pulmonary vascular resistance} = \frac{\text{pulmonary artery pressure - pulmonary artery wedge pressure}}{\text{cardiac output}}$$

This gives a result in mmHg/L/min or Wood units. The normal is 1.7 mmHg/L/min.

Treatment

1. Treatment of pulmonary hypertension that is secondary to an underlying respiratory or cardiac condition begins with an attempt to optimise treatment or fix the underlying condition.
   (a) **COPD:** bronchodilators, steroids, continuous oxygen.
   (b) **ILD:** oxygen. Aggressive treatment of an underlying connective tissue disease may halt or slow progression of the pulmonary pressures.
   (c) **Pulmonary embolus:** anticoagulation, vena caval filter and occasionally pulmonary embolectomy.
   (d) **Mitral stenosis:** valvotomy or replacement.

Echocardiography Report

Reason for study: ?Pulmonary hypertension
Study quality: Good <u>Satisfactory</u> Poor

RV	32	(mm) (N 10–26)
Sept.	8	(mm) (N 7–11)
LVEDD	51	(mm) (N 36–56)
LVESD	30	(mm) (N 20–40)
LVPW	10	(mm) (N 7–11)
Aorta	22	(mm) (N 20–35)
LA	36	(mm) (N 24–40)
FS	41	% (N 27–40)
EF	72	% (N 55–70)

Valves

Mitral	Mild MR
Tricus.	Moderate TR
Aortic	Appears normal
Pulm.	Appears normal

Doppler—2D
The right ventricle is dilated. There is paradoxical septal motion. The LV is not dilated. The cardiac valves appear normal. The main pulmonary artery was not dilated. No ASD was seen.

Doppler—colour flow mapping
Moderate tricuspid regurgitation was detected. The TR flow velocity was 4 m/s. Estimated RV pressure 70 mmHg. Mild MR is present. No ASD flow or intracardiac shunting was detected.

Conclusions
Severe pulmonary hypertension. RV dilated, abnormal septal motion. No intracardiac shunting detected.

Comment
The most important signs of pulmonary hypertension on 2D echocardiographs are RV dilatation and abnormal septal motion. The septum normally behaves as part of the left ventricle and contracts inwards, towards the lateral wall of the left ventricle. Significant increases in RV pressure cause the septum to move away from the left ventricle during systole. Measurement of the velocity of the regurgitant tricuspid valve jet enables estimation of RV pressures. It is difficult to exclude an ASD on a transthoracic echocardiogram unless it is of very good quality. A transoesophageal echocardiograph may be required if there is any doubt about the cause of pulmonary hypertension.

Key
ASD = atrial septal defect; EF = ejection fraction; FS = fractional shortening; LA = left atrium; LVEDD = left ventricular end-diastolic dimension; LVESD = left ventricular end-systolic dimension; LVPW = left ventricular posterior wall; MR = mitral regurgitation; Pulm. = pulmonary; RV = right ventricle; Sept. = septal thickness; TR = tricuspid regurgitation; Tricus. = tricuspid.

Figure 6.8 Echocardiography report in a patient with pulmonary hypertension.

(e) **Mitral regurgitation:** repair or replacement if left ventricular function remains reasonable.

(f) **Atrial septal defect:** surgery or, if suitable, closure in the catheter laboratory (e.g. with an Amplatzer closure device). There must be evidence of reversibility of the pulmonary pressure if it is close to systemic.

(g) **Eisenmenger's syndrome:** repair of the defect responsible for the shunt is not usually possible once reversal of shunting has occurred. Consider heart and lung transplant if conservative treatment (diuretics, digoxin and sometimes ACE inhibitors) has failed.

2. General measures include continuous oxygen, diuretics, digoxin and spirono-lactone for problems with right heart failure. Use of the newer endothelin receptor antagonists (bosentan), prostoglandins (iloprost) or phosphodiesterase inhibitors (sildenafil) is generally indicated for IPH and pulmonary hypertension secondary to connective tissue disease and pulmonary embolism. These expensive drugs can improve symptoms and prognosis.

Idiopathic (primary) pulmonary hypertension
Treatment of this progressive and debilitating condition involves the general measures outlined above. Untreated patients have a poor survival rate: two to three years median survival from the time of diagnosis.

1. Bosentan has been approved for use for patients with IPH. This drug is an endothelin receptor antagonist. Endothelin-1 is a potent vasoconstrictor whose levels have been shown to be elevated in patients with IPH. Modest improvements in functional capacity and pulmonary artery pressures have been demonstrated after treatment of patients with IPH and those with underlying connective tissue disease. The drug is only available for patients with class III symptoms and a right atrial pressure of >8 mmHg. Its side effects include teratogenicity, an increase in liver enzyme levels and possibly male infertility.

2. Prostacyclin analogues, such as iloprost, which are taken by inhalation, can also be effective. Continuous IV epoprostenol has been shown to improve symptoms and prognosis in a number of small randomised trials for IPH patients at least.

3. Sildenafil (a phosphodiesterase inhibitor) is a vasodilator that must not be used in combination with nitrates because of the risk of severe and prolonged hypotension.

4. Warfarin is usually recommended because of the demonstrated risk of the formation of in situ thrombus in the pulmonary arteries.

5. Suitable patients (severe unresponsive disease, right heart failure, young patient) should be considered for transplant. Successful outcomes have been shown with heart–lung, double lung or single lung transplants. IPH has not been found to recur in the transplanted lung. The prognosis depends on the NYHA-WHO functional class: class I–II, 6 years; class III, 2.5 years; class IV, 6 months.

Sarcoidosis

This chronic, systemic, granulomatous disease is relatively common and patients occasionally require admission to hospital for investigation or treatment. It is an unusual lung disease in that it is less common in smokers. Although most patients present between the ages of 20 and 40 years, children and elderly people are sometimes affected. There are cases of familial sarcoidosis. The disorder results from an exaggerated T-helper lymphocyte response that occurs for unknown reasons and is responsible for granuloma formation and fibrosis.

The history

1. Ask whether the patient has been admitted to hospital and if so, why. The patient may already know the diagnosis and be in hospital for further investigations or treatment, or the diagnosis may be suspected because of lymphadenopathy or changes on chest X-ray (see Fig 6.9). Most patients present with asymptomatic hilar adenopathy (see Table 6.14).

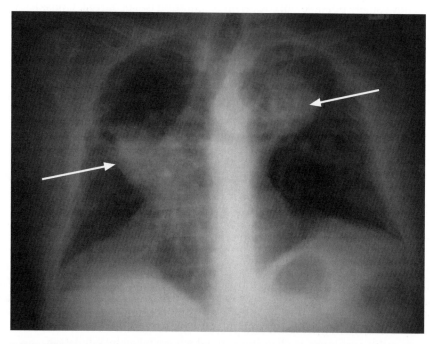

Figure 6.9 Massive bilateral hilar lymphadenopathy (arrows).
Figure reproduced courtesy of The Canberra Hospital.

TABLE 6.14 Clinical presentation of sarcoid
1. Abnormal chest X-ray (30%)
2. Fever, weight loss, malaise, cough or dyspnoea (20%)
3. Arthralgia and erythema nodosum (20%)
4. Eye symptoms (10%)
5. Palpable lymphadenopathy (5%)
6. Skin abnormalities (5%)
7. Rare: cardiac arrhythmias, hypercalcaemia or cranial nerve palsies

2. Ask about acute or subacute symptoms, as sarcoidosis develops in this way in about one-third of cases. The patient may have fever, weight loss, loss of appetite and malaise. The occurrence of erythema nodosum, joint symptoms and bilateral hilar adenopathy on chest X-ray suggests an acute presentation. A combination of fever, facial nerve palsy, parotid enlargement and anterior uveitis may occur.

3. Symptoms suggesting a more insidious onset include persistent cough and dyspnoea. If the patient has chronic sarcoidosis, it is still important to find out how he or she originally presented, as the insidious onset is more often

associated with chronic sarcoidosis and the development of damage to the lungs (up to 15% develop progressive pulmonary fibrosis—ILD) and other organs.

4. Ask about skin eruptions (e.g. erythema nodosum, plaques, maculopapular lesions and subcutaneous nodules). Erythema nodosum, fever and migratory polyarthralgias, when found in combination with hilar lymphadenopathy, may indicate Lofgren's syndrome.

5. Eye symptoms occur in about one-quarter of patients. The patient may have noticed blurred vision, excess tears and light sensitivity as a result of uveitis. Involvement of the lacrimal glands can cause the sicca syndrome, resulting in dry, sore eyes.

6. Ask about nasal stuffiness, as the nasal mucosa is involved in about one-fifth of patients. Occasionally, a hoarse voice or even stridor may result from sarcoid involving the larynx.

7. Renal involvement is uncommon but occasionally nephrolithiasis can result because of hypercalcaemia.

8. Ask about neurological symptoms—facial nerve palsy is the most common manifestation, but psychiatric disturbances and fits may occur.

9. Almost half the patients at some time in the course of the disease have arthralgia; even frank arthritis can occur.

10. The patient may be aware of cardiac abnormalities. Conduction problems, including complete heart block and ventricular arrhythmias, occur in about 5% of patients.

11. If the patient is female, ask about pregnancies. Sarcoidosis tends to abate in pregnancy but then flare up in the postpartum period.

12. Enquire about gastrointestinal symptoms (e.g. dysphagia from hilar adenopathy), although these are very rare. Liver involvement is common but rarely causes symptoms. The patient may know about abnormal liver function tests (usually a cholestatic picture).

13. Ask how the diagnosis was made. Specifically determine whether a lymph node biopsy or closed or open lung biopsy has been performed. Sometimes a skin or conjunctival biopsy may have been obtained to make the diagnosis. Bronchial or transbronchial lung biopsies are used to make the diagnosis in most cases. Occasionally, mediastinoscopy with lymph node biopsy is needed to make the diagnosis. The CT scan has a characteristic appearance and may have been the only investigation performed, although in most cases the diagnosis is confirmed by biopsy.

14. Ask about treatment. Find out whether the patient has been receiving steroids and what dose is currently being taken. Various other treatments may have been tried, including NSAIDs, cyclosporin and cyclophosphamide.

The examination

1. Begin with an examination of the skin.
   (a) You might be lucky enough to find erythema nodosum. These raised red or purple lesions are most commonly found on the lower limbs. They resolve spontaneously after three or four weeks.
   (b) Look at the face, back and extremities for maculopapular eruptions. These are elevated spots less than 1 cm in diameter that have a waxy, flat top. There may also be lupus pernio on the face. These are purple swollen nodules with a shiny surface, which affect particularly the nose, cheeks, lids and ears. They may make the nose appear bulbous; occasionally the mucosa of the nose may be involved and the underlying bone can be destroyed. Lupus pernio sometimes also involves the fingers and knees. Pink nodules may be found in old scars.

2. Examine the eyes for signs of uveitis. Yellow conjunctival nodules may be present. Examine the fundi for papilloedema. Feel the parotids. Uveoparotid fever presents with uveitis, parotid swelling and seventh cranial nerve palsy.
3. Next examine the respiratory system (see p 291). Most commonly, physical examination of the chest reveals no abnormality. Look particularly for signs of interstitial lung disease; basal end-inspiratory crackles may be present. Pleural effusions occur rarely.
4. Next examine all the lymph nodes. Lymphadenopathy is sometimes generalised.
5. Now examine the abdomen for hepatomegaly (20%) and splenomegaly (up to 40%).
6. Examine the joints for signs of arthritis, which is almost always non-deforming.
7. Examine the nervous system (see p 349). Look particularly for facial nerve palsy.
8. Feel the pulse (heart block or arrhythmia) and look for signs of right ventricular failure or cardiomyopathy. Note the presence a pacemaker or defibrillator box.

Investigations

1. A full blood count may reveal lymphocytopenia and sometimes eosinophilia.
2. The ESR is often raised. There may be hyperglobulinaemia.
3. The ACE level is raised in about two-thirds of patients with active sarcoidosis but unfortunately is not diagnostic; ACE is also sometimes elevated (5%) in healthy persons or those with primary biliary cirrhosis, leprosy, atypical mycobacterial infection, miliary tuberculosis, silicosis, acute histoplasmosis and hyperparathyroidism. ACE is not elevated in patients with malignancies (e.g. lymphoma). Hypercalcaemia and, more commonly, hypercalciuria may be present.
4. The chest X-ray is usually abnormal (see Table 6.15) and the changes can be classified into three stages:
   • *Stage 1* Bilateral hilar lymphadenopathy alone
   • *Stage 2* Bilateral hilar lymphadenopathy and pulmonary infiltration
   • *Stage 3* Pulmonary infiltration without hilar lymphadenopathy
   Patients with stage 1 X-rays are considered to have an acute reversible form of the disease, whereas the other stages tend to be more chronic. The chest X-ray may show paratracheal lymphadenopathy; cavitation and pleural effusions are rare. Cavities may become colonised with *Aspergillus*. CT scans of the chest may show a ground-glass appearance when active alveolitis is present. Always think about excluding tuberculosis and histoplasmosis.
5. If there is parenchymal granulomatous involvement, respiratory function tests reveal the changes that are typical of interstitial lung disease, with reduced lung volumes and diffusing capacity, but a normal FEV_1/FVC ratio. Occasionally, a mixed pattern of obstruction and restriction is seen.
6. Blood gas estimations may show mild hypoxaemia.

TABLE 6.15 Chest X-ray changes in sarcoidosis
1. Hilar lymphadenopathy—up to 90%
2. Paratracheal lymphadenopathy—less than 80%
3. Reticulonodular changes—70%
4. Peripheral nodules—less than 5%
5. Cavitation—less than 5%
6. Pleural effusion—less than 5%
7. Linear atelectasis—less than 1%

7. A gallium-67 lung scan usually shows a pattern of diffuse uptake, but increased uptake in the lacrimal and parotid glands (panda sign) or in the right paratracheal and left hilar areas (lambda sign) is more specific for sarcoidosis. Enlarged nodes also tend to show up on the scans.
8. Bronchoscopy with transbronchial biopsy will usually establish the pathological diagnosis. Bronchioalveolar lavage will show an increase in the number of CD4$^+$ T-helper lymphocytes. However, this is not diagnostic of the condition.
9. Biopsy of lymph nodes, skin or liver may be diagnostic. The non-caseating granulomas found in sarcoidosis are non-specific; they are also found in berylliosis, leprosy, hypersensitivity pneumonitis and granulomatous infection, and in lymph nodes that drain adjacent carcinomas.

Treatment
Indications for treatment are lack of resolution of active pulmonary sarcoidosis with increasing symptoms or worsening lung function; neurological, renal or cardiac complications; major eye disease; and occasionally severe systemic symptoms (e.g. fever and weight loss).
1. The drug of choice is prednisolone. This is begun in high dose (1 mg/kg) for up to six weeks and then tapered over the following few months. Treatment is continued for 12 months. The prognosis is good. About 50% of patients develop some permanent organ damage but, in most, this is mild.
2. Patients who require longer treatment may be offered steroid-sparing drugs, including chlorambucil, methotrexate or azathioprine.
3. Hydroxychloroquine may be useful for skin disease.
4. Infliximab (a monoclonal antibody directed at tumour necrosis factor [TNF]) has been shown to improve lung function for patients already being treated with steroids and cytotoxics.

Cystic fibrosis
The survival of children with cystic fibrosis into adult life is now common. More than 50% of patients reach the age of 30 years and the prognosis is improving all the time. Although paediatricians are often reluctant to give up these patients, they are increasingly coming under the care of adult physicians. A small number of cases are diagnosed in adult life. They, unfortunately, tend to spend long periods in hospital and are thus readily available for clinical examinations.

Cystic fibrosis is a common, serious, congenital inherited defect in Caucasian people. It has an autosomal recessive inheritance and the gene has been identified. The mutation is in the cystic fibrosis transmembrane conductance regulator protein gene on chromosome 7. The trait is present in about 1 in 25 Caucasians and 1 in 2000 has the condition. It is very rare in other races. It is a chronic disease that can affect the lungs, pancreas, bowel, liver and sweat glands.

The history
1. Ask about presentation:
   (a) age at diagnosis—milder forms are sometimes not diagnosed until adult life
   (b) presenting symptoms—the patient may have been told that he or she had meconium ileus as a baby or recurrent respiratory infections in early life; failure to thrive may suggest the diagnosis
   (c) pulmonary symptoms—cough and sputum, haemoptysis, wheeze, dyspnoea
   (d) nasal polyps and sinusitis—relatively common
   (e) gastrointestinal symptoms—problems maintaining weight; diarrhoea and steatorrhoea (pancreatic malabsorption); constipation and abdominal distension and bowel obstruction (defective water excretion into the bowel)

(f) heat exhaustion in hot weather—patients with cystic fibrosis can lose large amounts of salt in their sweat, which sometimes causes problems, particularly in the tropics

(g) cardiac symptoms—the patient may know of cardiac involvement (cor pulmonale is a late development)

(h) jaundice and variceal bleeding—focal biliary cirrhosis and portal hypertension occur occasionally

(i) diabetes mellitus—occurs in 10% of patients with cystic fibrosis.

2. Ask about diagnosis. The patient may know whether a sweat test was performed. Collection of sweat and measurement of the chloride concentration is still the accepted method of diagnosing the condition. A sweat chloride concentration of more than 70 mmol/L suggests cystic fibrosis in an adult. Otherwise, a combination of respiratory and malabsorptive problems may be considered enough to make the diagnosis. A list of the major and minor diagnostic criteria is presented in Table 6.16. DNA markers are likely to be used increasingly in the diagnosis. At the moment this is difficult because there are a large number (over 1200) of abnormal genotypes that can result in the disease. Screening for the most common mutations is especially helpful for those patients who have the clinical syndrome but a negative sweat test (1–2%).

TABLE 6.16 Diagnosis of cystic fibrosis

Major criteria

1. Elevated chloride sweat test (98%)—pilocarpine iontophoresis on 100 mg of sweat

    >70 mmol/L diagnostic in adults

    >60 mmol/L diagnostic in children

    50–60 mmol/L suggestive

    <50 mmol/L normal

2. Azoospermia in males (95%)

3. Family history of cystic fibrosis (70%)

Minor criteria

1. Nasal polyps

2. Meconium ileus equivalent (distal bowel obstruction from inspissated secretions)

3. Rectal prolapse

4. Focal biliary cirrhosis

5. Diabetes mellitus (uncommon)

3. Ask about family history—the autosomal recessive inheritance means siblings and other close relatives may be affected.

4. Ask about treatment. Pulmonary disease is the main determinant of mortality. Aggressive treatment of the pulmonary complications has had the greatest effect on the improvement in life expectancy. The patients are usually well aware of this and are largely responsible for their own treatment. The condition is a chronic suppurative progressive one causing bronchiolitis, bronchitis, pneumonia and eventually bronchiectasis. The pathology is probably the result of the formation of viscous mucous plugs, which lead to distal infection and lung damage.

(a) The mainstay of treatment is physiotherapy, which the patient, with help from family and a physiotherapist, performs. Ask about deep breathing, percussion, postural drainage, the use of a flutter valve and the forced expiratory technique called 'huffing'.

(b) Mucolytic drugs are of doubtful benefit and may even be harmful.

(c) The patient should also know what antibiotics have been used and whether continuously or intermittently. Nebulised bronchodilators and antibiotics are commonly prescribed. *Staphylococcus aureus* and *Pseudomonas aeruginosa* are common pathogens because of their ability to grow on the abnormal bronchial mucus of cystic fibrotic lungs. The patient may know if the pseudomonas is antibiotic resistant.

(d) Ask whether treatment for complications, such as haemoptysis, cor pulmonale or pneumothorax, has been required. Minor haemoptysis, where less than 250 mL of blood is lost, occurs in about 60% of patients. Major haemoptysis occurs in about 7% of patients and bronchial artery embolisation may be required. Cor pulmonale may require treatment with diuretics, spironolactone and possibly vasodilators, but aggressive treatment of the lung disease and supplementary oxygen are more important in the long term. Pleurodesis used to be the treatment of choice for recurrent pneumothorax, but this may result in a contraindication to lung transplantation. Macrolide antibiotics, especially azithromycin, are being used because of their anti-inflammatory properties.

5. Enquire about gastrointestinal symptoms. These tend to be less of a problem, but malabsorption may make weight gain very difficult for these patients. Ask what pancreatic enzyme replacement the patient uses and how often.

6. Ask about the number of admissions to hospital over the past 12 months and the length of each stay. There is some evidence that routine admission to hospital three or four times a year for intensive physiotherapy and nebulised antibiotics and bronchodilators will be beneficial.

7. Enquire about social support. Ask whether the patient knows about or belongs to the local cystic fibrosis association and whether he or she has been in touch with other affected patients. Try to find out tactfully whether the patient understands the inheritance of the disease; male patients may know that azoospermia is usually present due to destruction of the vas deferens by abnormal secretions (95%). Eighty per cent of women are fertile, and pregnancy and breastfeeding are often successful. Find out in some detail how a young adult copes with this debilitating and life-shortening disease.

The examination

1. Look at the patient's size and physique. Muscle bulk is considered a good indicator of the severity and prognosis in a particular patient. Measure the patient's height and weight.

2. Ask the patient to cough. Listen for a loose cough and examine any sputum for the degree of purulence.

3. Now examine the respiratory system carefully. Note clubbing, which is present in the majority of patients. Look for abnormal chest wall development. Estimate forced expiratory time and examine the chest, listening particularly for crackles, wheezes and reduced breath sounds.

4. Examine the heart for signs of cor pulmonale and right ventricular failure.

5. Examine the abdomen for signs of faecal loading, especially in the right iliac fossa.

Investigations

1. Sputum culture is most important. Colonisation with *H. influenzae* and *S. aureus* tends to occur in young patients and this is often followed by nosocomial *E. coli* and *Proteus* spp. By the age of 10 years, *Pseudomonas* is the main pathogen in most patients, but usually it does not cause systemic infection.
2. A full blood count should be asked for to look for anaemia, which may be caused by malabsorption or chronic disease; the white cell count may indicate acute infection. Polycythaemia is rare, despite chronic hypoxia.
3. The electrolyte levels and liver function tests should be looked at. There may be evidence of deficiencies of fat-soluble vitamins (A, D, E and K). The creatinine level should be known before aminoglycosides are used.
4. The chest X-ray (see Fig 6.10) should be looked at carefully and should be compared with previous films if these are available. Increased lung markings are present in 98% of patients. These occur particularly in the upper lobes. Cystic bronchiectatic changes occur in more than 60% of patients. Mucous plugs may be seen in one-third and atelectasis occurs in just over 10% of patients. Look also for pneumothorax and pleural changes at the site of previous pneumothoraces or pleurodesis.
5. Chest CT is not routine but may help define focal areas of bronchiectasis that are amenable to resection.
6. Spirometry readings may fluctuate because of airway inflammation. An FEV_1 that is persistently less than 40% indicates a poor prognosis.

Management

Try to form an idea of the patient's ability to cope with the illness, as so much of the management depends on this.

1. Intensive and repetitive physiotherapy is the mainstay of treatment.
2. Intravenous antibiotics may be indicated for acute exacerbations of pulmonary disease if these are severe or fail to respond to oral antibiotic treatment. Intravenous options include tobramycin and ceftazimide for *Pseudomonas*. Inhaled tobramycin seems useful and bronchodilators can help airway clearance. Nebulised anti-pseudomonas antibiotics improve lung function and prognosis.
3. Malabsorption may require aggressive treatment with pancreatic enzyme supplements, including lipase, and frequent small meals as well as vitamin supplements.
4. Double lung transplantation and sometimes combined heart and lung transplantation is now an accepted, although still uncommon, treatment in patients with advanced disease. Cystic fibrosis does not recur in the transplanted lung. The two-year survival rate is only about 60%.
5. Human recombinant DNAase seems effective in degrading the concentration of DNA in sputum, reducing sputum viscosity and improving the patient's ability to clear pulmonary secretions. Gene therapy may be the treatment of choice in the future.

Tuberculosis

The increased incidence of pulmonary tuberculosis (TB) over the past 10 years or so and its association with HIV infection have made it a possible long case. Protection from *Mycobacterium tuberculosis* is via cell-mediated immunity involving $CD4^+$ T-helper lymphocytes. The defects of these cells in number and effectiveness, which is characteristic of HIV infection, explain this susceptibility. It may be a difficult diagnostic or management problem, or both. It also has important social and public health implications.

Figure 6.10 Cystic fibrosis PA (a) and lateral (b) films in a young patient. Note increased lung markings in the right middle lobe with 'tram tracking'—increased bronchial wall thickness (arrows).

Figures reproduced courtesy of The Canberra Hospital.

The history

The patient is likely to know that the diagnosis has been made or is suspected.

1. Find out whether the patient is a recent immigrant and, if so, from where.

2. Ask whether there has been a previous diagnosis of any other serious medical problem that might interfere with cell-mediated immunity, such as malnutrition, alcoholism or HIV infection.

3. Establish how the diagnosis was made and how long ago.

4. Ask about some of the important symptoms—weight loss, sweats and fever, cough with purulent and blood-stained sputum, and pleuritic chest pain from pleural lesions or uncontrolled coughing.

5. Ask what investigations have been performed or are planned. TB may have been suspected after a chest X-ray was performed because of respiratory symptoms or as a routine screening test. The patient may remember having to give early morning sputum specimens on a number of occasions or having had a bronchocospy with washings, if sputum was not being produced. Bronchoscopy may have been performed to exclude other causes of an abnormal chest X-ray, such as carcinoma of the lung.

   A tuberculin (Mantoux) skin test may have been performed as a screening test or to support the diagnosis where cultures have been negative. A positive tuberculin test is still significant, even if the patient has received a bacille Calmette-Guérin (BCG) vaccination in the past. Remember, if the patient is in a high-risk group (HIV positive, immunosuppressed, in close contact with a clear-cut case of TB or has evidence of prior TB on chest X ray), the Mantoux test is considered positive with just 5 mm of induration (vs 15 mm in low-risk patients).

6. Find out what treatment regimen the patient is receiving. Considerable detail must be sought about the drugs themselves—doses (if known), how long treatment will continue, how the drugs are administered (supervised or unsupervised) and what side effects have occurred (see Table 6.17 on p 109). Remember that rifampicin and rifabutin colour body fluids, including urine, orange.

7. Ask whether there has been a trigger for reactivation of previous infection (diabetes mellitus, old age, HIV infection).

8. Find out what effect this serious and chronic disease has had on the patient's life. Has the patient been able to work or go to school? Do friends and workmates know the diagnosis? Does the patient's occupation involve a public health risk?

9. Establish how the problem has been handled from a public health aspect. What screening has been done on the patient's family and friends? Are any of the family also being treated?

The examination

Early in the course of the illness there may be no specific signs. Of those patients without HIV infection who have TB, 80% have only pulmonary disease. However, the majority of patients with HIV and TB have extrapulmonary and pulmonary disease.

1. Note the patient's general appearance. Look for wasting and cachexia that may be associated with the risk factors for TB (HIV, alcoholism) or may be a result of the disease (which is also known as consumption for this reason).

2. Examine the lungs for signs of the aggressive primary infection that can occur in immunocompromised patients. These include a pleural effusion or tuberculous empyema and lobar collapse (as a result of lymphadenopathy and bronchial obstruction).

3. Post-primary disease is more common in adults. There is almost always a loose cough and often haemoptysis. There may be no abnormal findings, but you should look especially for upper lobe signs, including coarse crackles and

wheezes owing to partial bronchial obstruction caused by lymphadenopathy, and the rare amphoric breath sounds that occur over a cavity.

4. Extrapulmonary disease most commonly involves the lymph nodes (especially in HIV patients). Examine all the palpable lymph node groups. The most often affected are the cervical and supraclavicular. There is usually painless swelling.

5. Involvement of the genitourinary tract can be associated with haematuria and tenderness over the flanks.

6. The bones are involved in a small number of cases. The lumbar spine (Pott's disease), hips and knees are most affected. Collapse of the vertebral bodies may cause kyphosis and even paraplegia.

7. Tuberculous pericarditis can cause symptoms and signs of pericarditis and occasionally tamponade.

8. Abdominal TB can cause various gastrointestinal signs. There may be a palpable abdominal mass. Severe abdominal tenderness suggests tuberculous peritonitis.

Investigations

1. The diagnosis depends on microscopy of a specimen that shows mycobacteria (e.g. send three sputum specimens on separate days, followed by confirmation by culture of the organism). Traditionally, specimens of sputum or gastric or bronchial washings, or a lymph node biopsy, are stained with the Ziehl-Neelsen stain. Modern laboratories are more likely to use auramine-rhodamine stains and fluorescence microscopy. Only about 60% of patients with eventually proven TB have positive microscopy. Culture of the organism takes about six weeks, but is needed for the definitive diagnosis. These organisms should then be tested for sensitivity to the main antituberculous drugs. This takes up to eight more weeks. If multidrug resistance (MDRTB) is suspected, the *rpo* gene can be tested: it is responsible for 95% of rifampicin resistance. Polymerase chain reaction (PCR) testing can now provide rapid identification of *M. tuberculosis*, but is not available everywhere and does not distinguish between viable and non-viable organisms.

2. A chest X-ray showing the typical pattern of infiltrates and cavities in the upper lobe strongly suggests the diagnosis, but many other patterns are consistent with TB (see Figs 6.11 and 6.12).

3. Tuberculin testing is useful for screening. The test may be negative in severe disease (e.g. in up to 50% of cases of miliary TB). IFNλ release assays use a specific tuberculosis antigen to stimulate release of IFNλ from T cells in vitro. These tests are more specific than tuberculin testing and may be useful where rates of TB are low.

4. Biopsies of the pleura, lymph nodes or bone marrow may be needed. Bronchoscopy is sometimes necessary to exclude other causes of X-ray changes.

5. The fasting blood sugar level should be taken to rule out diabetes mellitus.

6. HIV patients may have TB despite a completely normal chest X-ray. They may also have less typical chest X-ray findings—often lower lobe changes without cavities. They are more likely to have infection with other mycobacteria, such as MAC. Remember that the diagnosis can be made even when the organism is not isolated.

Treatment

There are four first-line drugs for the treatment of TB: isoniazid, rifampicin, ethambutol and pyrazinamide. These are all given orally. Second-line drugs tend to be more toxic and are used only for organisms resistant to the first-line drugs. They include streptomycin, quinolone, kanamycin and amikacin (parenteral), and cycloserine,

Figure 6.11 CT scan of the thorax in a patient with TB; note the destructive changes and cavitation.
Figure reproduced courtesy of The Canberra Hospital.

Figure 6.12 Pulmonary tuberculosis. Two small rounded areas of shadowing are seen in the right upper zone (black arrow). The right hilum is enlarged by the enlarged draining lymph nodes (open arrow). This combination of focal shadowing and enlarged lymph nodes is the primary (Ghon) complex of tuberculosis. With healing, calcification may occur in the parenchymal and nodal lesions. In contrast, in tuberculosis reactivation or re-infection, cavitation may occur and there is no lymphadenopathy.

ethionamide and PAS (para-aminosalicylic acid). The initial isolate should undergo drug susceptibility testing, especially if treatment seems to have failed or there is a relapse of symptoms.

1. Treatment begins with a combination regimen of three drugs (usually isoniazid, rifampicin and pyrazinamide) for two months. A fourth drug (usually ethambutol) is often given until the organism's sensitivities are available. The aim here is to kill the majority of the organisms, improve the patient's symptoms and render him or her non-infectious. This is followed by four months of treatment with two drugs (isoniazid and rifampicin).

2. Adherence to the full course of treatment is very important, but difficult to ensure. Complicated public health arrangements, with monitoring of compliance, may be needed to enforce treatment. Direct observed treatment (DOT) is insisted on by public health authorities if compliance seems doubtful. These patients present as required to be observed taking their treatment.

3. The response to treatment is monitored by repeat sputum cultures until they become negative. Persisting positive cultures after three months suggest resistance of the organism or non-compliance on the part of the patient. Patients are probably not an infectious risk if no sputum is produced or if the sputum is consistently acid-fast bacilli (AFB) negative.

4. Patients need to be aware of the most important side effects of treatment, which include hepatitis (up to 5% in the general population and 30% in HIV patients), deafness and visual disturbance (see Table 6.17). Small increases in the transaminases (to three times normal) are no cause for alarm and are poor predictors of significant hepatotoxicity. Treatment should be reviewed immediately if jaundice develops.

5. Multiple drug resistance is increasingly common and should be expected if the infection was acquired from a patient with a known resistant organism or if the infection was acquired in parts of Asia or South America. The addition of a fluoroquinolone to the regimen should be considered while resistance studies are underway.

6. Prevention of infection by vaccination with BCG is not widely practised in Australia; its effectiveness is uncertain. The Mantoux test should be interpreted as usual regardless of previous BCG vaccination (15 mm is a positive skin test for low-risk individuals). If the Mantoux test is positive (≥5 mm) in a high-risk group (patients with exposure to TB (especially household contacts) or who are HIV infected, on prolonged steroid treatment (≥15 mg ≥1 month) or have undergone organ transplant) prescribe treatment with isoniazid for latent TB (5 mg/kg/day for nine months). If close (e.g. household) contacts are negative on the tuberculin test, treat for 12 weeks and repeat the skin test: this reduces the chance of the development of open TB by 90%. If the test is ≥10 mm in an intermediate-risk group (IV drug abusers, prisoners, healthcare workers, nursing-home patients, homeless people or those with diabetes), also treat with isoniazid. Screening of contacts and high-risk patients with tuberculin testing is an important public health measure.

TABLE 6.17 Common antituberculous drugs and their side effects

Drug	Main side effects	Usual dose/day
Rifampicin	Hepatitis, flu-like illness	600 mg
Isoniazid	Hepatitis, fever, peripheral neuropathy	300 mg (reduced to 2 or 3 doses a week in renal failure)
Streptomycin	Ototoxicity, renal impairment	1 g (not safe in pregnancy)
Ethambutol	Optic neuritis	15 mg/kg
Pyrazinamide	Hepatitis	1.5–2 g
PAS	Hepatitis, diarrhoea, hypersensitivity	12 g
PAS = para-aminosalicylic acid.		

Lung transplantation

Although lung transplantion is an uncommon procedure, transplant patients have chronic management problems that make them very suitable long cases. The examiners will have the opportunity to ask questions about the patient's underlying pulmonary problem, the general indications for lung transplant, management of the complications of transplant and, of course, the types of social problems associated with a severe chronic illness. Occasionally, patients who are being assessed for possible transplant may be suitable for the clinical examinations.

The history

1. Find out why the patient is in hospital (it may just be for the clinical examinations).
2. Obtain some basic information about the transplant: how long ago, how many lungs were transplanted and whether the patient's heart was also originally someone else's.
3. Enquire what the original lung disease was. Emphysema (including that caused by alpha$_1$-antitrypsin deficiency) is the most common indication, accounting for about half the unilateral transplants and one-third of the bilateral transplants. Idiopathic pulmonary hypertension, cystic fibrosis and Eisenmenger's syndrome are the main indications for heart/lung transplants.
4. Ask how successful the procedure has been from the patient's point of view. Lung function tests should be normal after bilateral transplant and nearly so after unilateral transplant. A decline in lung function test measurements of more than 10% usually is important.
5. Find out what complications the patient can remember. Ask about known rejection episodes and how they were managed. Have there been difficult infections? The patient may know what organisms have been detected. Stenosis of a bronchial anastomosis site is an occasional early problem. This is often treated with dilatation and stenting.
6. Ask what medications the patient is taking. If necessary, prompt for prednisolone, cyclosporin, mycophenolate, azathioprine and tacrolimus. Find out whether blood levels of tacrolimus and cyclosporin are measured regularly. Remember that these two drugs are metabolised via the cytochrome P450 pathway in the liver and blood levels may be affected by other medications (so make sure you review all of the drugs being taken).
7. If the patient is being assessed for transplant, try to find out whether the patient fits the current guidelines for transplant (see Tables 6.18 and 6.19). In general, suitable patients are sick enough to require the operation but not too sick to present an intolerable operative risk.
8. Establish how the patient has coped with the procedure, its complications and the immunosuppressants. What regular follow-up is carried out? Many transplant units have a transplant nurse available after hours whom the patient can contact directly if there are problems.

The examination

Perform a thorough respiratory examination.

1. Look especially for thoracotomy scars and attempt an assessment of the patient's functional capacity (e.g. look for signs of breathlessness while the patient is undressing and, if the room is big enough, get the patient to walk backwards and forwards).
2. Listen for end-inspiratory pops and squeaks (bronchiolitis obliterans at an advanced stage can be associated with the development of bronchiectasis).
3. Note signs of infection—fever and areas of bronchial breathing or crackles.

TABLE 6.18 Age criteria for lung transplant

	Unilateral	Bilateral	Heart/lung
Age (years)	<65	<60	<55

TABLE 6.19 Indications and contraindications for lung transplant

Indications	Contraindications
COPD—FEV$_1$ <25% predicted, $PaCO_2$ >55 mmHg **Cystic fibrosis, bronchiectasis**—FEV$_1$ <30% or complications (e.g. cachexia, severe haemoptysis) or $PaCO_2$ >50 mmHg, PaO_2 <55 mmHg **ILD**—progressive symptoms, VC, DLCO <60% **Pulmonary hypertension**—NYHA class III or IV, pulmonary artery pressure >55 mmHg, cardiac index <2 L/min **Eisenmenger's syndrome**—severe symptomatic impairment. The two-year prognosis is not improved for these patients	**Relative** Diabetes Osteoporosis Alcohol excess Still smoking Likely compliance problems Atypical mycobacterial colonisation of lungs Weight >130% of ideal or <70% of ideal **Absolute** HIV, hepatitis B, hepatitis C and liver disease, malignancy, other organ failure

DLCO = diffusion capacity for carbon monoxide; VC = vital capacity; ILD = interstitial lung disease.

4. Look for sputum and assess the cough.
5. Is the patient Cushingoid?

Management

The detection of complications and their management is likely to dominate the discussion.

1. **Rejection.** Early rejection episodes are common and treated with boost doses of prednisone. Symptoms of acute rejection include malaise, fever, dyspnoea and cough. Clinical assessment may reveal crackles, decreasing FEV$_1$, hypoxia and a raised white cell count. The chest X-ray may show infiltrates and pleural effusions. A transbronchial biopsy tends to be performed if there is any suspicion of rejection and allows an accurate diagnosis. In some places, routine biopsies are performed to detect asymptomatic rejection. It is not clear, however, whether these should be treated.

2. **Infection.** Most lung transplant patients develop infections requiring treatment. Infection is the most common cause of death. A combination of immunosuppression and local problems, such as impaired ciliary activity, are relevant. Infections with cytomegalovirus (CMV), adenovirus, influenza A and paramyxovirus are common and associated with a significant mortality. Invasive fungal organisms, such as *Aspergillus*, result in an even worse prognosis. Patients now receive at least three months of routine prophylactic antibiotic, antiviral and antifungal treatment. This approach has improved the early postoperative prognosis.

3. **Immunosuppression.** The usual problems with immunosuppressive drugs occur in lung transplant patients. Renal impairment, hypertension and hyperlipidaemia are frequent problems. Osteoporosis and peripheral neuropathy are also possible problems. Five per cent of lung transplant patients develop post-transplant lymphoproliferative disorders.

4. **Bronchiolitis obliterans.** The gradual onset of small airways obstruction is a manifestation of chronic rejection. It does not usually begin until two or more years after transplant but is detectable in at least half of transplant patients within five years. It may occur more often in those who have had more frequent acute rejection episodes and in those with a human leucocyte antigen (HLA) mismatch with the donor. There tends to be a very gradual onset of dyspnoea, fatigue and cough. Patients have a slowly decreasing FEV_1 but chest X-rays are often normal. CT scans may show a central mottling opacity. Biopsy will establish the diagnosis. The prognosis is not good. Sometimes an aggressive increase in immunosuppression may stabilise the condition, but it cannot be reversed and often the patient deteriorates rapidly.

5. **Disease recurrence.** Sarcoidosis and some forms of idiopathic ILD can recur in the transplanted lungs.

Chapter 7

The gastrointestinal long case

One finger in the throat and one in the rectum
makes a good diagnostician.
Sir William Osler (1849–1919)

Peptic ulceration

This long case is usually a straightforward management problem. The most important causes of chronic peptic ulcer disease are *Helicobacter pylori* infection and traditional NSAIDs, including low-dose aspirin. The COX-2-specific NSAIDs have a lower incidence of peptic ulceration. Idiopathic ulcers (*H. pylori* negative, NSAID negative) are increasingly being reported. The Zollinger-Ellison syndrome (gastrinoma) is a very rare but important cause. Since peptic ulcer disease affects 10% of the population, a history of this condition is not uncommon in the long case. Patients are usually admitted to hospital with peptic ulcer disease because of complications—typically haemorrhage, but more rarely perforation.

The history

1. Determine whether the patient currently has dyspepsia or a past history of dyspepsia (i.e. epigastric pain or discomfort, early satiation or postprandial full-ness). Typical ulcer symptoms include burning or sharp epigastric pain related to meals that may wake the patient from sleep at night and is relieved by antacids or antisecretory drugs. However, many patients with these symptoms do *not* have peptic ulcer disease and ulcers are often associated with atypical symptoms. Duodenal and gastric ulcers cannot be distinguished from one another on the basis of symptoms. The differential diagnosis of dyspepsia includes gastro-oesophageal reflux disease (usually also causing heartburn or acid regurgitation), gastric cancer (especially in older patients with new onset of symptoms or with alarm features such as weight loss), biliary pain (typically severe, constant pain in the right upper quadrant or epigastrium that occurs episodically and unpredictably and lasts at least 20 minutes, but usually hours), chronic pancreatitis, pancreatic cancer or intestinal angina (chronic mesenteric ischaemia, which causes severe postprandial pain such that the patient is afraid to eat and loses weight).

   Diabetes mellitus, thyroid dysfunction, hyperparathyroidism and connective tissue diseases can also cause dyspepsia.
2. Ask about the course of the symptoms and, if intermittent, the number of recurrences and treatments given. Ask about alarm symptoms, such as weight loss (which suggests the possibility of malignancy) or recurrent vomiting (e.g. gastric outlet obstruction).

3. Ask about the types of investigations the patient has had undertaken in the past. If an ulcer was apparently documented, determine whether this was by endoscopy (the most sensitive and specific test) or barium meal, or just by symptoms alone (which is inadequate). Determine whether the patient knows if *H. pylori* status was determined from gastric biopsies or by non-invasive tests, such as serology, urea breath testing or stool antigen testing.

4. A history of past ulcer surgery is important because of the associated complications (e.g. pain or bloating owing to bile reflux gastritis or an afferent loop syndrome, recurrent ulceration, early or late dumping, post-vagotomy diarrhoea, anaemia as a result of iron, vitamin B12 or folate deficiency and osteomalacia or osteoporosis).

5. Ask about the family history: a strong family history of peptic ulcer may reflect the multiple endocrine neoplasia (MEN) I syndrome.

6. Enquire carefully about medication use—medications (e.g. digoxin, potassium, iron, oral antibiotics) can induce dyspepsia, which can be confused with peptic ulcer. *All* NSAIDs are an important cause of dyspepsia with or without chronic ulceration. Alcohol can also induce acute dyspepsia (but not chronic ulcers). Patients with an ulcer history may be taking maintenance acid suppression. Treatment for *H. pylori* usually includes a proton pump inhibitor (PPI) plus two antibiotics for seven days.

7. Determine why the patient is in hospital on this occasion. If the admission is because of acute gastrointestinal bleeding, then the treatment applied needs to be documented (e.g. blood transfusion, injection of a bleeding visible vessel in a peptic ulcer base with adrenaline, or surgical oversewing of an ulcer).

The examination

Physical examination in patients with suspected peptic ulcer disease is usually unhelpful. Epigastric tenderness is not a specific sign. An upper abdominal scar may indicate past ulcer surgery. Look for alarm signs, including evidence of anaemia (e.g. from bleeding) or current bleeding (melaena, tachycardia, postural hypotension) or an abdominal mass (e.g. gastric or pancreatic carcinoma).

Investigations

1. **Endoscopy.** This is the standard test for determining that an active peptic ulcer is present. It is also the key test in a patient with upper gastrointestinal bleeding to determine whether the patient is at high risk of rebleeding and also to provide endoscopic therapy where required. Patients with active bleeding or a visible vessel at endoscopy need endoscopic therapy (e.g. injection with adrenaline followed by coagulation with a heater probe). Patients with a low risk of rebleeding (i.e. a clean ulcer base) can be discharged if stable. For patients with upper gastrointestinal tract bleeding, it is also important to exclude other causes, including variceal bleeding, erosions, angiodysplasia, a Mallory-Weiss tear or a Dieulafoy's lesion (rupture of a large submucosal artery). Where possible, biopsies should be obtained at a diagnostic endoscopy in ulcer patients to determine the *H. pylori* status.

2. **Abdominal imaging.** In the patient with unexplained dyspepsia where endoscopy is normal, ultrasound can be useful in certain clinical circumstances to investigate for biliary tract pathology. CT scanning is more sensitive for pancreatic disease.

3. **Atypical peptic ulcer.** Peptic ulceration in an unusual location, peptic ulcers resistant to therapy, an ulcer relapse after operation, or frequent or early ulcer recurrence can occur in the Zollinger-Ellison syndrome. This syndrome can also be associated with enlarged duodenal or gastric folds, or diarrhoea or

steatorrhoea. The diagnosis is made by measuring the fasting serum gastrin level: >300 pg/mL is suggestive and >1000 pg/mL is almost diagnostic. Acid secretion can be confirmed by testing the pH of gastric juice obtained at endoscopy. The next diagnostic test of choice in uncertain cases is the secretin test, where a paradoxical increase in gastrin of >200 pg/mL above basal levels is highly specific. Preoperative localisation of the tumour is then attempted by CT scanning and, if necessary, angiographic venous sampling. In patients with metastatic or multifocal disease, surgery is avoided, but all other cases require surgical exploration. High-dose PPIs are used to control the disease medically.

Remember that hypergastrinaemia also occurs in hypochlorhydria (gastric pH is not acidic; e.g. in type A atrophic gastritis and pernicious anaemia, following vagotomy or in renal failure). Other causes of hypergastrinaemia with acid hypersecretion include a retained gastric antrum after peptic ulcer surgery, massive small bowel resection, gastric outlet obstruction and thyrotoxicosis. If hypercalcaemia is present in patients with ulcer disease, this may suggest MEN I (autosomal dominant) (with hyperplasia, adenoma or carcinoma of the parathyroid, pituitary and pancreatic islets; hyperparathyroidism and pituitary adenoma are most often associated with the Zollinger-Ellison syndrome in MEN I). In MEN I (autosomal dominant with variable penetrance), there is often a strong family history of peptic ulcer disease.

Treatment

1. There is now consensus that if peptic ulcer disease is documented and *H. pylori* is present, this infection should be treated. Almost all duodenal ulcers will be cured by this approach, as will most gastric ulcers, unless associated with NSAID use.
2. Therapy with acid suppression alone for peptic ulcer disease is now obsolete unless no cause is identified. The optimal approach for curative treatment of *H. pylori* is currently three drugs (e.g. PPI plus amoxycillin plus clarithromycin), which give cure rates of approximately 70% if given for one week. Side effects occur with such treatment in up to 20% of cases. PPIs cause an increase in gastrin secretion and may predispose the patient to the development of atrophic gastritis, particularly in the setting of continued *H. pylori* infection, but the risk is probably small.
3. Patients with gastric ulcers may be advised to have a repeat gastroscopy to confirm healing and exclude carcinoma. However, 98% of cancers will be detected at the initial gastroscopy and biopsy. Therefore, repeat endoscopy is usually recommended only if symptoms have not been relieved.
4. In peptic ulcer disease, confirm that *H. pylori* infection has been cured (e.g. by repeat endoscopic biopsy or urea breath testing at least one month after completing treatment).
5. NSAID ulcers should initially be treated with a PPI, which is effective even if the NSAID is continued (although this does delay healing).
6. PPIs are more effective than histamine H2-receptor antagonists in promoting ulcer healing. NSAID use is an independent risk factor for peptic ulcer and therefore eradication of *H. pylori* in this situation may not prevent ulcer disease if NSAIDs are continued.
7. Certain patients taking traditional NSAIDs have a higher risk of ulcer complications. These include elderly patients, those having their first three months of treatment, those on higher doses, those with a past history of peptic ulcer, those taking concomitant corticosteroid therapy or anticoagulants, and those with other serious medical illnesses. NSAID ulcers often present with complications without a history of dyspepsia because these drugs are analgesic

agents that may mask symptoms. The prostaglandin E1 analogue misoprostol and PPIs both substantially reduce the risk of NSAID-induced gastric and duodenal ulcers; histamine H2-receptor antagonists in standard doses do not prevent NSAID-induced gastric ulcers. *H. pylori* eradication before treatment reduces, but does not eliminate, the risk of aspirin-induced ulcer development. *H. pylori* eradication alone provides insufficient protection from gastroduodenal complications arising from non-selective NSAID use in high-risk patients, who will still require a PPI.

Malabsorption

This can be a difficult long case. It is usually a diagnostic problem. Coeliac disease (see Table 7.1), chronic pancreatitis and previous gastric surgery account for 60% of cases of malabsorption.

TABLE 7.1 Coeliac disease
Diagnostic criteria for coeliac disease
1. Evidence of malabsorption
2. Abnormal jejunal biopsy
3. Clinical, biochemical and histological improvement on a gluten-free diet (no wheat, rye or barley)
4. Relapse on reinstitution of gluten (rarely done today except in children)
Note: Splenomegaly in coeliac disease usually indicates that lymphoma has complicated the disease because otherwise splenic atrophy is characteristic and manifests with Howell-Jolly bodies in the peripheral blood smear.
Causes of lack of response to a gluten-free diet
1. Incorrect diagnosis
2. Patient not adhering to the diet
3. Collagenous sprue
4. Intestinal lymphoma
5. Diffuse ulceration
6. Other intercurrent disease
Complications of coeliac disease
1. T-cell lymphoma
2. Ulceration of the small bowel
3. Incidence of carcinoma of the gastrointestinal tract is generally slightly increased

The history

1. Ask about presenting symptoms:
   (a) pale, bulky, offensive stools (steatorrhoea)
   (b) weight loss
   (c) weakness (potassium deficiency)
   (d) anaemia (megaloblastic, iron deficiency etc.)
   (e) bone pain (osteomalacia)
   (f) glossitis and angular stomatitis (vitamin B group deficiency)
   (g) bruising (vitamin K deficiency)
   (h) oedema as a result of protein deficiency

(i) peripheral neuropathy (owing to vitamin B_{12} or B_1 deficiency)

(j) skin rash (eczema, dermatitis herpetiformis)

(k) amenorrhoea (owing to protein depletion).

2. Ask about the time of onset of symptoms and their duration.

3. Ask aetiological questions concerning:

(a) gastrectomy, other bowel surgery

(b) history of liver or pancreatic disease

(c) drugs (e.g. alcohol, neomycin, cholestyramine)

(d) history of Crohn's disease

(e) previous radiotherapy

(f) gluten-free diet treatment at any stage

(g) history of diabetes mellitus

(h) risk factors for HIV infection.

4. Ask about current treatment (e.g. diet, pancreatic supplements, vitamin supplements, cholestyramine, antibiotics).

5. Enquire about family history (e.g. coeliac disease, inflammatory bowel disease).

6. Ask about social problems related to the chronic illness.

The examination

Pay particular attention to the current weight and nutritional status (e.g. BMI), the presence of abdominal scars, skin lesions (e.g. bruising, dermatitis herpetiformis, erythema nodosum, pyoderma gangrenosum, stomatitis, pigmentation, perianal lesions), signs of anaemia, signs of chronic liver disease, signs of peripheral neuropathy and lymphadenopathy.

Investigations *(see Table 7.2)*

1. Demonstrate malabsorption:

(a) **the 'big six' laboratory screen tests**—look for a low serum iron, prolonged prothrombin time, low calcium, low cholesterol, low carotene and a positive Sudan stain of the stool for fat (which is a good screening test for steatorrhoea)

(b) **faecal fat estimation over three days**—more than 7 g per day is abnormal; note that patients with severe small bowel diarrhoea of any cause without fat malabsorption may lose up to 14 g per day; this gold standard test is very useful if you strongly suspect fat malabsorption based on the screening evaluation

(c) **xylose test for jejunal disease**—a normal result in the setting of steatorrhoea suggests diffuse small bowel disease is unlikely and points to pancreatic pathology, but the test is rarely ordered

(d) **glucose or lactulose breath hydrogen test** for bacterial overgrowth (think about this possibility in the setting of macrocytosis with a high folate and low B_{12} level, or in patients with structural, motility or immunoglobulin deficiency disorders that predispose to bacterial overgrowth)

(e) **Schilling test** for ileal disease causing vitamin B_{12} deficiency (rarely ordered).

2. Evaluate the consequences:

(a) blood count with particular attention to red cell indices

(b) serum iron and ferritin, serum and red cell folate, and vitamin B_{12} studies

(c) serum albumin estimation

(d) vitamin D level (25-OH vitamin D), serum calcium, phosphate and alkaline phosphatase estimations

(e) clotting profile—international normalised ratio (INR)

(f) cholesterol and carotene.

3. Find the cause.
   (a) Check small bowel X-ray films for localised disease (e.g. Crohn's disease or anatomical causes of bacterial overgrowth such as diverticula or blind loops).
   (b) Check gastroscopy and small bowel biopsy (four biopsies) and duodenal aspirate for histology, parasites and bacterial overgrowth; look for multiple duodenal ulcers (e.g. as a result of Zollinger-Ellison syndrome, lymphoma, jejunoileitis).

   Subtotal villous atrophy may be present histologically in:
   - coeliac disease
   - tropical sprue
   - giardiasis
   - lymphoma
   - hypogammaglobulinaemia
   - Whipple's disease.

   Note that tissue transglutaminase (or anti-endomysial antibodies) is the most useful screening test for sprue. Remember that 2% of the population is IgA deficient and will have negative serology, so check IgA levels if testing is negative. Do not rely on antigliadin antibodies. Serology is not a substitute for small bowel biopsy, which remains the gold standard test if coeliac disease is suspected.
   (c) Vitamin B_{12} absorption may be abnormal in ileal disease, bacterial overgrowth, pernicious anaemia and pancreatic disease.
   (d) Greatly raised faecal fat levels (>40 g per day) strongly suggest pancreatic disease—this is investigated by plain abdominal X-ray films (for calcification), CT scan, magnetic resonance cholangiopancreatography (MRCP) and endoscopic ultrasound; pancreatic function testing is not performed routinely.

TABLE 7.2 Typical results of investigations in malabsorption

Investigation	Coeliac disease	Bacterial over-growth	Whipple's disease	Terminal ileal disease	Chronic pancreatitis
Stool fat	High	High	High	High	Very high
d-xylose*	Low	Low	Low	Normal	Normal
Folate (serum)	Low (in >50%)	High to normal	Low	Normal	Normal
Small bowel biopsy (proximal)	Subtotal or total villous atrophy	Abnormal culture (>10⁵ organisms on quantitative jejunal fluid culture) Histology often normal	Clubbing and flattening of villi, PAS-positive macrophages	Normal	Normal

* This is a test of proximal small bowel function. Falsely low values occur in patients with chronic renal failure, dehydration, ascites or hyperthyroidism and in the elderly.
PAS = periodic acid-Schiff technique.

Treatment

Treatment depends on the cause and also involves the replacement of essential nutrients (see Table 7.3).

TABLE 7.3 Causes and treatment of malabsorption
1. Lipolytic phase defects
Possible causes
(a) Chronic pancreatitis
(b) Cystic fibrosis
Treatment
(a) Reverse causes
(b) Pancreatic enzyme supplements
(c) Medium-chain triglycerides
2. Micellar phase defects
Possible causes
(a) Extrahepatic biliary obstruction
(b) Chronic liver disease
(c) Bacterial overgrowth
(d) Terminal ileal disease (e.g. Crohn's disease or resection)
Treatment
(a) Reverse causes (e.g. antibiotics for bacterial overgrowth)
(b) Cholestyramine if bile acid cathartic effect is important (e.g. <100 cm of ileum resected)
(c) Medium-chain triglycerides for steatorrhoea (e.g. >100 cm of ileum resected)
(d) Fat-soluble vitamin supplements
3. Mucosal and delivery phase defects
Possible causes
(a) Coeliac disease (see Table 7.1)
(b) Tropical sprue
(c) Lymphoma, intestinal lymphangiectasia
(d) Whipple's disease
(e) Small bowel ischaemia, resection
(f) Amyloidosis
(g) Hypogammaglobulinaemia
(h) HIV infection (Kaposi's sarcoma, idiopathic)
Treatment
(a) Reverse causes—gluten-free diet (coeliac disease), antibiotics (Whipple's disease)
(b) Fat-soluble vitamin supplements

Management of coeliac disease

Coeliac disease is a commonly missed diagnosis! Have a low threshold for ordering serology; patients may present with no gastrointestinal symptoms. Remember to consider the possibility in patients with osteoporosis or osteomalacia, abnormal transaminases, new neuropsychiatric symptoms and unexplained iron deficiency.

1. The management of coeliac disease includes a gluten-free diet (exclusion of wheat, rye and barley; there is controversy about oats). Symptoms usually

improve in weeks and the histology in months; tissue transglutaminase antibody also normalises in three to six months.

2. A strict diet may reduce complications. It is reasonable to re-biopsy the duodenum in three months to confirm histological healing.
3. Lack of response to a gluten-free diet may be caused by inadvertent gluten exposure, the presence of another problem (e.g. lactose intolerance, pancreatic insufficiency, bacterial overgrowth), refractory sprue (which may respond to corticosteroids) or lymphoma (T cell enteropathy: unresponsive to steroids).
4. Pneumococcal vaccine is recommended because of the hyposplenism of coeliac disease.
5. Osteoporosis must be looked for and corrected.
6. Latent coeliac disease can be diagnosed if the small bowel biopsy appears normal but there is a positive serology. For these patients, a gluten-free diet is not usually recommended, but follow-up with repeat biopsy is indicated if the symptoms recur.

Inflammatory bowel disease

Both ulcerative colitis and Crohn's disease are common conditions in hospitals and outpatient clinics. They present both diagnostic and treatment problems. Mutations in the *NOD2* gene (also called *CARD 15*) increase the risk of Crohn's disease (ileal and fibrostenosing). The patient will usually know the diagnosis but you may have to decide which type of inflammatory bowel disease (IBD) is present.

The history

1. Find out about symptoms at presentation and, if relevant, the current reason for admission. Ulcerative colitis typically presents in young adults with relapsing bloody diarrhoea, malaise, fever and weight loss. Crohn's disease has a variable presentation, including an insidious onset of pain, diarrhoea, weight loss, malabsorption, intestinal obstruction and 'appendicitis'.
2. Ask about local complications and extracolonic manifestations of the disease (see Table 7.4).
3. Enquire about sexual preference (infective proctitis in men who have sex with men must be considered in the differential diagnosis).
4. Ask about medications—NSAIDs, retinoic acid and possibly oral contraceptives can cause a similar picture. Ascertain the patient's smoking history (smoking increases the risk of Crohn's disease but decreases the risk of ulcerative colitis).
5. Determine the investigations at the time of presentation and subsequently (and particularly whether infectious causes were considered).
6. Ask about the number of hospital admissions.
7. Ask whether regular follow-up colonoscopy has been performed in patients with longstanding ulcerative colitis.
8. Find out about treatment, including medications—such as sulfasalazine, 5-aminosalicylic acid preparations (mesalazine, olsalazine), local or systemic steroids, budesonide, metronidazole, immunosuppressants (e.g. azathioprine), other antibiotics (consider pseudomembranous colitis), infliximab or adalimumab (tumour necrosis factor antibody)—and a detailed surgical history.
9. Enquire about family history of inflammatory bowel disease or bowel carcinoma.
10. Ask about smoking—a greater proportion than average of Crohn's disease patients are smokers and the risk of developing ulcerative colitis rises when people give up smoking.
11. Enquire about the patient's domestic arrangements and employment.

TABLE 7.4 Complications of inflammatory bowel disease

Ulcerative colitis

Local

1. Toxic megacolon (diameter of colon >6 cm on plain abdominal X-ray film)

2. Perforation

3. Massive haemorrhage

4. Strictures

5. Carcinoma of the colon—often multicentric and related to disease extent and duration

Extracolonic

1. Liver disease
   (a) fatty liver
   (b) primary sclerosing cholangitis (large duct or small duct [pericholangitis])
   (c) cirrhosis
   (d) carcinoma of the bile duct
   (e) amyloidosis

2. Blood disorders
   (a) anaemia (owing to chronic disease, iron deficiency, ileal involvement, haemolysis from sulfasalazine or microangiopathy)
   (b) thromboembolism (as a result of antithrombin III deficiency, stasis, dehydration)

3. Arthropathy
   (a) peripheral (large joints)
   (b) ankylosing spondylitis

4. Skin and mucous membranes
   (a) erythema nodosum (coincides with active disease)
   (b) pyoderma gangrenosum
   (c) aphthous ulcers

5. Ocular—uveitis, conjunctivitis, episcleritis

Crohn's disease

Local

1. Anorectal disease (including anal fissures or fistulas, pararectal abscess or rectovaginal fistula)

2. Obstruction (usually terminal ileum)

3. Fistula

4. Toxic megacolon and perforation (rare)

5. Carcinoma of the small and large bowel (incidence increased only slightly)

Extracolonic

Similar to ulcerative colitis, except for the following:

1. Liver disease—primary sclerosing cholangitis is less common

2. Gallstones are more common (owing to decreased bile salt pool)

3. Renal disease includes urate and calcium oxalate stones, pyelonephritis (owing to fistulas), hydronephrosis (ureteric obstruction), amyloidosis

4. Malabsorption as a result of small bowel involvement

5. Osteomalacia

The examination

A thorough gastrointestinal system examination is important (see p 310). Evaluate the general state of nutrition and hydration. Feel for any tenderness or abdominal masses and look for anal lesions externally. Always ask for the results of a rectal examination. Look for the signs of Cushing's syndrome if the patient is taking steroids. Search for the other extracolonic manifestations, being guided by the history (e.g. arthropathy, skin lesions, uveitis, anaemia, liver disease).

Investigations

It is important to exclude other causes of colitis (see Table 7.5). For the investigation of inflammatory bowel disease, the following should be considered.

TABLE 7.5 Causes of colitis
1. Inflammatory bowel disease
2. Infections, including pseudomembranous colitis
3. Radiation
4. Ischaemic colitis
5. Diversion colitis (colonic loops excluded from the faecal stream)
6. Toxic exposure (e.g. peroxide or soapsud enemas, gold-induced colitis)
7. Microscopic or collagenous colitis
8. Lymphocytic colitis

1. **Infection must be excluded.** The causes include amoebiasis (diagnosed by rectal mucosal scraping or warm stool examination), *Shigella*, *Salmonella*, *Yersinia*, *Campylobacter*, *Escherichia coli* 0157:H7 and pseudomembranous colitis (*Clostridium difficile* toxin). Lymphogranuloma venereum (a chlamydial disease that is sexually transmitted), gonorrhoea and syphilis (particularly in men who have sex with men), and other infections in immunocompromised hosts (e.g. herpes, cytomegalovirus, cryptosporidium, *Isospora belli*) should be considered in patients at risk.

   Remember that TB can, uncommonly, mimic Crohn's disease. Also, reactivation of TB is a major risk with anti-tumour necrosis factor therapy: a chest X-ray and tuberculin skin test are mandatory before starting this therapy.

2. **Sigmoidoscopy (and biopsy).** Note decreased mucosal translucency, loss of vascular pattern, granular and friable mucosa, hyperaemia, ulceration and pseudopolyps.

3. **Plain abdominal X-ray film.** It is important to look for bowel wall thickening (oedema), gaseous distension and evidence of toxic megacolon in ulcerative colitis. In Crohn's disease also look for loops of matted bowel and small bowel obstruction.

4. **Blood count.** Check for anaemia (caused by chronic disease, blood loss, macrocytic anaemia in ileal disease, or haemolytic anaemia from an autoimmune process, microangiopathic disease or sulfasalazine). Check the white cell count (e.g. leucopenia from azathioprine). Look at the ESR (or CRP) for evidence of active disease.

5. **Liver function tests and blood levels of electrolytes, urea and creatinine.** These patients may develop liver disease. Crohn's disease may lead to renal stones, pyelonephritis, hydronephrosis or amyloidosis. Remember that hypo-albuminaemia is a sign of severe disease.

6. **Barium enema.** This is only rarely used to make a diagnosis. It is contraindicated in very active colitis and with toxic megacolon because of the risk of perforation. This investigation will help distinguish ulcerative colitis from Crohn's disease—in ulcerative colitis the rectum is nearly always involved and there are no skip lesions. Look for loss of haustrations, mucosal irregularity and ulceration, spasm, pseudopolyps and bowel shortening. Also look for evidence of strictures and carcinoma. In Crohn's colitis, look for thickening, 'cobblestoning', luminal narrowing, skip lesions, fistulas and transverse fissures (sinus tracts).

7. **Colonoscopy.** This is a very useful investigation to assess whether disease is patchy or not and to assess its extent; the test is more sensitive than a barium enema. Mucosal biopsies may not differentiate ulcerative colitis from Crohn's disease. Mucus depletion and prominent crypt abscess formation are more suggestive of ulcerative colitis. Granulomas (in 25%) or focal inflammation are found in Crohn's colitis (but, note, granulomas also occur in biopsies from *Chlamydia trachomatis* and syphilitic proctitis or in cases of tuberculosis). Patients with ulcerative or Crohn's colitis who have had pancolitis for more than seven years or left-sided colitis for 15 years or more should have colonoscopic screening with biopsy offered every one or two years to look for high-grade dysplasia and carcinoma. If high-grade dysplasia is confirmed in the absence of severe inflammation, colectomy is indicated. If severe inflammation is present, assessment for dysplasia may be misleading.

8. **Antibody testing.** The presence of perinuclear antineutrophil cytoplasmic antibodies (p-ANCA) and anti-*Saccharomyces cerevisiae* antibodies (ASCA) does not make the diagnosis, but p-ANCA-negative and ASCA-positive patients are more likely to have Crohn's disease than ulcerative colitis (the test is specific but not sensitive).

Treatment
Ulcerative colitis
In ulcerative colitis, grade the severity of the disease:
- **mild**—fewer than four bowel motions per day, minimal bleeding, normal temperature and pulse
- **severe**—more than six motions per day, profuse bleeding, temperature >37.5°C, pulse >90 beats/min, abdominal tenderness
- **fulminant**—more than 10 motions per day, continuous bleeding, fever and tachycardia as above, abdominal tenderness and distension.

Other useful indices of severity are anaemia, hypoalbuminaemia and acute phase reactants (e.g. ESR, CRP).

1. In an acute attack, remember to correct hypokalaemia and avoid barium enema to prevent toxic megacolon or perforation. Do not prescribe opiates or anticholinergic agents for the same reason. In severe colitis, intravenous broad-spectrum antibiotics (including metronidazole) are usually given. Intravenous steroids are the mainstay of treatment in patients with moderate-to-severe disease. Cyclosporin may be given intravenously as a short-term alternative to colectomy for patients who do not respond to steroid treatment. Infliximab is an alternative. Close cooperation with a surgeon who is interested in this field is important in severe disease.

2. In mild-to-moderate disease, sulfasalazine is useful; mesalazine is the active agent, while sulfapyridine is the cause of most intolerance (allergic reactions such as skin rash—including Stevens-Johnson syndrome—and Heinz body haemolytic anaemia; and side effects such as nausea, headache, folate deficiency and reversible male infertility). The minimum dose is 4 g per day. Sulfasalazine decreases the relapse rate and administration should be continued indefinitely.

Mesalazine is as effective as sulfasalazine but has fewer side effects and higher doses may be given. Mesalazine is useful for patients with sulfasalazine intolerance. Note that the alternative, olsalazine, may cause diarrhoea in patients with active ulcerative colitis (because of ileal secretion)—as a result, it is normally used as maintenance treatment. Chronic steroid use does *not* reduce relapse rates. Remember to correct iron and folate deficiency if necessary.

3. If proctitis is the problem, first-line treatment is topical (steroid or mesalazine enemas twice daily) plus sulfasalazine or mesalazine orally for more active disease.

4. Azathioprine or 6-mercaptopurine is useful if there are repeated episodes of ulcerative colitis. Side effects include pancreatitis in 3% of patients and reversible bone marrow suppression in <10% of patients. The use of methotrexate is controversial.

5. It is important to try to differentiate ulcerative colitis from Crohn's disease using the clinical presentation, X-ray, endoscopic and histological findings. This is because ulcerative colitis that does not respond to medical management can be cured by colectomy; patients with extensive ulcerative colitis are at an increased risk of developing colorectal cancer. In up to 10% of patients, a specific distinction cannot be made.

Colectomy in ulcerative colitis is curative. Indications for surgery include chronic ill-health and severe disease, complications (e.g. perforation, massive bleeding) and severe disease not responding to optimal medical treatment in 7–10 days.

Patients with a very high risk of carcinoma (confirmed high-grade dysplasia on biopsy or dysplasia in a lesion or mass) should be advised to undergo a colectomy. All manifestations of the disease are cured by colectomy, but ankylosing spondylitis, liver disease and occasionally pyoderma gangrenosum do *not* respond.

While the standard Brooke ileostomy is the simplest procedure, the ileal pouch anal anastomosis is increasingly being used as it maintains intestinal continuity, although it does leave the patient with four to eight bowel movements daily and sometimes with minor incontinence (20%), and is often complicated by pouchitis (in up to 50% of patients). The latter usually responds to treatment with metronidazole.

Crohn's disease

For active disease, treatment is similar to ulcerative colitis. Always advise the patient to stop smoking!

1. Sulfasalazine or mesalazine is more effective in colonic disease, whereas steroids are more effective in small bowel disease.

2. Budenoside (a steroid derivative that acts locally and is 90% inactivated by the liver) is useful in ileocolonic disease.

3. In quiescent disease, mesalazine only modestly reduces the frequency of relapse in the postoperative setting.

4. Azathioprine (or 6-mercaptopurine) is useful for those who cannot cease steroids and to reduce relapse (including post resection surgery). Methotrexate is an alternative if azathioprine fails.

5. Oral cyclosporin is largely ineffective. With extensive ileal disease, diarrhoea may respond to a bile-salt-sequestering drug (cholestyramine or colestipol).

6. Metronidazole is modestly useful for severe perianal disease and fistulae, which tend to recur once treatment is stopped; azathioprine may be tried in difficult severe cases.

7. Infliximab (tumour necrosis factor [TNF] alpha monoclonal antibody) and

adalimumab heal fistulae and suppress underlying inflammatory disease, but relapse is common and therefore maintenance treatment is now indicated. A positive antinuclear antibody occurs in half the patients. Infusion reactions, infection (including miliary tuberculosis), lymphoproliferative diseases and demyelination can occur. These drugs are very expensive, but TNF antibody therapy is becoming the standard of care for fistulas and refractory disease.

8. Surgery is reserved for the complications of Crohn's disease (e.g. internal fistula with abscess, intestinal obstruction not responding to medical management). The best operation is resection. Strictureplasty may allow relief of localised obstruction without the deleterious effects of multiple resections.

9. When a total colectomy is needed, a standard ileostomy is the procedure of choice. The recurrence rate of the disease is unchanged by surgery.

Colon cancer

This is a particularly common tumour that usually develops in those 50 years of age or older, although patients at risk with hereditary syndromes will present at a younger age. Because early disease is curable, there has been increased interest recently in colon cancer screening. Hence, a history of polyps or colon cancer is increasingly likely to be encountered in the examination.

The history

1. The patient may have been diagnosed recently as having a colon cancer. In this case, ascertain the reasons for diagnostic testing. A recent change in bowel habit or bright red blood per rectum (from a rectal or left-sided colon cancer), symptoms of anaemia, new-onset abdominal pain or symptoms suggestive of small bowel obstruction (with a slow-growing caecal cancer) may be the presenting complaint. There may be symptoms from involvement of the bladder or female genital tract owing to local invasion. Sacral plexus pain is a very late manifestation.

2. If colon cancer was identified, determine the staging tests and treatment undertaken. If radiotherapy was given to the pelvis, enquire about any ongoing proctitis or cystitis.

3. Determine whether the patient understands the prognosis and ascertain the social support network.

4. If the patient has a history of polyps, try to determine from the patient whether these were adenomatous polyps, their approximate size and number. Patients are often rather unclear about these matters and when discussing with the examiners you may need to request information from the medical record. Adenomatous polyps may be tubular or villous (or tubulovillous); invasive cancer is more likely in larger polyps (10% of those >2.5 cm are malignant). If polyps were detected, ask the patient whether surveillance colonoscopy has been conducted in the past, when this began and how often. A repeat colonoscopy after three years in those patients without previously documented colonic cancer who have a documented large (>1 cm) adenomatous polyp or multiple (3–10) polyps is generally recommended, although surveillance needs to be tailored to other risk factors, including the family history.

5. The family history needs to be carefully obtained for any patient with a history of polyps or colon cancer in the past. If the patient describes having had thousands of adenomatous polyps throughout the large bowel, then familial adenomatous polyposis (FAP) is the diagnosis (until proven otherwise). These polyps usually occur after puberty and most individuals are affected by the age of 25 years. If the colon is not removed, almost all will have colon cancer before the age of 40. In this type of clinical case, ask about the presence of any

soft-tissue or bony tumours (Gardiner's syndrome) or tumours in the central nervous system (Turkot's syndrome), which are variants of FAP.

Most patients with FAP will have undergone a total colectomy with ileoanal anastomosis. Ask about continence and stool frequency if this operation has been performed. Screening for duodenal and periampullary cancers every one to three years by endoscopy is generally recommended.

Ask whether any offspring of a patient with this condition have been screened. Flexible sigmoidoscopy on an annual basis is recommended. DNA testing of peripheral blood mononuclear cells for the presence of the mutated *APC* gene at puberty is also useful (after first testing affected relatives to validate the *APC* mutation presence) in screening offspring.

If there is a strong family history of colon cancer, consider the possibility of Lynch syndrome (see below). There is a 70% lifetime risk of colon cancer in this autosomal dominant disease.

There is often also a family history of either ovarian or endometrial carcinoma. Members of such families are typically screened by colonoscopy biennially beginning at the age of 25 years, as well as undergoing pelvic ultrasonography and endometrial biopsies.

6. Enquire about any history of documented inflammatory bowel disease. The risk of colorectal cancer in a patient with ulcerative colitis is small during the initial 7–10 years after pancolonic disease development, but then increases approximately 1% per year. Ask whether colonoscopic surveillance has been undertaken or not. Patients with Crohn's colitis should now also be offered similar surveillance.

7. Ask whether there has been any history of possible septicaemia. *Streptococcus bovis* or *Clostridium septicus* bacteraemia indicates an underlying high risk of occult colon cancer and requires aggressive investigation.

8. Haematomas of the gastrointestinal tract with mucocutaneous pigmentation (Peutz-Jeghers syndrome) increase the risk of both large and small bowel cancer, as well as breast, uterine and ovarian cancers. Affected patients should undergo surveillance by colonoscopy and gastroscopy every three years from 18 years of age.

9. Determine whether there is any history of a ureterosigmoidostomy for correction of congenital exstrophy of the bladder, which increases the risk of colon cancer 15–30 years later.

10. Diabetes mellitus and acromegaly may be associated with an increased risk; regular full-dose aspirin use may reduce the risk of colon cancer.

The examination

1. Look for evidence of jaundice or anaemia.
2. If the patient is currently undergoing fluorouracil-derived chemotherapy, look at the palms and soles for evidence of hand–foot syndrome (very tender, symmetrical erythema).
3. Carefully examine the abdomen, in particular looking for any evidence of malignant deposits in the liver or other intraperitoneal masses or skin changes that are consistent with radiotherapy. Record any scars on the abdomen.
4. Results of a rectal examination need to be obtained.
5. Other lymph node groups should be examined and evidence of metastatic malignancy elsewhere (e.g. the lungs, bones or brain) should be sought.
6. Look for the pigmentation of Peutz-Jeghers syndrome.
7. Multiple skin lesions (e.g. sebaceous adenomas and carcinomas, basal cell and squamous cell carcinomas, keratoacanthomas) occur in a variant of hereditary non-polyposis colorectal cancer (Torres syndrome).

Investigations

1. **Screening.** The possibility of hereditary non-polyposis colon cancer (HNPCC, or Lynch syndrome) should be considered for certain patients. This includes patients who have three or more relatives with a history of colon cancer where one of these is a first-degree relative of the other two; those who have one or more cases of colorectal cancer in family members younger than 50; and those who have colorectal cancer diagnosed in at least two generations of the family. Screening starts at age 25 in affected families. In most kindreds with HNPCC, germ-line mutations have occurred in one of six DNA mismatch repair genes. Commercial testing is available for *hMSH2* and *hMLH1* mutations and these have a high sensitivity. 'Microsatellite instability' (MSI) is the expansion or contraction of short repeated DNA sequences. MSI has been observed in more than 90% of samples of tumour tissue from patients with HNPCC who fulfil the clinical (Amsterdam) criteria for this disease and also in up to 15% of tumours from patients with sporadic colorectal cancer. The presence of MSI may indicate a better prognosis and better response to adjuvant chemotherapy. Testing for the presence of MSI in a tumour or adenoma should be an initial screening test for patients suspected of having HNPCC, and positive cases should undergo genetic screening.

2. **Symptomatic patients.** Most will have had the cancer identified by colonoscopy or barium enema examination. With the increasing introduction of screening measures in asymptomatic patients (e.g. faecal occult blood testing), earlier stage colon cancers will be detected in average-risk patients. The prognosis depends on the stage of disease. Survival is decreased if the bowel wall is penetrated (Dukes' B2 stage) or with lymph node involvement (Dukes' C stage).

Treatment

1. For colon cancer, total tumour resection in local disease is the treatment of choice undertaken either endoscopically or surgically. Before surgery, patients should be evaluated for the possibility of metastatic disease, including a careful physical examination. Many physicians would also order a chest X-ray and liver function tests and measure the baseline carcinoembryonic antigen (CEA) level. If possible, a complete colonoscopy should be undertaken to look for evidence of synchronous cancers or polyps. If colonoscopy was not performed before the operation, it should be carried out as soon as practicable after the operation.

2. Following a resection, patients are often followed up for five years with annual physical examinations and surveillance colonoscopy every three years. Measuring CEA levels every three months for two years after surgery for Dukes' B or C stage disease, as a test for tumour recurrence, is often recommended but remains controversial.

3. If metastatic disease is present, resection of the primary colorectal tumour does not change prognosis and should be done only for symptomatic reasons. The exception is metastases to the liver only, where 25% may be cured by resection.

4. Determine whether the patient has had radiation therapy to the pelvis, which may have been offered with a rectal cancer. Some patients may have received chemotherapy; in particular, patients with Dukes' C stage often have had adjuvant leucovorin modulated 5-fluorouracil for six months. Oxaliplatin may be added.

Chronic liver disease

Cirrhosis alone or in combination with other disease will often crop up, particularly in repatriation hospitals. (*Warning:* You may be exposed to prolonged war stories and discussions about shrapnel.) It is a pathological diagnosis. This discussion will be limited to aspects of cirrhosis and chronic hepatitis, which tend to be most frequent in the examination.

The history

Cirrhosis can present with jaundice, ascites, abdominal pain, acute bleeding or encephalopathy. Occasionally patients present with only weakness, lassitude or loss of libido. There may be no symptoms (incidental cirrhosis).

1. Ask about length of history of liver disease:
   (a) past history of hepatitis or jaundice, including contacts
   (b) alcohol intake (in men, 80 g per day for more than 10 years is usually necessary; women need less exposure)
   (c) history of drug addiction (intravenous), sexual orientation, transfusions, tattoos etc.
   (d) drug history (e.g. for chronic hepatitis: methyldopa, isoniazid, nitrofurantoin)
   (e) history of diabetes mellitus, cardiac failure or arthropathy (haemochromatosis)
   (f) overseas travel (e.g. acute hepatitis).
2. Ask about treatment (e.g. protein restriction, fluid restriction, alcohol abstinence, steroids, lactulose, neomycin).
3. Ask about complications, such as any history of encephalopathy, any history of portal hypertension (ascites or bleeding from varices), recent abdominal pain (gallstones—usually pigment stones, acute alcoholic hepatitis etc.).
4. Ask about investigations (e.g. liver biopsy).
5. Ask about operations (e.g. transjugular intrahepatic portosystemic shunt—TIPS).
6. Enquire about erectile dysfunction, loss of libido.
7. Enquire about social problems (e.g. employment, family).

The examination

1. Note the patient's racial origin. Hepatitis B and C viruses are endemic in Southeast Asia, Italy and Egypt. Look for tattoos—tattoo needles are a source of infection. Examine carefully for the signs of chronic liver disease. Also note any hepatic encephalopathy, signs of portal hypertension, including splenomegaly, ascites, oedema and signs of bleeding (e.g. melaena).
2. Consider hepatocellular carcinoma (particularly in haemochromatosis and cirrhosis as a result of hepatitis B or C virus infection). In patients with decompensated cirrhosis, examine for a hard mass and liver bruit (hepatoma).
3. Look for the signs of haemochromatosis. In young patients, consider Wilson's disease and look carefully for Kayser-Fleischer rings. If there is deep jaundice with scratch marks and xanthelasma, particularly in a woman, consider end-stage primary biliary cirrhosis.
4. Exclude severe right heart failure, tricuspid regurgitation or constrictive pericarditis clinically in all patients. Search for other causes and sequelae (see Tables 7.6 and 7.7).

Investigations

Management of cirrhosis depends on the aetiology, morphology and hepatic function. It is important to make a diagnosis and exclude potentially reversible causes of further liver deterioration.

TABLE 7.6 Causes of cirrhosis in adults

1. Alcohol
2. Postviral (hepatitis B, delta, C)
3. Non-alcoholic steatohepatitis (NASH)
4. Drugs (e.g. methyldopa, chlorpromazine, isoniazid, nitrofurantoin, propylthiouracil, methotrexate, amiodarone)
5. Autoimmune chronic hepatitis
6. Haemochromatosis
7. Wilson's disease
8. Primary sclerosing cholangitis
9. Primary biliary cirrhosis
10. Secondary biliary cirrhosis
11. Alpha$_1$-antitrypsin deficiency
12. Cystic fibrosis
13. Budd-Chiari syndrome
14. Cardiac failure, chronic constrictive pericarditis
15. Cryptogenic (idiopathic)

TABLE 7.7 Sequelae of cirrhosis

1. Portal hypertension and ascites
2. Portal vein thrombosis (rare)
3. Spontaneous bacterial peritonitis
4. Hepatic encephalopathy
5. Hepatorenal syndrome
6. Hepatocellular carcinoma

1. **Liver function tests.** These should be used to confirm abnormalities, follow progress and give an idea of prognosis (particularly a low albumin level and prolonged INR). An aspartate aminotransferase (AST) to alanine aminotransferase (ALT) ratio of >2.0 suggests alcoholic liver disease.
2. **Full blood count.** This is helpful because anaemia may be caused by chronic disease, blood loss, folate deficiency, bone marrow depression, hypersplenism, haemolysis or sideroblastic anaemia. Round macrocytes are common in alcoholics. Remember that leucopenia and thrombocytopenia occur in hypersplenism.
3. **Renal function tests.** These are important to exclude the hepatorenal syndrome. Hyponatraemia is common in cirrhosis.
4. **Ascitic tap** (see Tables 7.8 and 7.9).
5. **Ultrasound or abdominal CT scan** (see Fig 7.1). This may help exclude biliary obstruction and infiltration. The texture of the liver may suggest infiltration (e.g. fat) or nodularity (cirrhosis).
6. In the setting of dyspnoea, consider hepatopulmonary syndrome. Platypnoea (dyspnoea that is worse when the patient sits up and is relieved by lying down) and orthodexia (arterial desaturation when upright) are strongly suggestive; a diagnosis of intrapulmonary vascular dilatation may be possible by contrast echocardiography.

TABLE 7.8 Causes of ascites and interpretation of ascitic fluid studies
Causes
1. Related to portal hypertension (serum-to-ascites albumin gradient [SAAG] ≥11 g/L):
(a) cirrhosis
(b) alcoholic hepatitis
(c) cardiac ascites (right heart failure)
(d) fulminant hepatic failure
(e) veno-occlusive disease
(f) Budd-Chiari syndrome (hepatic vein thrombosis) or inferior vena caval obstruction (see Table 7.9)
(g) myxoedema
2. Not related to portal hypertension (SAAG <11 g/L):
(a) peritoneal carcinomatosis
(b) peritoneal tuberculosis
(c) pancreatitis
(d) nephrotic syndrome (see Table 11.2)
Examination of ascitic fluid following a diagnostic paracentesis
1. *SAAG*—≥11 g/L in portal hypertension (e.g. cirrhosis)
2. *Blood*—suggests malignancy or a recent invasive test
3. *Turbid or white fluid*—suggests infection or chylous ascites
4. *Cell count*—0–300 × 10^6/L mononuclear cells is normal; >500 cells or >250 polymorphs × 10^6/L suggests spontaneous bacterial peritonitis
5. *Lactate*—increased in spontaneous bacterial peritonitis
6 *Amylase*—elevated in pancreatic ascites
7. *Cytology*—for malignant cells
8. *Culture*—for spontaneous bacterial peritonitis

7. Always assess for possible causative factors (see Table 7.6).
   • Obtain hepatitis B and C serologies.
   • Screen for antimitochondrial antibody (AMA) if primary biliary cirrhosis is suspected. In suspected chronic hepatitis (e.g. young woman with raised globulins) test for antinuclear antibody (ANA), smooth muscle antibody, and anti-liver and kidney microsomes type 1 (anti-LKM1) antibody. In type I autoimmune chronic hepatitis there is marked hyperglobulinaemia, and ANA and anti-smooth muscle antibody (ASMA) are present. In type II, ANA is negative, but anti-LKM1 is present in high titre and liver cytosol antigen may be present (this antibody also occurs in low titre in hepatitis C). In the rare overlap syndromes, the only serological abnormality may be AMA, but the histology shows autoimmune hepatitis or the patient is ANA or ASMA (but not AMA) positive and has primary biliary cirrhosis (autoimmune cholangiopathy) on histology.
   • Order iron studies and, in a young patient, caeruloplasmin levels. Alpha₁-antitrypsin deficiency should be considered; absence of the alpha₁ fraction on a protein electrophoresis is a useful clue.

TABLE 7.9 Budd-Chiari syndrome

Typically young adults who have pain (owing to hepatic congestion), hepatomegaly and ascites

Causes

1. Idiopathic (thrombosis or fibrous obliteration of hepatic vein)

2. Myeloproliferative disease, especially polycythaemia rubra vera

3. Malignant disease (e.g. renal, pancreatic, hepatoma, adrenal, testicular, thyroid)

4. Oral contraceptives or pregnancy

5. Paroxysmal nocturnal haemoglobinuria (PNH)

6. Drugs (e.g. azathioprine, adriamycin)

7. Fibrous membrane, trauma, schistosomiasis, amoebiasis

Diagnosis

1. *Liver function tests*—non-specific, but serum alkaline phosphatase level may be high

2. *Ascitic tap*

3. *Ultrasonography with Doppler flow studies*—less sensitive than angiography but diagnostic in >85% of cases

4. *Technetium sulfur colloid liver scan (increased caudate lobe uptake)*—less useful

5. *Magnetic resonance angiography (and venography)*—diagnostic

6. *Liver biopsy*—highly suggestive ('nutmeg' liver)

Figure 7.1 CT scan of abdomen showing a hepatocellular carcinoma (arrow), confirmed on biopsy.
Figure reproduced courtesy of The Canberra Hospital.

- Evaluate for evidence of inflammatory bowel disease if there are colonic symptoms. Perinuclear antineutrophil cytoplasmic antibodies (p-ANCA) occur in up to 80% of patients with ulcerative colitis and are a marker for primary sclerosing cholangitis (60% of cases).
- Screening for hepatocellular carcinoma (HCC) is recommended for patients with cirrhosis secondary to hepatitis B or C. Screening is by six-monthly measurement of alpha-fetoprotein and liver ultrasound.
- Assess the hepatic functional reserve of patients with known or suspected cirrhosis (see Table 7.10).

8. **Liver biopsy.** This is a definitive test and probably should be done if the diagnosis is uncertain, unless there are specific contraindications (e.g. coagulopathy).

TABLE 7.10 Child's classification of patients with cirrhosis in terms of hepatic functional reserve

	A	B	C
Degree of impairment	Minimal	Moderate	Severe
Serum bilirubin (mmol/L)	<35	35–50	>50
Serum albumin (g/L) (mmol/L)	>35 (>507)	30–35 (435–507)	<30 (<435)
Ascites	None	Easily controlled	Poorly controlled
Encephalopathy	None	Minimal	Advanced; 'coma'
Nutrition	Excellent	Good	Poor; 'wasting'

Treatment

Decide whether the patient has acute or acute-on-chronic disease and decide whether the disease is compensated or decompensated. Management includes treating hepatocellular failure (synthetic function) and portal hypertension (plumbing). Cirrhosis is irreversible. However, removing causative factors, such as alcohol, iron overload and drugs, or treating viral infection is of value.

Hepatocellular failure

Acute hepatic encephalopathy is precipitated by bleeding into the gastrointestinal tract or electrolyte disturbances (alkalosis increases the ammonia crossing the blood–brain barrier, whereas hypokalaemia increases renal ammonia production). Hypokalaemia may be caused by recent diuretic use. Infection (e.g. spontaneous bacterial peritonitis), drugs (e.g. sedatives), a high-protein diet, constipation, deteriorating liver function (e.g. alcoholic binge, hepatoma) and rarely metabolic disturbances (e.g. hypoglycaemia, hypoxia) may also precipitate encephalopathy.

Management

1. Management consists of removing the precipitating factors. This means removing blood from the gut (e.g. enemas), giving a low-protein diet, treating infection, correcting electrolyte disturbances, avoiding sedatives and attacking the urea-splitting organisms with lactulose (or lactitol; these decrease the pH inhibiting the flora) or antibiotics (e.g. neomycin, metronidazole or rifaximin), or both.
2. Chronic hepatocellular failure should be managed by treating the cause where possible and manipulating the protein diet as required.
3. Control encephalopathy and ascites.
4. Watch for gastrointestinal bleeding and renal failure.
5. In cases of autoimmune chronic hepatitis, steroids are helpful in patients without viral markers.

Portal hypertension
Clinical features include splenomegaly, the presence of collaterals, ascites and fetor hepaticus. Investigations include endoscopy for oesophageal varices, ascitic tap and abdominal ultrasound with Doppler arterial and venous flow studies.

Management
1. An attempt should be made to assess the bleeding risk for a patient with varices. High-risk patients (75% risk of haemorrhage over one year) are those with Child's class C cirrhosis, gross ascites and large varices. All patients with large varices should be recommended prophylactic treatment—usually with beta-blockers or, if contraindicated, variceal band ligation.
2. Bleeding varices should be managed acutely by replacing blood and correcting coagulation abnormalities. Intravenous octreotide (or vasopressin combined with glyceryl trinitrate) is first-line therapy but only a temporary measure. Oesophageal variceal banding therapy is effective (and superior to sclerotherapy) in stopping acute bleeding. Balloon tamponade at the gastro-oesophageal junction with the gastric balloon is now rarely required; oesophageal balloon tamponade may worsen the prognosis. To prevent recurrent variceal bleeding, elective endoscopic banding to obliterate varices may be effective. Beta-blockers (propranolol) can reduce portal pressure and may be useful in patients with good liver function. TIPS is preferable to shunt surgery. Mortality is high for 'crash' shunts.
3. Treatment of ascites consists of gentle diuresis (maximum weight loss of 500 g per day). Begin with bed rest, salt restriction and spironolactone but increase the dose slowly. If the urinary sodium to potassium ratio is >1, a dose of 150 mg/day is usually adequate; if the ratio is less than 1, higher doses are needed. Frusemide is given if necessary. A combination of frusemide 40 mg daily and spironolactone 25 mg daily may be the most helpful, although there is evidence that spironolactone alone may be as effective. Therapeutic paracentesis is a safe alternative in patients with tense ascites, especially when there is also peripheral oedema. Intravenous salt-poor albumin is given to replace the protein lost in ascitic fluid and 5–10 L can be removed; the procedure can be repeated if necessary. Therapeutic paracentesis is contraindicated in renal failure or severe coagulopathy.
4. In resistant ascites, alternatives include the TIPS.
5. Liver transplantation is the definitive treatment in suitable patients (in the absence of hepatorenal syndrome).

Hepatitis B
Hepatitis B virus (HBV) may be transmitted parenterally (intravenous drug users, infected blood products etc.) or sexually. Most infected individuals seroconvert and develop immunity; however, a small proportion become chronic carriers or progress to chronic hepatitis and ultimately cirrhosis. The risk of developing HCC in the latter group is high.

The diagnosis of hepatitis B is made by positive serology (HBsAg-positive) and active disease is usually associated with the HBeAg-positive state, as well as elevated serum transaminase levels, particularly the serum ALT level. Measuring for HBV-DNA provides a more accurate assessment of viral load. Precore mutants of HBV are usually diagnosed in patients who are HBeAg-negative and HBeAb-positive, but have elevated transaminase and HBV-DNA levels.

The most accurate method of staging the disease is by means of a liver biopsy. The liver biopsy is important to assess the extent of the inflammation and fibrosis in those with chronic hepatitis.

Treatment

1. The aim of antiviral therapy is to stop viral replication (i.e. seroconversion from positive HBeAg to negative HBeAg and HBV-DNA levels), as well as normalising ALT levels and histology. 'Inactive carriers' (normal transaminases, HBV-DNA $<10^5$ copies/mL and normal biopsy) do not need antiviral therapy.

2. Treatment is with subcutaneous interferon, most commonly 5 million units thrice weekly for two to six months, or lamivudine or entecavir for as long as necessary. Interferon produces a response rate of approximately 30% with loss of HBeAg status and no resistance. Younger patients and women contemplating pregnancy are offered interferon. Nevertheless, the drug has many debilitating side effects and is contraindicated in decompensated liver disease. Lamivudine has minimal side effects, with a seroconversion rate after two years of about 30%. Lamivudine is an orally active nucleoside analogue that interferes with HBV replication. Long-term use of lamivudine may be associated with the development of a *YMDD* mutant form of HBV. To date these variants have not been shown to cause any additional liver damage. Patients should be maintained on lamivudine, despite the presence of the variant, because re-emergence of wild-type virus may have a worse outcome. Drug resistance to entecavir is low. Adefovir is active against lamivudine-resistant HBV.

3. Liver transplantation can be considered in patients with decompensated HBV liver disease, but without proper preparation HBV infection recurs in the transplanted liver and may cause very aggressive liver disease. Fortunately, strategies are available to overcome this problem. Currently, antiviral drugs are used prior to transplantation to lower HBV-DNA levels and then large doses of hepatitis B immunoglobulin are used in the peritransplantation period. This strategy is extremely effective in preventing recurrence after liver transplantation.

Hepatitis C

Hepatitis C virus (HCV) is predominantly parenterally transmitted and is particularly common in intravenous drug users. If HCV antibody positive, confirm the diagnosis with HCV RNA. The virus is also commonly found in migrants from endemic regions, including Southeast Asia, Egypt and Italy. The majority of patients are incidentally found to be infected and are usually asymptomatic, although fatigue is a common symptom.

Extrahepatic manifestations are listed in Table 7.11. The disease process is insidious in onset.

TABLE 7.11 Extrahepatic manifestations of hepatitis C

- Mixed cryoglobulinaemia
- Porphyria cutanea tarda
- Cutaneous necrotising vasculitis
- Membranoproliferative glomerulonephritis
- Lichen planus
- Hashimoto's thyroiditis
- B-cell lymphoma
- Polyarthralgias and polyarthritis

Approximately 80% of infected individuals go on to develop chronic hepatitis over a 20-year period. It is estimated that 20–30% of patients with chronic hepatitis C develop cirrhosis, but the process is generally slow and insidious. Once cirrhosis develops, symptoms are more common and the signs of end-stage liver disease can appear with jaundice, weakness, wasting and gastrointestinal bleeding. After 25 years of infection about 4% of patients with cirrhosis develop HCC.

Diagnosis is based on a positive HCV antibody ELISA test and then active virus is checked with HCV-polymerase chain reaction (PCR) testing. Quantitative HCV-PCR is useful in monitoring the response to treatment. A liver biopsy is necessary to stage the disease and estimate the extent of fibrosis. Patients with cirrhosis respond poorly to antiviral therapy and are also at risk of developing HCC.

Management

1. Currently, therapy is prescribed for chronic hepatitis C patients with abnormal transaminases and is based on a combination of oral ribavirin *and* weekly injections of pegylated interferon for 12 months (if genotype 1) or six months (if genotype 2 or 3), unless there is no response to therapy at three months (less than a 2 log unit decrease by HCV RNA testing suggests treatment is futile). Sustained response rates can be achieved in approximately 55% of patients. Watch for depression (interferon) and haemolytic anaemia (ribavirin). Do *not* treat with interferon if there is cirrhosis.
2. Vaccination against hepatitis A and B is recommended for patients who are not already immune.
3. Patients who develop end-stage liver disease may be transplant candidates. Hepatitis C-related liver disease is the most common reason for liver transplantation today.
4. Surveillance for hepatoma is recommended if there is cirrhosis (ultrasound every six to 12 months).

Haemochromatosis

This is an autosomal recessive disease marked by progressive iron loading of parenchymal cells of the liver, pancreas, heart and other organs. The diagnosis is often made before symptoms develop (the result of routine iron studies) and is much more common in men (menses protect women).

Symptomatic patients usually present with hepatomegaly and abdominal pain. HCC occurs in up to 30% of patients with cirrhosis. Diabetes mellitus is a classical presentation, as is grey skin pigmentation ('bronzed diabetes'), dilated cardiomyopathy, arthropathy (second and third MCP joints) and impotence (owing to iron pigmentation in the pituitary gland).

Hereditary haemochromatosis is a common genetic disorder in Caucasians, with a prevalence of at least 1 in 250. Diagnosis is suggested by an increased transferrin saturation (>62% men, >50% women) and a raised ferritin level (>300 µg/L in men and >200 µg/L in women is suggestive). The serum ferritin level is an acute-phase reactant and may be elevated in other chronic inflammatory conditions, notably those involving the liver, including non-alcoholic steatohepatitis (NASH), alcoholic liver disease and chronic viral hepatitis.

Liver biopsy is useful to measure the amount of iron overload and the extent of liver disease (fibrosis, cirrhosis etc.). There are specific features on biopsy; a Perl's Prussian blue stain visually demonstrates the extent of iron overload. It is important to determine the hepatic iron concentration and index (usually >1.9) on liver biopsy specimens.

The genetic defect has been localised to the short arm of chromosome 6. The gene has been termed *HFE*. Two mutations have been described: *C282Y* and *H63D*. Better identification of family members is now able to be undertaken, based on documenting the presence of these two mutations. Patients with phenotypic haemochromatosis are usually homozygous for the *C282Y* mutation; a few are compound heterozygotes (*C282Y* and *H63D* mutation). Homozygotes for *H63D* may not be at risk; 5% of those with haemochromatosis have none of these mutations. Genetic testing is recommended for all first-degree relatives of the proband. In those cases homozygous for *C282Y*, there is a one in four chance of the siblings being homozygous. The children's chance of developing haemochromatosis depends on the other parent (homozygous normal indicates no risk).

Management
1. Treatment is through regular venesection (weekly) for approximately two years and then once every three months. The optimal regimen is not established, but the aim is to reduce iron stores as quickly as possible: 50 units of blood contain 12.5 g of iron. Patients with iron overload as a result of mutations of the iron export protein ferroportin may not tolerate this rate of removal.
2. The avoidance of alcohol is important.
3. Arthropathy and endocrine changes do not respond to treatment.
4. Hepatocellular carcinoma is not prevented by venesection in patients with established cirrhosis, but life expectancy is normal in those without end-organ damage whose iron stores are reduced.

Non-alcoholic steatohepatitis

Non-alcoholic steatohepatitis is defined by histological features, resembling those of alcoholic hepatitis, which are present in patients who have not consumed excessive quantities of alcohol. The majority of patients present because they are inadvertently found to have abnormal liver function tests or steatosis detected on imaging. Even though clinical findings are uncommon, hepatomegaly is the most frequent sign detected. The typical liver function abnormalities are a two- to threefold elevation of the serum aminotransferase levels, with the serum ALT greater than the serum AST level (the opposite of alcoholic liver disease). The serum gamma-glutamyl transferase (GGT) levels are also similarly elevated. Viral markers are absent.

NASH is more common in women and the most frequently associated underlying clinical conditions are obesity, type 2 diabetes mellitus and hyperlipidaemia, particularly hypertriglyceridaemia. Look for evidence of the metabolic syndrome (including hypertension, increased waist circumference and high lipids). Nevertheless, studies have documented lean men with NASH. Although the peak age of presentation is the fifth and sixth decades of life, NASH is now the most common cause of liver disease in adolescents.

Exclude drug causes such as steroid use and amiodarone. The definitive diagnostic test is a liver biopsy. The histopathological features should be evaluated in conjunction with a detailed history of alcohol and drug intake (e.g. methotrexate). Where relevant, other liver disease must be excluded (e.g. haemochromatosis, chronic viral hepatitis) (see Table 7.12). The typical histological features are macrovesicular steatosis with an associated necroinflammatory infiltrate (usually mononuclear) and a variable degree of fibrosis.

Another group of patients has fatty liver disease without inflammation and with normal transaminase levels—non-alcoholic fatty liver disease (NAFLD).

A proportion of patients will progress to more chronic liver disease with fibrosis and ultimately cirrhosis. NASH may explain many cases previously labelled as cryptogenic. Studies have documented elevations in both cardiovascular and hepatic mortality.

TABLE 7.12 Causes of hepatic steatosis	
Metabolic disorders	**Drugs and toxins**
Obesity	Alcohol
Diabetes mellitus	Methotrexate
Hyperlipidaemia	Organic solvents
Jejunoileal bypass	Amiodarone
Total parenteral nutrition	

Management
Management options are limited to treating the underlying clinical condition, with slow weight loss recommended for obese patients and strict control of hyperlipidaemia and hyperglycaemia. Alcohol should be avoided.

Liver transplantation
Liver transplantation is now an important therapeutic option in patients with irreversible, progressive liver disease for which there is no acceptable alternative therapy and no absolute contraindication. The one-year survival rate overall is 75%. In the examination setting, a patient will either have chronic liver disease and be a candidate for transplantation or be a transplant recipient who has a problem.

The history
1. Obtain details of the patient's liver disease, including diagnosis and duration. Candidates for liver transplantation include patients with cirrhosis, primary sclerosing cholangitis, autoimmune chronic hepatitis, chronic portal-systemic encephalopathy, Budd-Chiari syndrome, inherited metabolic diseases (e.g. Wilson's disease, alpha$_1$-antitrypsin deficiency) and acute or subacute hepatic failure.
2. The timing of the transplantation is crucial. This should be considered when the patient is invalided but before complications have occurred that may preclude proceeding (e.g. preterminal variceal bleeding, irreversible hepatorenal syndrome, development of a catabolic state, irreversible coagulopathy, vascular instability with ascites or incapacitating osteopenic bone disease). Those with end-stage liver disease who have had a life-threatening episode of decompensation or whose quality of life has become unbearably reduced are potential candidates. Accepted criteria include a Child-Pugh score >6, an episode of variceal bleeding or spontaneous bacterial peritonitis, or stage II encephalopathy in acute liver failure. A model for end-stage liver disease (MELD), which has been developed at the Mayo Clinic and is based on three parameters (serum bilirubin, INR and creatinine), helps predict survival and is widely used (transplant candidates have a score >10).
3. If the patient may be a candidate for liver transplantation, enquire about potential contraindications. Relative contraindications include active sepsis outside the liver, metastatic malignancy, cholangiocarcinoma, continuing alcohol consumption, HIV, diffuse portal vein thrombosis and advanced cardiopulmonary or renal disease, a prior portacaval shunt (TIPS is not a contraindication), intrahepatic or biliary infection, localised portal vein thrombosis, prior complex hepatobiliary surgery, severe hypoxaemia as a result of intrapulmonary shunting (patients with the hepatopulmonary syndrome and hypoxia can benefit, but a PaO_2 of <50 mmHg is a relative contraindication) and renal impairment.
4. Ask about tests that have been done in preparation for transplant. These typically include cardiac and pulmonary tests (electrocardiogram, echocardiogram,

stress test, chest X-ray, pulmonary function tests), renal tests (urine protein and creatine, and glomerular filtration rate estimation) and liver tests (imaging to exclude a hepatoma and to define the vascular anatomy).

5. Enquire about complications of the patient's liver disease (e.g. previous haemorrhages, ascites, pre-coma, hypoxaemia caused by hepatopulmonary syndrome etc.).

6. If the patient has had a transplant, enquire about the postoperative course, including whether further surgery was carried out (e.g. drainage of abscesses, reconstruction of the biliary tract for control of bleeding, retransplantation for graft failure and for hepatic arterial thrombosis). Also ask about postoperative infections.

7. Ask about complications of liver transplantation. Early on (in the first five days), primary graft failure, technical problems (e.g. bleeding, hepatic arterial thrombosis, bile leaks, portal vein thrombosis), renal failure and pulmonary complications (atelectasis, pleural effusion, infection) may occur. Major problems after discharge from hospital include rejection, infection, biliary complications, hypotension, recurrent disease, bone disease, nutrition and de-novo cancer. Infections occur in most patients, largely related to immunosuppression; chronic opportunistic infections usually occur from four weeks after transplantation. Biliary strictures may also occur from four weeks after transplantation. Acute liver rejection is rarely seen after the initial six months. Chronic rejection usually occurs six weeks to nine months after transplantation; there is progressive cholestasis and diagnosis is best made by liver biopsy. Bone disease and ectopic calcification may occur some months after transplantation.

8. Ask about current medications and related complications with their use. Cyclosporin may induce cholestasis (dose-dependent), hypertension, nephro-toxicity, gum hypertrophy, seizures (controlled by phenytoin, which itself induces cyclosporin metabolism) and central nervous system effects, including tremor and central pontine myelinolysis. Patients with a low serum cholesterol level are at increased risk of central nervous system toxicity. Steroids in high doses may induce a number of problems, including aseptic necrosis of long bones, cataracts and psychosis. Enquire about drug compliance.

9. Ask about the specific complications of immunosuppression. Systemic and local infections are frequent problems and can be rapidly fatal if not treated aggressively. Opportunistic infections include *Pneumocystis jirovecii* and *Candida albicans*. Cytomegalovirus infection remains a major problem. Try to find out tactfully whether there has been any problem with malignancy. The incidence of skin cancers and lymphomas (especially in the central nervous system) is increased with immunosuppression.

The examination

1. The pre-transplant patient should be examined for signs of chronic liver disease and complications of liver disease.

2. The post-transplant patient should be examined for liver tenderness (e.g. acute rejection) and jaundice (e.g. vanishing bile ducts in chronic rejection, biliary stricture). Examine the chest for infection and the mouth for candidiasis. The temperature must be taken (see Table 7.13). Examine the central nervous system (e.g. cyclosporin toxicity or cerebral infarction from perioperative hypotension or air embolism). Tap the spine for tenderness (e.g. vertebral collapse). Take the blood pressure (hypertension may occur at any time after transplantation; it is often caused by cyclosporin).

TABLE 7.13 Causes of fever in the outpatient with a liver transplant

Biliary tract (stricture and cholangitis)
Pneumonia (e.g. *Pneumocystis*, bacterial, fungal)
Urinary tract sepsis
Hepatitis (acute or recurrent)
Central nervous system infection (especially fungal)
Viral infection (e.g. cytomegalovirus, herpes, varicella-zoster)

Investigations

Pre-transplant patients need tests to confirm the diagnosis, determine current liver synthetic function (e.g. serum albumin, INR) and rule out contraindications. Ultrasound and CT scanning are routine. In patients with possible or definite malignancy, metastases must be sought. Assess bone density; osteopenia is common in liver disease and increases following transplant. Cardiopulmonary and psychiatric evaluation are important.

Management

Routine outpatient monitoring after transplantation should include a full blood count, electrolyte levels, renal and liver profile, and trough cyclosporin levels. Remember drug interactions with cyclosporin. Diabetes mellitus may supervene as a result of treatment with tacrolimus or steroids. Hypertension should be treated. Diseases that can recur in the graft include hepatitis B and C, Budd-Chiari syndrome and primary biliary cirrhosis.

Chapter 8

The haematological long case

> The modern haematologist, instead of describing in English what he can see, prefers to describe in Greek what he can't.
>
> *Richard Allan John Asher (1912–69)*

Haemolytic anaemia

This is an uncommon but important long case. It is usually a diagnostic problem. Coombs' positive haemolytic anaemia is most often encountered in the examination.

The history

1. Ask about the symptoms of anaemia (e.g. fatigue, shortness of breath on exertion) and whether the patient has noticed or been told about jaundice.
2. Determine whether there is a history of known haemolytic episodes. Onset at an early age or a family history suggests an intrinsic red cell defect (e.g. hereditary spherocytosis or elliptocytosis [both autosomal dominant], sickle cell anaemia).
3. Ask about symptoms of connective tissue disease. Joint pain or swelling may also occur in acute sickle cell crisis and especially affect the knees and elbows. Refractory leg ulcers occur in hereditary spherocytosis and sickle cell syndromes. Systemic lupus erythematosus (SLE) and other connective tissue disorders may be associated with warm antibody immunohaemolytic anaemia. Lymphoma is associated with both warm and cold antibodies and anaemia.
4. A history of pain in the abdomen, back and elsewhere suggests sickle cell anaemia or paroxysmal nocturnal haemoglobinuria. Congenital haemolytic anaemias can result in pigment gallstones that can cause symptomatic cholelithiasis and even acute cholecystitis; these episodes can be confused with acute crises.
5. Ask about neurological problems. Spinal cord lesions can occur with hereditary spherocytosis. Paraspinal masses (extramedullary haemopoiesis) may be seen in any hereditary haemolytic anaemia or lymphoma. Acute sickle cell crisis can also result in neurological impairment, particularly stroke. Tertiary syphilis may cause paroxysmal cold haemoglobinuria. In thrombotic thrombocytopenic purpura (TTP) there are often fluctuating neurological abnormalities. For other features of TTP, remember the mnemonic FAT RN:

> **F**ever
> **A**naemia (microangiopathic haemolytic)
> **T**hrombocytopenia
> **R**enal failure
> **N**eurological abnormalities

6. List all drugs that have been taken. For example, methyldopa, penicillin and quinidine can cause warm antibody immunohaemolytic anaemia, and anti-malarials, sulfonamides and nitrofurantoin cause haemolysis in subjects deficient in glucose-6-phosphate dehydrogenase (G6PD). *Note:* Between 10% and 20% of people taking methyldopa have a positive direct Coombs' test, but only a small minority of these develop haemolysis. The drug alters Rh antigens so that antibodies are produced against them, which then cross-react with normal Rh antigens. The indirect Coombs' test is therefore positive, even when the drug is not added to the test. The other drugs produce an indirect Coombs' test result only when the drug is added to the mixture, because in that case the antibodies are directed against a combination of drug and cell membrane. Fludarabine, which is increasingly used as second-line treatment of chronic lymphatic leukaemia and non-Hodgkin's lymphoma, may cause exacerbation of warm autoimmune haemolytic anaemia.

7. Enquire about any operations, particularly mechanical heart valve replacement (10% of those with aortic valve prostheses have significant haemolysis; this percentage is lower with mitral valve prostheses unless a paravalvular leak is present, as the pressure gradient is lower). Severe haemolysis in these patients suggests a paravalvular leak. Consider the other occasional cause of haemolysis within the circulation—external trauma, such as occurs in joggers who wear thin-soled shoes, and the traditional group, bongo drummers.

8. Determine the patient's ethnic background (e.g. Greeks or Italians may inherit the beta-thalassaemia trait; black men may have G6PD deficiency).

9. The patient may have an underlying medical problem associated with the risk of developing microvascular fragmentation of red cells. These conditions include: disseminated intravascular coagulation (DIC), which is usually caused by vessel wall changes related to an underlying disease, such as disseminated malignancy, renal graft rejection or malignant hypertension; TTP, which is of unknown aetiology; and haemolytic uraemic syndrome (HUS, with similar features to TTP), which can follow gastroenteritis caused by *E. coli 0157:H7* infection (do not treat these cases with an antibiotic, since this increases the risk of HUS!).

The examination

1. A careful haematopoietic system examination is required. The characteristic 'chipmunk' facies in a young person with thalassaemia is caused by maxillary marrow hyperplasia and frontal bossing.

2. Look for pallor and icterus.

3. Examine the heart for a valve prosthesis or severe aortic stenosis (traumatic haemolysis). Profound anaemia may be associated with high-output cardiac failure. An iron overload state in thalassaemia major from repeated transfusions may cause skin pigmentation, cardiac failure and hepatomegaly.

4. Carefully palpate for the spleen; splenomegaly from any cause (see Table 15.21) may result in haemolysis. Lymphadenopathy may indicate lymphoma (associated with warm or cold antibody haemolysis), chronic lymphocytic leukaemia or in practice glandular fever (cold agglutinin haemolysis).

5. Signs of chronic liver disease should be noted—in severe cirrhosis spur-cell (acanthocyte) anaemia is occasionally observed.

6. Examine for focal neurological signs. Look in the fundi—retinal detachment, retinal infarcts and vitreous haemorrhages can be manifestations of sickle cell anaemia; Kayser-Fleischer rings may be present in the cornea when haemolysis is caused by Wilson's disease.

7. Joint swelling and tenderness, and occasionally aseptic necrosis of bone (e.g. neck of femur), also occur in sickle cell anaemia; bony infarcts may become infected (e.g. *Salmonella* osteomyelitis).

8. Look for leg ulceration. Note any signs of connective tissue disease.
9. Test the urine—urobilinogen may be present with haemolysis; it may be dark from haemoglobin in intravascular haemolysis and the sediment may be abnormal (e.g. TTP).
10. Fever may occur with septicaemia or malaria-associated haemolysis, with acute crises in sickle cell anaemia and in TTP.

Investigations

It is important to confirm that haemolysis is present, exclude intravascular haemolysis and perform tests to determine the aetiology. The history and physical examination may have provided hints about the likely aetiology.

1. Ask for the results of a blood count, reticulocyte count, serum bilirubin and lactate dehydrogenase. Haemolysis is likely to be present if there is a normochromic normocytic anaemia with an increased reticulocyte count (but reticulocytosis also occurs with blood loss or partially treated anaemia) and release of red blood cell components (increased unconjugated bilirubin and, more variably, lactate dehydrogenase).
2. Usually serum haptoglobin is absent and haemosiderin is present in the urine. Intravascular haemolysis is documented by the presence of methaemalbumin in the plasma (Schumm's test) and, less often, of haemoglobin in the urine.
3. The presence of fragmented red cells (schistocytes) suggests valve haemolysis, DIC and TTP (or HUS). TTP (or HUS) is very likely when fragmented red cells occur in association with thrombocytopenia and normal coagulation studies; look for renal and neurological impairment.
4. The blood film usually shows polychromasia; it may show other red cell changes (see Tables 8.1 and 8.2). In thalassaemia, the anaemia is often hypochromic and microcytic.
5. If a congenital intracorpuscular defect seems unlikely, ask for a Coombs' test to determine whether the anaemia is immunohaemolytic. The polyspecific direct Coombs' test measures the ability of anti-IgG and anti-C3 to agglutinate the patient's red blood cells. Warm antibodies (80% of cases) react at body temperature and may occur with lymphoma (usually non-Hodgkin's), chronic lymphocytic leukaemia, solid tumours (lung, colon, kidney and ovary), SLE and drugs, or may be idiopathic. They are usually IgG antibodies directed at the Rh antigens. Cold reactive antibodies are precipitated by exposure to room temperature ('cold')—cold agglutinin disease (IgM antibodies) may occur acutely with glandular fever, mycoplasma infection or hepatitis C, and chronically may be caused by lymphoma or may be idiopathic; paroxysmal cold haemoglobinuria (IgG antibodies) is rare.
6. If the haemoglobinuria occurs usually at night and there is pancytopenia and venous thrombosis, paroxysmal nocturnal haemoglobinuria (PNH) should be strongly suspected (an acquired stem cell disease secondary to a defective *PIG-A* gene). The disease may also complicate recovery from aplastic anaemia, in which the neutrophil alkaline phosphatase score is low (but this test is now rarely performed). The sucrose lysis and acid haemolysis (Ham's) test used to be performed. The most reliable test now is analysis by flow cytometry for glycosylphosphatidylinositol (GPI)-linked proteins (e.g. *CD55* or decay-accelerating factors [DAF] on the red cell surface, and *CD59* or homologous restriction factor). PNH, which is an acquired clonal disease, is a result of a mutation that causes faulty or absent production of the GPI anchor molecule. Various linked proteins are missing from the red cell surface and, as a result, the cells are not protected from lysis by complement.

   Tests for other causes of haemolysis are presented in Table 8.2.

TABLE 8.1 Full blood count and liver function tests from a female patient with autoimmune haemolytic anaemia

Parameter	Value	Normal range
Haemoglobin	63 g/L	115–165 g/L (female)
Mean corpuscular volume (MCV)	100 fL	80–100 fL
White cell count (WCC)	15.0×10^9/L	$4.5–13.5 \times 10^9$/L
Platelet count	350×10^9/L	$150–400 \times 10^9$/L
Erythrocyte sedimentation rate (ESR)	58 mm/h	3–19 mm/h (female <50 years)
Reticulocyte count	18%	0.2–2.0% of red cell count
Bilirubin (total)	45 mmol/L	<20 mmol/L
Aspartate aminotransferase (AST)	30 U/L	<45 U/L
Alanine aminotransferase (ALT)	40 U/L	<40 U/L
Lactate dehydrogenase (LDH)	451 U/L	110–230 U/L
Protein (total)	72 g/L	62–80 g/L
Albumin	42 g/L	32–45 g/L
Haptoglobin	< 0.2 g/L	0.3–2.0 g/L

- *Blood film:* moderate anisocytosis, numerous spherocytes, prominent polychromasia. Nucleated red cells, neutrophilia and band forms.
- *Direct Coombs' test positive:* reaction grade 8–12.

Comment

The patient has a severe normochromic anaemia with marked reticulocytosis. The very high reticulocyte count suggests haemolysis rather than blood loss. The polychromasia, nucleated red cells and reticulocytosis are signs of increased marrow erythroid activity. The raised bilirubin and reduced haptoglobin levels are consistent with haemolysis. The classical triad suggesting haemolysis is a raised LDH level, reduced haptoglobin level and unconjugated hyperbilirubinaemia. The presence of spherocytes suggests hereditary spherocytosis or immune haemolysis. If there were fragmented red cells, mechanical haemolysis or microangiopathic haemolysis would be likely. Normal red cell morphology would suggest hypersplenism or paroxysmal nocturnal haemoglobinuria. The presence of 'bite' cells would suggest G6PD deficiency.

In this case the candidate should ask for a Coombs' test to distinguish autoimmune haemolytic anaemia from hereditary spherocytosis.

Treatment

This depends on the underlying disease process, which should be reversed if possible (e.g. drug withdrawal, treatment of transplant rejection, adoption of another musical instrument) (see Table 8.2).

1. Steroids are useful in immunohaemolytic anaemia caused by warm-reactive antibodies. The usual approach is to commence at a starting dose of 1 mg/kg/day of prednisolone. The haemoglobin level will usually rise within the first week. Concurrent use of folate is often recommended. Once a normal haemoglobin level has been achieved, the steroid dose must be tapered slowly. Splenectomy works as well as steroids, and is indicated in poorly responsive or resistant disease. Immunosuppressive treatment is reserved for those who do not respond to steroids and splenectomy. Azathioprine and cyclophosphamide have each been used with some benefit. Response takes two to three months. Normal human immunoglobulin is occasionally effective.

2. Transfusion is not usually indicated unless there is symptomatic anaemia with a haemoglobin level <90 g/L; it may exacerbate haemolysis. The antibody in

TABLE 8.2 Haemolytic anaemia

Classification	Peripheral blood morphology	Diagnostic test	Treatment
Extracorpuscular			
1. Immune haemolysis (a) 'Warm' antibody (i) autoimmune (lymphoma, connective tissue disease, idiopathic) (ii) drug-induced	Spherocytes	Coombs' (antiglobulin) test; differential Coombs' test (IgG, complement)	Clinically significant haemolysis—steroids; if steroids not tolerated or do not control disease—splenectomy; if still refractory—azathioprine, cyclophosphamide or danazol Discontinue drugs
(b) 'Cold' antibody (i) cold agglutinin (post-infection, lymphoma, idiopathic)	Red cell agglutination in cold	Cold agglutinins Coombs' test—C3 on red cell surface Anti-I (e.g. mycoplasma) or anti-i (e.g. glandular fever)	Maintain warm environment; immunosuppressives only if severe disease
2. Mechanical haemolysis (a) Microangiopathic (DIC, TTP, vasculitis etc.)	Schizocytes, microspherocytes	Evidence of intravascular haemolysis, evidence of underlying disease state	TTP: plasmapheresis DIC: treat the underlying cause
(b) Heart valve			Correct iron deficiency; replace valve if indicated
(c) March haemoglobinuria (e.g. marathon runners)			Avoid marathons
3. Infection (a) Septicaemia (b) Parasitic (e.g. malaria)	Spherocytes, fragments, intraerythrocyte parasites	Blood cultures, thin and thick smears	Treat infection
4. Acquired membrane abnormalities (a) Cirrhosis	Spur-cells (acanthocytes)	Liver function tests	Splenectomy if severe haemolysis

(Continues)

TABLE 8.2 Haemolytic anaemia (Continued)

Classification	Peripheral blood morphology	Diagnostic test	Treatment
Extracorpuscular (Continued)			
(b) Uraemia	Burr cells (echinocytes)	Renal function tests	Treat renal failure Correct iron deficiency
(c) Paroxysmal nocturnal haemoglobinuria	Spherocytes, microcytes	Flow cytometry (CD55, CD59)	Steroid or androgen therapy may reduce haemolysis; transfuse with washed red cells
Intracorpuscular			
1. Haemoglobinopathies (a) Amino acid substitutions (e.g. sickle cell)	Sickle forms, hypochromic	Sickle preparation, Hb electrophoresis	Detect infection early and treat, maintain adequate folic acid levels, acute crises—analgesia, oxygen if hypoxic, erythrocyte exchange (for priapism, stroke, acute chest syndrome)
(b) Thalassaemias—beta-thalassaemia, alpha-thalassaemia	Microcytic, target cells, tear drops	HbA$_2$ and HbF levels, globin synthesis study, gene mapping, family study of HbS	Beta-thalassaemia major—supportive: transfusion, iron chelating therapy
(c) HbH disease: inherited or acquired (myeloproliferative, myelodysplastic)	Heinz bodies on incubation	Hb electrophoresis, brilliant cresyl blue preparation	Folic acid, avoid oxidant drugs, treat underlying disease, bone marrow transplant
2. Inherited membrane abnormalities (e.g. spherocytosis)	Spherocytes	Osmotic fragility (increased), red cell membrane protein study	Splenectomy corrects the anaemia
3. Metabolic abnormalities (e.g. G6PD deficiency)	'Bite' cells, spherocytes	G6PD assay, G6PD electrophoresis	Prevent haemolytic episodes (avoid oxidant drugs, broad beans)

DAF = decay accelerating factors; DIC = disseminated intravascular coagulation; G6PD = glucose-6-phosphate dehydrogenase; Hb = haemoglobin; HbH = haemoglobin H; TTP = thrombotic thrombocytopenic purpura.

immunohaemolytic anaemia is likely to react with all normal donor cells so that standard cross-matching is not possible.

3. When cold-reactive antibodies are responsible, steroid treatment is less effective. Avoidance of cold can be helpful. The disease tends to progress unless the underlying malignancy can be treated.

4. The chimeric antibody, rituximab, which attaches to the CD20 binding site on B lymphocytes and induces their destruction, may be useful in severe cases of resistant autoimmune haemolytic anaemia.

5. The acute haemolytic episodes of patients with G6PD deficiency are self-limiting (only older red blood cells are affected) and require no specific treatment. Hydration should be maintained to protect renal function. Patients should be warned to avoid precipitating factors (e.g. broad beans, antimalarials and sulfonamides).

6. Valve haemolysis may be improved by iron supplements and an increase in haemoglobin (reduced cardiac output). Paravalvular leaks often need to be repaired and occasionally the prosthetic valve may have to be replaced with a larger one.

7. TTP is now treated with plasmapheresis, which improves the mortality rate from almost 100% to 10%. Twice-daily treatment is combined at first with high-dose steroids. Even severe neurological deficit, including coma, may be reversible. Anti-platelet drugs are of uncertain benefit. Cyclophosphamide and vincristine are used when plasmapheresis has been unsuccessful. Relapse (10%) can usually be treated successfully. Platelet transfusions must be avoided as they exacerbate thrombosis. The preferred replacement solution is cryosupernatent or fresh frozen plasma (FFP).

8. Splenectomy is virtually curative for patients with hereditary spherocytosis and elliptocytosis (only 10% have severe haemolysis), and may be useful in selected patients with massive splenomegaly, immunohaemolytic anaemia, certain haemoglobinopathies and enzymopathies. All patients undergoing splenectomy should receive pneumococcal vaccine preoperatively if possible. Sometimes, prophylactic treatment with penicillin is recommended for two years following splenectomy (see Table 8.3). Failure of splenectomy to control haemolysis may be caused by an accessory spleen (which can be detected by a liver–spleen scan).

9. PNH can be treated with washed red cell transfusions and steroids. Heparin and warfarin should be used for thrombotic episodes. Bone marrow transplant may be curative. Trials of the monoclonal antibody eculizimab, which blocks the complement cascade below C5, have been very encouraging; the drug prevents the complement-driven haemolysis in PNH.

TABLE 8.3 Treatment advice for patients having a splenectomy

1. Vaccinate for pneumococcus, *Haemophilus influenzae* type B, group C meningococcus and influenza two to three weeks before splenectomy if possible.

2. Consider continuous prophylactic penicillin V 250 mg b.d.

3. Patients should wear an alert bracelet. Overwhelming sepsis may present as obtundation and antibiotics should be given immediately.

4. Animal bites should be treated aggressively with local disinfection and systemic antibiotics.

5. Patients with possible septicaemia should have antibiotics to cover encapsulated organisms (pneumococcus, meningococcus and *Haemophilus influenzae*).

Thrombophilia

The discovery of new thrombophilic factors has made the patient with recurrent or even a single thrombotic episode a very suitable long case. Suspect this possibility if the patient is under 50 or has a family history of recurrent thromboses (see Table 8.4).

TABLE 8.4 Occurrence of, and risk associated with, the thrombophilic factors

	Deep venous thrombosis	Normal population	Relative risk	Arterial thrombosis
APC resistance	50%	4%	8 times	–
Antiphospholipid antibodies	Common	Sometimes— at low titre	8 times	+
AT III, protein, C & S	10%	1%	20 times	–
Prothrombin gene mutation	15%	3%	4 times	–
High homocysteine	15%	5%	3 times	+
Factor V Leiden	20%	3–7%	5–10 times	–
APC = activated protein C; AT = antithrombin.				

The history

1. Ask about the reason for the patient's current admission to hospital. There may have been a recent episode of venous or arterial thrombosis or the patient may have been admitted to hospital for a procedure that has a high risk of thrombosis.
2. Ask about the nature of thrombotic episodes. These may have been arterial or venous, or both. Find out how often the problem has occurred and what part of the body was involved.
3. Ask whether a thrombotic tendency has been identified and how this was done (the patient may know).
4. Ask what anticoagulation therapy is currently being used. The possibilities include intravenous unfractionated heparin, fractionated heparin given sub-cutaneously, low-molecular-weight heparin, warfarin, aspirin or (less likely) clopidogrel or dipyridamole.
5. If the patient is or has been on treatment with warfarin, find out how much he or she understands about the drug, including the importance and necessary frequency of international normalised ratio (INR) testing and the target INR. The patient should probably know the most recent INR result and have some understanding of food and drug interactions with warfarin. For a patient on warfarin, ask about the usual frequency of blood tests and whether practical difficulties have been encountered in getting to the pathology laboratory. Ask who usually relays INR results and dose changes to the patient, and whether the patient has ever used a home INR tester.
6. Enquire about a family history of thrombosis and whether the patient's own problem has led to the testing of other family members. In general, 50% of first-degree relatives will inherit the mutation if there is an identified autosomal dominant hereditary factor (e.g. protein C, protein S and antithrombin deficiency). Remember, a family history of thrombosis greatly increases a patient's risk. Patients with a thrombophilic defect, but without a family history of thrombosis, have only a slightly increased risk. The absence of a family history may make thrombophilia testing irrelevant, as positive tests will not likely change management.
7. Ask about other factors that may increase thrombotic risk, including smoking, oestrogen-containing oral contraceptives, pregnancy, malignancy, recent surgery and immobility. Long-aeroplane flights are controversial as a risk factor but have received extensive discussion in the popular press.

8. If the event has followed a surgical operation, ask what prophylaxis was used to try to prevent thrombosis.

9. In women, ask about previous unexplained miscarriages. This can be associated with the presence of antiphospholipid antibodies, which are autoantibodies against various platelet surface molecules, including phospholipids. These include lupus anticoagulant (which prolongs the aPTT), anticardiolipin and anti-β_2 glycoprotein antibodies. Consider this possibility too if there is a history of unusual thromboses or eclampsia and preeclampsia.

10. Specifically ask about previous myocardial infarction. The occurrence of myocardial infarction in young women with normal coronary arteries has been associated with factor V Leiden mutation.

11. Ask whether there have been chronic venous problems in the legs. Damage to the venous system can cause chronic oedema and ulceration that can be quite disabling. If there have been chronic problems, asking detailed questions about their effect on the patient's life is essential.

12. Ask about the congenital abnormality, homocysteinuria, which is associated with a Marfanoid habitus and premature strokes and coronary artery disease. Homocysteine is a thrombophilic agent.

13. Ask about features of PNH—recurrent episodes of dark urine, anaemia and pancytopenia.

The examination

1. Note the presence or absence of an intravenous heparin infusion. If present, look at the infusion rate.

2. Note the presence of obesity and look for signs of venous insufficiency from previous venous thromboses.

3. Examine the legs for oedema, venous ulceration and venous valvular insufficiency.

4. Check the peripheral pulses for evidence of arterial obstruction.

5. Note the presence of abdominal wall bruising from subcutaneous low-molecular-weight heparin injections.

6. There may be evidence of a myeloproliferative disorder, SLE or a malignancy.

Investigations

There is a case now for testing anyone with a significant arterial or venous thrombosis for thrombophilic factors (see Tables 8.4 and 8.5), especially those with a family history of thromboembolic disease. Certainly, unusual or repeated thromboses should be investigated, as set out below. The currently available routine screening tests are listed in Table 8.6.

TABLE 8.5 Indications for thrombophilia investigations
1. Recurrent venous thromboses
2. Venous thrombosis before the age of 45

3. Thrombosis at an unusual site:
  • portal vein
  • cavernous sinus
  • hepatic vein

4. Adverse family history of venous thrombosis

TABLE 8.6 Tests for thrombophilia
Full blood count and ESR (and tests for myeloproliferative disorders and possibly malignancy)
Factor V Leiden (APC resistance)
Antiphospholipid antibodies, including lupus anticoagulant
Antithrombin III
Protein C and S (off warfarin for two weeks)
Prothrombin gene mutation
Plasma homocysteine

1. **Factor V Leiden** is an abnormal factor V molecule. The abnormality is caused by a point mutation that affects the cleavage site on the activated molecule. The abnormal factor V is resistant to neutralisation by activated protein C (APC), which forms part of the natural anticoagulation pathway. The condition is also called APC resistance. The mutation occurs in 4% of the general population in Australia and in up to 50% of people with a family history of recurrent venous thrombosis. The condition is autosomal dominant. The heterozygous state is associated with an eightfold increase in venous thrombotic risk; the homozygous state also occurs and these people have 100 times the average risk.

   The thrombotic risk is higher for women with this condition because of the additional risk associated with pregnancy and the use of oral contraceptives containing oestrogen. Use of these drugs causes a 35 times increased risk of a thrombotic event (approximately a 3% risk over 10 years). The mechanism is probably that of lowering antithrombin III levels.

2. **Antithrombin III deficiency** is present in a mild form in about 1 in 2000 of the population. The thrombotic risk is somewhat unpredictable, but the occurrence of a first thrombotic event in these patients is a relative indication for lifelong anticoagulation therapy with warfarin.

3. **Proteins C and S** are natural anticoagulants. Their deficiency is associated with recurrent venous thrombosis and pulmonary embolism, but the level of increased risk is less clear than that for the abnormalities above. There is overlap between the serum levels in people with, and apparently without, an increased risk of thrombosis. Testing must occur after at least two weeks without warfarin treatment. In homozygotes with protein C deficiency, warfarin may induce skin necrosis.

4. **Prothrombin gene mutation** is present in about 3% of the Australian population. This point mutation leads to an increased plasma level of prothrombin. Its detection requires DNA PCR analysis. It is an autosomal dominant trait and leads to a fourfold increase in the risk of venous thrombosis.

5. Homocysteine levels are increased in patients with venous thrombosis and are also an independent risk factor for coronary artery disease. The test is now widely available.

6. Combined thrombophilic abnormalities are relatively common and further increase the thrombotic risk.

7. **Antiphospholipid syndrome** is diagnosed if there is clinical evidence of thrombosis or a suggestive history of miscarriage plus an abnormal test on two occasions. *Anticardiolipin* antibodies and *lupus anticoagulant (IgG or IgM antiphospholipid)* antibodies are associated with an increased risk of venous thrombus and arterial embolus. In most cases, both are abnormal. The transient presence of these antibodies at low titres is common, is often associated with infection and is probably not of clinical significance. They may be present as part of SLE or occur alone (primary antiphospholipid syndrome).

8. Consider investigations for other illnesses that are 'prothrombotic'. These include malignancy, cardiac failure and haematological conditions such as PNH, polycythaemia rubra vera and thrombocythaemia.

Management

Try to identify transient and continuing risk factors.

1. In general, an initial episode of thrombosis is treated in the usual way, with low-molecular-weight heparin or intravenous non-fractionated heparin. This should be followed by at least six months of treatment with warfarin for idiopathic above-knee DVTs or for pulmonary embolism. Patients with antithrombin III deficiency will still respond to treatment with heparin because of the presence of small amounts of antithrombin III. Tests for the vitamin K-dependent proteins C and S should be performed before the patient is begun on warfarin.

2. Patients with protein C and S deficiency or heterozygous APC resistance do not need long-term anticoagulation until after their second thrombotic event. Homozygous APC deficiency is an indication for long-term warfarin treatment.

3. All patients with thrombophilia and their affected asymptomatic relatives need aggressive prophylaxis before surgery or during periods of immobilisation, such as long aeroplane flights. Surgical prophylactic treatment should include heparin, compressive stockings and foot pumps, and early mobilisation. Long aeroplane flights may be an indication for prophylactic subcutaneous fractionated heparin. Aspirin is of unproven benefit for the prevention of venous thrombosis.

4. Pregnant women with a history of DVT require prophylaxis (with heparin) throughout pregnancy and until the puerperium. Warfarin is contraindicated in pregnancy.

5. The detection of antiphospholipid antibodies in women with miscarriages is an indication for treatment with low-molecular-weight heparin with or without low-dose aspirin during pregnancy. Patients should be advised strongly against smoking and should avoid oestrogen-containing oral contraceptives. Progesterone-only preparations appear to be safe.

6. There is still controversy about the long-term treatment of patients with antiphospholipid syndrome and their relatives, but recurrent unexpected thrombosis may be an indication for long-term anticoagulation with warfarin maintaining a high INR (3.5). Remember that treatment with warfarin involves a 1–2% risk annual risk of serious bleeding. Relatives should be tested for the appropriate defect and offered prophylaxis, if affected.

Polycythaemia

The myeloproliferative disorders (see Table 8.7) often occur in the clinical examination. They present a diagnostic and management problem. Polycythaemia rubra vera (erythraemia or increased red cell mass) is the most common myeloproliferative disease encountered. This disease occurs in later middle life and is slightly more common in males. No specific gene defect has been isolated, but the condition is a clonal disease. Secondary causes of polycythaemia (erythrocytosis) must be excluded.

TABLE 8.7 Myeloproliferative disorders
1. Polycythaemia rubra vera
2. Myelofibrosis
3. Essential thrombocythaemia
4. Chronic myeloid leukaemia

The history

The patient will probably know the diagnosis. If you suspect polycythaemia, ask about:

1. symptoms of polycythaemia or polycythaemia rubra vera:
   (a) vascular problems, such as transient ischaemic episodes, angina, peripheral vascular disease (thrombosis and digital ischaemia); intra-abdominal venous thrombosis, including the Budd-Chiari syndrome
   (b) bleeding from the nose
   (c) symptoms of peptic ulceration (increased four to five times in polycythaemia rubra vera)
   (d) abdominal pain or discomfort from gross splenomegaly or urate stones
   (e) pruritus after showering ('aquagenic pruritis')
   (f) gout
2. symptoms owing to disease causing secondary polycythaemia (see Table 8.8), such as chronic respiratory diseases, chronic cardiac or congenital heart diseases, renal diseases (especially polycystic kidneys, hydronephrosis or carcinoma); ask about the use of coal tar derivatives, which can cause the production of abnormal haemoglobin such as methaemoglobin, since secondary polycythaemia may occur as a result
3. investigations performed and how the diagnosis was made (e.g. blood counts abdominal imaging, and renal, pulmonary and cardiac investigations); the patient may know if the erythropoietin level has been measured
4. the treatment initiated (e.g. phlebotomy [how often and for how long], radioactive phosphorus, treatment of renal, pulmonary or cardiac disease)
5. resolution of symptoms with treatment
6. social problems related to chronic disease.

The examination

1. Stand back and look at the patient. Note plethora, the state of hydration, cyanosis and any cushingoid features.
2. Examine the patient's hands for nicotine stains, clubbing and signs of peripheral vascular disease. Note any gouty tophi.
3. Look for scratch marks and bruising on the arms and take the blood pressure (systolic hypertension accompanies an increased red cell mass and phaeochromocytoma is associated with increased erythropoietin).
4. Look at the eyes for injected conjunctivae and examine the fundi for hyper-viscosity changes.
5. Examine the tongue for central cyanosis.
6. Examine the cardiovascular system for signs of cyanotic congenital heart disease, if appropriate, and the respiratory system for signs of chronic lung disease.
7. Examine the abdomen for hepatomegaly (hepatoma must be excluded) and more importantly splenomegaly, which occurs in 80% of cases of polycythaemia rubra vera, but not in secondary polycythaemia. Palpate for renal masses (polycystic kidneys, hydronephrosis, carcinoma). Rarely, uterine fibromas may be found, or very rarely virilisation may be noted.
8. Look at the legs for scratch marks (pruritus may be secondary to elevated plasma histamine levels), gout and evidence of peripheral vascular disease.
9. Auscultate over the cerebellar regions for a bruit (cerebellar haemangio-blastoma). Note any upper motor neurone signs (cerebrovascular disease owing to thrombosis or the hyperviscosity syndrome).
10. Check the urine for evidence of renal disease.

TABLE 8.8 Causes of polycythaemia

Absolute polycythaemia (increased red cell mass)

1. Primary—polycythaemia rubra vera

2. Secondary polycythaemia

   (a) increased erythropoietin:

      (i) renal disease (e.g. polycystic disease, hydronephrosis, tumour)

      (ii) hepatoma

      (iii) cerebellar haemangioma

      (iv) uterine myoma

      (v) virilising syndromes

      (vi) Cushing's syndrome

      (vii) phaeochromocytoma

      (viii) self-injection of erythropoietin (e.g. athletes)

   (b) hypoxic states (erythropoietin secondarily increased):

      (i) chronic lung disease

      (ii) hereditary haemorrhagic telangiectasia (because of pulmonary arteriovenous malformations)

      (iii) sleep apnoea

      (iv) cyanotic congenital heart disease

      (v) abnormal haemoglobins (high-affinity variants)

      (vi) carbon monoxide poisoning

Relative polycythaemia (decreased plasma volume)

1. Dehydration

2. Smokers' polycythaemia—carboxyhaemoglobinaemia (erythrocyte mass also increased)

3. Stress polycythaemia—Gaisbock's disease (? a distinct entity)

Investigations

Confirm the presence of polycythaemia (haematocrit >60% for men or >56% for women) and establish whether this is primary or secondary. Remember that erythrocytosis is an increase in the absolute red cell mass, which occurs as a result of some stimulus (usually hypoxia), and erythraemia (polycythaemia vera) is an increase in red cell mass of unknown aetiology (see Table 8.9).

Note: Red cell mass and plasma volume are no longer routinely measured.

TABLE 8.9 An approach to the diagnosis of polycythaemia rubra vera

1. *JAK2* mutation present (up to 95% of cases)

2. Splenomegaly

3. Normal PaO_2

4. Splenomegaly, or leucocytosis and thrombocytosis

5. Low or normal erythropoietin level

6. Rule out secondary causes (e.g. smoking, chronic lung disease, tumours)

1. In polycythaemia rubra vera the following are increased: haemoglobin value, haematocrit value, red cell count, white cell count (including the absolute basophil count), platelet count and more variably the neutrophil alkaline phosphatase (NAP) score. Check the mean corpuscular volume and red cell distribution width (RDW). Microcytic erythrocytosis can only be caused by polycythaemia rubra vera or hypoxic erythrocytosis (RDW usually elevated), or beta-thalassaemia (RDW normal).
2. The ESR is very low in both primary and secondary polycythaemia.
3. Assess for splenomegaly (and renal disease) with an abdominal ultrasound or CT scan.
4. Check the arterial blood gases (in polycythaemia rubra vera, 80% of patients have an arterial oxygen saturation >92% and in almost all it is >88%).
5. Serum erythropoietin level is usually substantially reduced or absent in polycythaemia rubra vera and elevated in secondary polycythaemia. Remember, however, that certain tumours (haemangioblastoma, renal cell carcinoma, renal sarcoma and carcinoma of the liver) cause polycythaemia by excreting erythropoietin.
6. The total vitamin B_{12} level is elevated in 75% of cases of polycythaemia rubra vera. The vitamin B_{12} level is raised owing to increased transcobalamin I and III, made by neutrophils, which have an increased turnover.
7. Rule out renal disease with abdominal ultrasound and CT scanning, if indicated.
8. In polycythaemia rubra vera there is significant panhyperplasia and iron stores are often reduced, but in secondary polycythaemia the bone marrow is usually normal. There are no consistent cytogenetic markers. Bone marrow biopsy is not essential for the diagnosis: it is only necessary if another myeloproliferative disorder is suspected. Fibrosis may be seen in the advanced stages of polycythaemia rubra vera.
9. Genetic testing is very useful. The *JAK2* mutation is present in most patients with polycythaemia rubra vera.

Treatment

1. The aim is to lower the haematocrit value to 0.42–0.45 (haemoglobin <140 g/L for men and <120 g/L for women) and maintain it at this level. Patients may die of thrombosis, which seems related entirely to the elevated red cell mass. The presence of thrombocytosis does not increase the risk of thrombotic events, and anticoagulation is not indicated. Thrombotic risk can usually be controlled with phlebotomy alone. Untreated cases have a median survival of two years because of the thrombotic risk. This is extended to more than 10 years with phlebotomy alone.
2. Polycythaemia rubra vera should be treated by phlebotomy. Frequent venesection is required until a state of iron deficiency has been produced. This will then limit red cell production and the frequency may be reduced to about three monthly.
3. Radioactive phosphorus (phosphorus-32) irradiates the bone marrow and is easy to use and effective, but it increases the incidence of acute myeloid leukaemia and should be avoided in patients under the age of 70 years (and perhaps in all patients). Alkylating agents (e.g. busulfan) must be monitored closely for the same reason and should not be given routinely. Hydroxyurea is a much safer drug in these circumstances.
4. Pruritus may not respond to antihistamines, and interferon alpha (IFNα) or PUVA therapy (combination drugs and ultraviolet light) may be required.
5. Hyperuricaemia should be treated with allopurinol.
6. Low-dose aspirin is recommended to prevent thrombosis in patients without excessive gastrointestinal bleeding (avoid high doses).

7. Secondary polycythaemia is treated by removal of the cause, and phlebotomy if the haematocrit exceeds 0.55.
8. Interferon alpha may help with the problem of symptomatic splenomegaly.

Idiopathic myelofibrosis

This is a rare form of chronic myeloproliferative clonal disorder. Patients are often asymptomatic at the time of diagnosis. The condition is frequently diagnosed following a routine full blood count or the discovery of splenomegaly. Myelofibrosis may also be the result of a number of malignant and non-malignant conditions (see Table 8.10).

Median survival is four to five years, but patients with severe anaemia (<100 g/L) have a worse prognosis (median survival about two years).

TABLE 8.10 Causes of myelofibrosis	
Non-malignant	**Malignant**
1. SLE	1. CML
2. HIV infection	2. Acute leukaemia
3. Renal osteodystrophy	3. Lymphoma
4. Tuberculosis	4. Multiple myeloma
5. Hyperparathyroidism	5. Metastatic carcinoma

Findings and investigations

1. Occasionally, there may be signs of aggressive extramedullary haematopoiesis: bowel or urethral obstruction, ascites, pericardial effusion, skin masses or spinal cord compression. Rapid splenic enlargement can cause splenic infarction (with the sudden onset of left upper quadrant pain and tenderness). The typical patient is over 50 years of age and has marked splenomegaly (>10 cm) and mild-to-moderate hepatomegaly.
2. The white cell counts may be normal, increased or decreased. The blood film will show teardrop poikilocytes and a leucoerythroblastic picture (presence of myelocytes, metamyelocytes and nucleated red blood cells). Any process that infiltrates the bone marrow may cause this picture (e.g. malignancy, TB, fungi).
3. Bone marrow biopsy (aspiration is usually impossible) may reveal karyotypic abnormalities on cytogenetic examination. This finding is associated with a worse prognosis.
4. The condition must be distinguished from myelofibrosis secondary to other conditions, such as lymphoma, leukaemia, myeloma, polycythaemia, chronic myeloid leukaemia (CML) and SLE. These may be amenable to specific treatment.

Treatment

Treatment is primarily supportive. Most patients are treated with repeated blood transfusions.

1. Hydroxyurea is helpful for symptomatic patients with organomegaly or marked thrombocytosis.
2. Folate and vitamin B_{12} may help if they are deficient; erythropoietin has not been particularly effective. Allopurinol is used when there is hyperuricaemia.
3. Splenectomy may be indicated if massive splenomegaly has occurred.
4. Alkylating agents are contraindicated.
5. Cure is possible only with allogenic bone marrow transplantation for the few patients who are young enough and for whom a suitable donor can be found.
6. Leukaemic transformation may occur in 10% of patients.

Essential thrombocythaemia

This is a relatively common form of chronic myeloproliferative clonal disorder. Many patients are asymptomatic and the diagnosis is made on a routine platelet count.

Patients usually present with symptoms related to a high platelet count ($>800^3 \times 10^9$/L)—especially thromboembolism, but also poor memory, erythromelalgia (painful red extremities) and migraine. Up to 50% of patients have haemorrhagic problems, especially from the gut, and easy bruising. A prolonged bleeding time and abnormal platelet aggregation may be present. An acquired deficiency of von Willebrand factor may occur when platelet numbers are very high; the large von Willebrand multimers are destroyed by the platelets. There are, however, no consistent platelet abnormalities.

Modest splenomegaly (<5 cm) is seen in 50% of patients.

Investigations

1. A definitive diagnosis requires exclusion of reactive thrombocytosis secondary to infection, polycythaemia, malignancy, inflammation, bleeding, recent surgery or an asplenic state.
2. Cytogenetic studies may be necessary to exclude CML (Philadelphia chromosome t(9;22) or its products: *BCR-ABL* fusion mRNA or *BCR-ABL* protein).

Treatment

1. Asymptomatic patients, even if they have a platelet count of more than one million, often need no treatment. Unexpectedly, bleeding tends to be more of a problem when the platelet count is over one million and thrombosis when it is less than one million.
2. Neurological symptoms and erythromelalgia should first be treated with aspirin. Failure of response is an indication to reduce platelet numbers, usually with hydroxyurea or interferon (IFNα). Anagrelide is a more specific anti-megakaryocyte agent that can be useful for symptomatic patients.
3. Bleeding problems may be improved with tranexamic acid; this may be useful if given before surgery.
4. Transformation to acute leukaemia is uncommon (<10%) and often the result of prior alkylating chemotherapy.
5. The condition usually runs an indolent and benign course and the continuing temptation to treat asymptomatic patients should be strongly resisted.

Chronic myeloid leukaemia

Some patients with CML are diagnosed from routine blood tests—symptoms tend not to be specific (see Table 8.11).

Investigations

1. The typical patient has moderate splenomegaly (6–8 cm) and a white cell count $>50 \times 10^9$/L. The white cell differential count will show two peaks, one at the neutrophil stage and the other at the myelocyte stage.
2. Basophilia is common.
3. A low NAP score is another typical laboratory feature. The blast phase has over 20% blasts.
4. Diagnosis depends on finding the Philadelphia (Ph) chromosome (>90%)—a shortened chromosome 22. Translocation of part of chromosome 22 to chromosome 9 results in a hybrid gene *BCR/ABL* rearrangement on chromosome 9.
5. The platelet count is usually elevated and there is mild normochromic anaemia.
6. There is no association with alkylating agents and no evidence of a viral cause.

TABLE 8.11 CML symptoms
Symptoms at presentation
1. Fatigue
2. Malaise
3. Loss of weight
4. Abdominal discomfort and fullness from splenomegaly
5. Infection
6. Thrombotic episodes (e.g. stroke, myocardial infarction, venous thrombosis)
Symptoms of progression of disease
1. Fever
2. Infections
3. Bone pain
4. Joint pain
5. Haemorrhage or thrombosis

Treatment

Untreated, the disease will eventually undergo blastic transformation.

1. A cure or long-term remission can be achieved with allogenic bone marrow transplantation from a compatible donor.
2. Imatinib (a tyrosine kinase inhibitor) has revolutionised treatment of CML. This drug causes aptosis of cells expressing *BCR/ABL*. It is now the first-line treatment for younger patients without a suitable donor and for older patients (>65 years). It may be an option even for patients who are suitable for bone marrow transplant. Its use can be associated with hepatotoxicity, myalgia and fluid retention.
3. Interferon alpha therapy is sometimes helpful in the chronic phase. It may induce differentiation of the immature cells.

Lymphomas

These diseases provide complicated diagnostic and management problems. Treatment in expert units is important, because many patients can be cured. Cure should be possible in more than 85% of patients with Hodgkin's disease and in up to 40% of those with non-Hodgkin's lymphomas.

Remember that the cell lineage is uncertain for Hodgkin's disease (although probably mostly B cell), but 80% of non-Hodgkin's lymphomas are of B cell origin. There are a number of slightly different classification systems. Some are based on the cell type (see Table 8.12), some are histopathological (see Table 8.13) and others are clinical staging (see Table 8.14).

Hodgkin's disease (see Table 8.13) presents either with discrete, rubbery, painless nodes or with generalised symptoms (fever, night sweats, weight loss and sometimes pruritus). Mediastinal adenopathy usually occurs in young people with nodular sclerosing disease. Older people with generalised symptoms, in whom the only enlarged nodes may be in the abdomen, often have lymphocyte-depleted Hodgkin's disease.

The majority of cases of non-Hodgkin's lymphomas (see Table 8.13) present with painless enlargement of peripheral lymph nodes (a lymph node of >1 cm diameter that has been present for six weeks or more for no obvious reason should be biopsied). The great majority of patients with peripheral lymph node enlargement do not

TABLE 8.12 World Health Organization (WHO) classification of lymphomas (lymphoid malignancies)—more common types

B cell	T cell	Hodgkin's disease
Precursor B cell neoplasm	**Precursor T cell neoplasm**	Nodular lymphocyte predominant
Precursor B cell lymphoblastic leukaemia/lymphoma	Precursor T cell lymphoblastic lymphoma/leukaemia	**Classic Hodgkin's disease**
Mature (peripheral) B cell neoplasms	**Mature (peripheral) T cell neoplasms**	Nodular sclerosis Hodgkin's disease
B cell chronic lymphocytic leukaemia/small lymphocytic lymphoma	Adult T cell lymphoma/leukaemia	Lymphocyte-rich Hodgkin's disease
Plasma cell myeloma/plasmacytoma	Mycosis fungoides	Mixed cellularity Hodgkin's disease
MALT lymphoma, mantle cell lymphoma	Peripheral T cell lymphoma	Lymphocyte-depleted Hodgkin's disease
Follicular lymphoma	Angioimmunoblastic T cell lymphoma	
Diffuse large B cell lymphoma	Anaplastic large cell lymphoma	
Burkitt's lymphoma		
Note: There is an overlap of cell types between leukaemias and lymphomas. Leukaemia is diagnosed when the malignant cells are primarily found in the blood and bone marrow, and lymphoma when there are solid tumours of the immune system.		
MALT = mucosa-associated lymphoid tissue.		

have a malignancy. Localised or generalised painless adenopathy with or without hepatosplenomegaly may also occur. It may present with just an abdominal mass. Presentation with mediastinal adenopathy is much less common than in patients with Hodgkin's disease. In some patients the disease may arise at an extranodal site (e.g. the gastrointestinal tract—5%). These patients may present with abdominal pain, obstruction or haemorrhage.

Most non-Hodgkin's lymphomas are diffuse and aggressive. Waldeyer's ring, mesenteric and epitrochlear node involvement are more common in non-Hodgkin's than in Hodgkin's disease. Systemic symptoms are less common in non-Hodgkin's lymphoma. In low-grade non-Hodgkin's lymphoma, lymphadenopathy has often been present for a long time.

Other uncommon presentations include skin infiltration and direct renal infiltration. Primary neurological infiltration is also uncommon. Low-grade gastrointestinal lymphomas (e.g. MALT [mucosa-associated lymphoid tissue] lymphomas) are less common.

The history

1. Ask about the presenting symptoms and causes of symptoms, such as palpable nodes, cough as a result of mediastinal node involvement, systemic symptoms, bone pain owing to marrow infiltration or pathological fractures, spinal cord compression, splenic pain and alcohol-induced pain (rare).
2. Determine the history of infection (as a result of decreased cell-mediated immunity

TABLE 8.13 Histopathological classification of lymphoma

Hodgkin's disease

1. Lymphocyte predominant
2. Nodular sclerosing
3. Mixed cellularity
4. Lymphocyte-depleted

Non-Hodgkin's lymphoma

The Rappaport classification has largely been replaced. There are a number of new classifications, including the International Working Formulation (this classification translates into the clinical setting better than the others).

International Working Formulation

I   Low-grade lymphoma

    1.   Small lymphocytic cell

    2.   Follicular, mixed cleaved cell

    3.   Follicular, mixed small cleaved and large cell

II Intermediate-grade lymphoma

    1.   Follicular large cell

    2.   Diffuse small cleaved cell

    3.   Diffuse mixed small cleaved cell

    4.   Diffuse large cell

III High-grade lymphoma

    1.   Large cell immunoblastic

    2.   Lymphoblastic cell

    3.   Small non-cleaved cell (Burkitt and non-Burkitt)

TABLE 8.14 Staging of lymphoma—Ann Arbor classification

Stage I	Disease confined to a single lymph node region or a single extralymphatic site (Ie)
Stage II	Disease confined to two or more lymph node regions on the same side of the diaphragm, plus or minus splenic involvement
Stage III	Disease confined to lymph node regions on both sides of the diaphragm (III_1 = upper abdomen; III_2 = lower abdomen), with or without localised involvement of the spleen (IIIs), other extralymphatic organ or site (IIIe), or both
Stage IV	Diffuse disease of one or more extralymphatic organs (with or without lymph node disease)

For any stage:

      A. No symptoms

      B. Fever, weight loss >10% in six months or night sweats

in Hodgkin's disease or depressed humoral immunity from chemotherapy or radiotherapy).

3. Ask about the history of the predisposing condition, such as Klinefelter's syndrome, HIV infection, congenital or acquired immune deficiency, use of immunosuppressive drugs or autoimmune disease (e.g. Sjögren's syndrome). Ask also about the use of phenytoin (pseudo-lymphoma).

4. Find out the investigations performed—particularly lymph node biopsy, CT and gallium scans, and bilateral bone marrow aspirations. MRI scanning may have been used for suspected spinal cord, brain or bone marrow involvement. Lymphangiography and staging laparotomy are rarely indicated now. Lumbar puncture is important in high-grade lymphoma investigation if central nervous system involvement is suspected.
5. Ask about the treatment undertaken, as this gives an indication of the stage and type of disease. Ask about the side effects of any treatment (e.g. mantle radiation can result in pneumonitis, hypothyroidism, pericarditis, myocardial fibrosis and spinal cord injury). Ask whether the patient has been informed about possible long-term complications of treatment.
6. Determine the prognosis given and what the patient's understanding of this seems to be.
7. Find out about the patient's social situation—dependent family members, social support, ability to work, reactions to disease (e.g. depression, coping mechanisms) etc. As for other malignancies, work out the ECOG (Eastern Co-operative Oncology Group) performance status (see Table 8.15).

TABLE 8.15 ECOG performance status

Grade	ECOG performance status
0	Fully active; no restriction on activities compared with before the disease.
1	Restricted, but only from strenuous activity. Able to perform light or sedentary work.
2	Able to look after self. Mobile but not able to work.
3	Only partly able to look after self. In bed or chair more than 50% of waking hours.
4	Completely confined to bed or chair. Unable to look after self at all.

The examination

1. Examine the haemopoietic system thoroughly. Particularly note any lymph nodes and assess carefully for splenomegaly.
2. Attempt to stage the disease clinically (see Table 8.14). Remember that staging is much less relevant for non-Hodgkin's lymphomas because spread is haematogenous and not contiguous. Fewer than 10% of even nodular non-Hodgkin's lymphomas are localised and suitable for local irradiation at the time of presentation.
3. Note any radiotherapy marks (and the field covered).
4. Look for evidence of infection (e.g. herpes zoster).
5. If the patient is clinically anaemic, consider a Coombs' positive autoimmune process in your differential.
6. Assess for any evidence of the hyperviscosity syndrome (Waldenström macroglobulinemia secondary to a monoclonal gammaglobulin): look in the fundi.

Investigations

Investigations are aimed at determining the grade and stage of the disease.
1. The first step is to obtain histological confirmation of disease. Ask to see the pathology report if excision lymph node biopsies have already been performed. Fine-needle biopsy is not good enough to define lymph node architecture. Reed-Sternberg cells are *not* pathognomonic of Hodgkin's disease, but may occur in cases of glandular fever, other viral diseases and with other malignancies.
2. The next step is to stage the disease further.

(a) Ask for a full blood count and ESR, a bilateral bone marrow aspirate and trephine, liver function tests, and abdominal, pelvic and chest imaging (usually chest X-ray [see Fig 8.1] followed by CT scan).

(b) If there is a major leukaemic component, order flow cytometry of the peripheral lymphocytes to aid in the diagnosis.

3. In Hodgkin's disease, agranulocytosis (sometimes with marked eosinophilia or a leukaemoid reaction), an elevated ESR, reversed CD4/CD8 ratio, skin test anergy and a mildly elevated alkaline phosphatase level are often present, but may *not* indicate widespread disease. The ESR remains the best indicator of disease activity. Lymphangiography is less often done these days, especially if the CT, single-photon emission CT (SPECT) and gallium scans are normal. PET scanning may be more sensitive than gallium scanning in staging the disease at diagnosis and in monitoring residual disease. Staging laparotomies are now only rarely performed, but previously treated patients may bear the scar. Staging in this invasive way is less relevant now that systemic treatment is more often used for all patients. Always re-stage after treatment!

Figure 8.1 Chest X-ray showing bilateral hilar lymphadenopathy (arrows).
Figure reproduced courtesy of The Canberra Hospital.

Treatment

Hodgkin's disease (80% of patients are curable)
Treatment depends on the stage of the disease (see Table 8.14). Histological type is less important.

- Stages IA, IIA and IIIsA—radiotherapy or abbreviated course of chemotherapy followed by radiotherapy.
- Stage IIIA (with para-aortic node involvement with or without radiotherapy to involved sites), IIIB and IV—combined chemotherapy (e.g. ABVD [adriamycin, bleomycin, vinblastine and dacarbazine]).

Salvage treatment

Relapse less than one year after initial treatment or failure to achieve complete remission is an indication for second-line therapy. For relapse after more than one year, retreatment can be given using the original regimen. Further radiotherapy can be used for relapse outside the radiation field if the patient has early stage disease. Autologous stem cell transplant after high-dose chemotherapy is an alternative.

Prognosis

This depends on the stage. In general, in:

- stage I, expect 85–95% 10 years' disease-free survival
- stage II, expect 80–90% 10 years' disease-free survival
- stage III and IV, expect 60% 10 years' disease-free survival.

Complications of treatment

1. The improvement in survival achieved with current treatment means that complications of treatment are more likely to cause death than the disease. Routine annual testing and review is recommended (see Table 8.16).
2. Secondary malignancies, including leukaemia and carcinomas, are associated with the use of alkylating agents.
3. Breast cancer risk is associated with chest irradiation.
4. Chest radiotherapy also increases the risk of coronary artery disease after 10 years or more, and of hypothyroidism.
5. Radiotherapy and chemotherapy increase the risk of carcinoma of the lung, which is significantly greater again for smokers.
6. Infertility can occur in men and women treated with chemotherapy. The chance of recovery of fertility is much greater for young patients. Sperm or ovarian tissue banking may be offered to patients.

TABLE 8.16 Routine annual tests for patients treated for Hodgkin's disease

1. Thyroid function tests and clinical examination of the thyroid

2. Full blood count—looking for leukaemia and myelodysplastic syndromes (maximum risk at 3–12 years)

3. Mammography and breast examination—increased risk of breast cancer from 10 years after treatment

Non-Hodgkin's lymphoma

Prognosis and treatment depend mainly on the histological type (particularly whether it is nodular or diffuse and based on the International Working Formulation—see Table 8.13); most cases of low-grade lymphomas are stage III or IV at presentation. The International Prognostic Index (see Table 8.17) has proved an accurate way of assessing the patient's likely course. More recently, treatment decisions have been based on the WHO classification (see Table 8.12).

Treatment protocols: International Working Formulation classification

1. **Low-grade lymphoma.** These are not curable and treatment does not increase survival. Follicular mixed cleaved cell low-grade lymphoma is indolent. Commonly it presents as stage IVA.
   (a) For asymptomatic low-grade lymphoma no treatment is indicated.
   (b) For symptomatic low-grade lymphoma, chlorambucil with or without prednisone, or CVP (cyclophosphamide, vincristine and prednisone), is the usual initial treatment.

TABLE 8.17 International Prognostic Index—clinical risk factors for a poor outcome

Age >60

Lactate dehydrogenase level elevated

Ann Arbor stage III or IV

>1 extranodal site

Physical performance, e.g. Karnosky score >70 (self-caring, mobile etc.)

0–1 risk factors = low risk

  2 risk factors = low-to-intermediate risk

  3 risk factors = intermediate-to-high risk

  4 or 5 risk factors = high risk

For stages I and II low-grade lymphoma (uncommon), extended field radiation may be used in younger patients with curative intent, but they must be very carefully staged first. More aggressive regimens (as for intermediate-grade) may produce more complete remissions but have not been shown to increase survival. Maintenance single-agent chemotherapy has not reduced the relapse rate.

2. **Intermediate and high-grade lymphoma.** These have a poor prognosis if untreated. Diffuse large cell lymphoma and high-grade lymphomas are potentially curable with treatment.
   (a) Stage I and some stage II: aggressive treatment to try for cure is essential, but careful staging must be carried out first.
   (b) Stages II, III and IV:
       (i) diffuse large cell lymphoma—combination chemotherapy, such as CHOP (cyclophosphamide, adriamycin, vincristine and prednisone); high-dose methotrexate and intrathecal methotrexate may be added if indicated
       (ii) diffuse well-differentiated lymphocytic lymphoma—this is the most indolent type and prognosis is indistinguishable from that for chronic lymphocytic leukaemia; no treatment is required unless symptomatic
       (iii) other diffuse types: combination chemotherapy
       (iv) salvage chemotherapy—failure of remission or relapse is an indication of a poor prognosis; salvage treatment is usually attempted with drugs such as cisplatin or cytosine arabinoside, but remission rates are only 20–30%.
   (c) AIDS-related lymphomas: these tumours tend to be of the large B cell or Burkitt's type and very aggressive. Results of combination chemotherapy, so far, have been poor. The best regimens, using central nervous system prophylaxis, granulocyte-macrophage colony stimulating factor (GM-CSF) (to limit neutropenia) and a modified chemotherapeutic combination, have produced 50% complete response rates. There is a high mortality from associated infection in these immunodeficient patients.

Treatment protocols: WHO classification
1. **Precursor B cell neoplasms.** Precursor B cell lymphoblastic leukaemia/lymphoma is usually the childhood malignancy acute lymphocytic leukaemia (ALL). The lymphoma is rare in adults and rapidly progresses to become leukaemia. Combination chemotherapy is used to induce remission and continuing treatment to attempt cure. The cure rate in adults is about 50%.

2. **Mature B cell neoplasms.** B cell chronic lymphoid leukaemia/small lymphocytic lymphoma is the most common lymphoid leukaemia and represents about 75% of non-Hodgkin's lymphomas. Patients with only bone marrow involvement and lymphocytosis are not usually treated. They have a median survival of more than 10 years. Once liver and splenic involvement have occurred, treatment is likely to be required at some stage but may not be recommended until bone marrow failure is present. Oral chlorambucil or the more potent intravenous drug, fludarabine, is most often recommended. Young patients may benefit from bone marrow transplant.

3. **MALT-type lymphoma (extranodal marginal zone B cell lymphoma—8%).** These gastric mucosal lymphomas are curable when localised. MALT is associated with *Helicobacter pylori* infection. Eradication of the infection will usually induce remission (75%). Otherwise, chlorambucil or radiation treatment is used. Endoscopic follow-up is important. Splenic MALT lymphoma may follow hepatitis C infection; once other causes are excluded, splenectomy can induce a long remission.

4. **Mantle cell lymphoma (6%).** The majority of these present as a systemic disease. Treatment is not very successful. The usual approach is combination chemotherapy followed by radiotherapy. Chemotherapy may be used with rituximab (the anti-CD20 antibody). Bone marrow transplant is offered to younger patients.

5. **Follicular lymphoma (22%).** Asymptomatic patients may require no treatment. Chlorambucil alone or combination treatment (CVP or CHOP) can achieve a 75% remission rate. Interferon alpha seems to prolong survival once remission has been achieved, and rituximab can be helpful for patients who have relapsed. Between 5% and 7% of patients per year develop histological transformation into diffuse large B cell lymphoma. Follicular lymphoma (low-grade) prognosis can be further estimated from Table 8.18:

TABLE 8.18 Follicular lymphoma survival rates

Risk factors

1. Age >60 years
2. Haemoglobin <12 g/dL
3. Ann Arbor stage III or IV disease
4. >4 lymph nodes or other sites of disease
5. Increased lactate dehydrogenase (LDH)

Number of risk factors	Five-year survival	10-year survival
0–1 risk factors (36% of patients)	91%	71%
2 risk factors (37% of patients)	78%	51%
≥3 risk factors (27% of patients)	53%	27%

6. **Diffuse large B cell lymphoma (30%).** Treatment is usually begun with combination chemotherapy (often CHOP). This may be followed by radiotherapy if there is bulky stage I or II disease. Six cycles of treatment will produce a cure in up to 70% of patients. Monoclonal antibody treatment with rituximab is used for most patients. Bone marrow transplant is more effective than further chemotherapy for patients who relapse: it can achieve up to 40% long-term disease-free survival. The International Prognostic Index (IPI), which is based on five pre-treatment characteristics (see Table 8.19), predicts survival.

TABLE 8.19 Cure rates and five-year survival rates for diffuse large B cell lymphoma based on the IPI

Pre-treatment characteristics (risk factors)

1. Age >60
2. Stage III or IV
3. >1 extranodal site involved
4. ECOG status ≥2
5. Serum LDH normal

Number of risk factors	Cure rate	Five-year survival
0–1 risk factors (35% of patients)	87%	73%
2 risk factors (27%)	66%	51%
3 risk factors (22%)	53%	27%
4–5 risk factors (16%)	34%	26%

7. **Burkitt's lymphoma.** This is a rare disease in Australia, but is more common in Africa. Intensive combination chemotherapy with attention to the central nervous system will produce a cure in about 70% of patients.
8. **Hairy cell leukaemia.** This is an indolent lymphoma with leukaemic features. The peripheral smear shows lymphocytes with hairy projections. Look for splenomegaly and cytopenia. It responds well to chemotherapy.
9. **Immunodeficiency-associated lymphoma.** The WHO classifies these lymphomas into four groups:
   (a) lymphoproliferative diseases associated with primary immune disorders
   (b) HIV associated lymphomas
   (c) post-transplant lymphomas
   (d) methotrexate-associated lymphoproliferative disorders.
      These are usually aggressive B cell, CNS and Hodgkin's lymphomas, and treatment is as for the type of lymphoma.

Bone marrow transplant
Disease resistant to standard-dose chemotherapy can be treated with bone marrow ablation using chemotherapy or radiotherapy, or both. Bone marrow transplant is then performed with autologous stem cells or, less often, from a compatible donor. The mortality rate associated with this procedure (now <5%) and the success of engraftment have improved with the use of haematopoietic growth factors. Long-term outcomes are uncertain, as are the indications for the use of this treatment in patients with less aggressive disease. Follow-up of treated non-Hodgkin's lymphomas is similar to that for Hodgkin's lymphoma patients.

Multiple myeloma (myeloma)
This is a disseminated malignant disease of plasma cells. It can present as a diagnostic or a management problem. Myeloma occurs more commonly in the elderly—the median age is 60 years—and more often in men. It is more common in people whose occupations involve exposure to petroleum and in people exposed to nuclear radiation. Chronic antigenic stimulation may play a role in B cell clonal transformation. A number of chromosomal deletions and translocations have been identified in myeloma patients. The most important of these is 13q. Its presence has prognostic significance. Some myeloma begin as monoclonal gammopathies of uncertain significance (MGUS). MGUS are much more common than myeloma—they are found in up to 10% of 80-year-olds—and they evolve to myeloma at a rate of 10% a year ('smouldering myeloma').

The history

1. Ask about presenting symptoms:
   (a) bone pain or pain with movement affects nearly three-quarters of patients, occurs particularly in the ribs or axial skeleton and may cause pathological fractures; the association with movement may distinguish it from the bone pain of metastatic malignancy, which can be worse at night (persistent pain suggests a pathological fracture)
   (b) bacterial infection is the presenting problem in one-quarter of patients—particularly pneumonia and urinary tract infections (total immunoglobulins are increased, but the level of normal functional immunoglobulins is reduced as a result of reduced production and increased destruction; in advanced marrow disease there is white cell depletion); the CD4 count is low; the most common organisms are *Streptococcus pneumoniae*, *Staphylococcus aureus* and *Klebsiella pneumoniae* in the lungs, and *E. coli* in the urinary tract
   (c) symptoms of anaemia (normochromic and normocytic)—as a result of bone marrow depression from infiltration, chronic disease, renal failure or treatment
   (d) bleeding tendency—caused by paraprotein inactivation of plasma procoagulants and reduced platelet function (coating of platelets with antibodies) and thrombocytopenia as a result of bone marrow suppression
   (e) renal disease symptoms (owing to stone formation secondary to hypercalcaemia, hyperuricaemia, tubular damage by light chains, therapy, urinary tract infection, contrast studies, plasma cell infiltration or amyloid)—renal failure affects one-quarter of patients and half develop renal impairment; renal impairment at the time of diagnosis means a poor prognosis
   (f) hypercalcaemic symptoms owing to bone lysis
   (g) hyperviscosity symptoms once plasma viscosity exceeds 5 (normal is about 1.8)
   (h) spinal cord compression or, rarely, diffuse sensorimotor neuropathy
   (i) skin changes, such as pruritus, purpura, yellow skin, hypertrichosis (rare), erythema annulare (rare)
   (j) systemic amyloid deposition (10–15%).
2. Find out how the diagnosis was made.
3. Ask about treatment—ask about drugs (e.g. bisphosphonates, thalidomide) and their side effects, radiotherapy and bone marrow transplant (actual or planned).
4. Enquire about the patient's social history, including dependants, work, ADLs etc.
5. Determine the patient's understanding of this life-threatening condition and its prognosis—how much information he or she has about possible further problems and treatment.

The examination

1. Inspect the patient for signs of weight loss, anaemia, chest infection and general debility.
2. Examine the haemopoietic system. Pay particular attention to a search for bony tenderness. Kyphosis may be caused by compression fractures. Splenomegaly and lymphadenopathy occur only very rarely.
3. Note signs of anaemia and purpura. Look for skin rash.
4. Look for signs of infection (e.g. pulmonary consolidation).
5. Check carefully for any signs of spinal cord compression.
6. Check the urine analysis and temperature chart.

Investigations

1. Once the diagnosis is suspected, check the full blood count (and film) for anaemia (and rouleaux) and a raised ESR. Obtain a protein electrophoretogram (EPG) of serum and urine and an immunoelectrophoretogram (IEPG). An 'M' component (monoclonal globulin peak) is found in 95% of cases (any immunoglobulin class may appear as the 'M' component). Light chains are present in the urine in 50–75% of patients (Bence-Jones proteinuria cannot be detected by dipstick urine analysis).

2. The bone marrow must be examined for plasma cells (>10% in myeloma). Check the beta$_2$-microglobulin level (see below).

3. Look at X-ray films of the skull (see Fig 8.2), chest, pelvis (see Fig 8.3) and proximal long bones for fractures, osteoporosis and lytic lesions. The latter is a result of the secretion of osteoclast-activating factors by the tumour cells. Since there is little osteoblastic activity, bone scans are much less sensitive than plain X-rays.

4. MRI scans may be the best way to investigate pain and possible nerve root or spinal cord compression.

5. Also check the serum calcium and urate levels and the renal function.

   The three major diagnostic features of multiple myeloma, in order of importance, are:
   • plasma cells in the bone marrow (>10% involvement is consistent with the diagnosis)
   • production of serum paraprotein (50% are IgG, 33% IgA, 5% IgM, 10% only light chains, 2% nil)
   • bone destruction (lytic lesions).

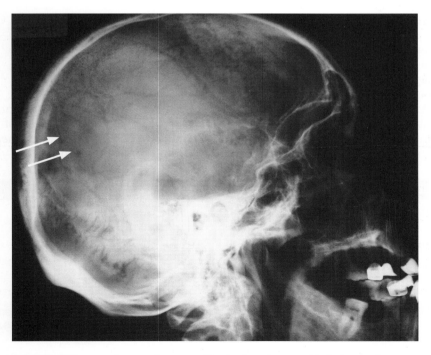

Figure 8.2 Skull X-ray of a myeloma patient showing multiple lucent areas— pepper-pot skull (arrows).
Figure reproduced courtesy of The Canberra Hospital.

Figure 8.3 X-ray of the pelvis showing destruction of the left superior ramus of the ischium (arrow).
Figure reproduced courtesy of The Canberra Hospital.

The disease can be staged according to certain criteria (see Table 8.20). On this basis, median survival can be estimated as follows:
- stage IA—61 months
- stage IIA or IIB—55 months
- stage IIIA—30 months
- stage IIIB—15 months.

An elevated serum beta$_2$-microglobulin level (which reflects the myeloma cell burden and renal functional impairment) indicates a median survival of 12 months. Other poor prognostic features include advanced age and cytogenetic abnormalities (e.g. any translocation, deletion of chromosome 13q).

TABLE 8.20 Staging of myeloma	
Stage I	(i) Haemoglobin near normal (>100 g/L)
	(ii) Calcium not elevated
	(iii) Low M component
	(iv) Up to one lytic bone lesion
Stage II	Intermediate between stages I and III
Stage III	Poor prognostic features include anaemia (haemoglobin <85 g/L), hypercalcaemia (>3 mmol/L), advanced lytic bone lesions, high M component production rates.
Subclassification:	
	A. serum creatinine <200 mmol/L
	B. serum creatinine >200 mmol/L

Treatment

1. Irradiation is helpful for localised bone pain and spinal cord compression. Patients with a single bone plasmacytoma will often get prolonged disease-free survival after treatment with local radiotherapy. Pamidronate or one of the other bisphosphonates should be given to patients with more than stage I disease. Bisphosphonates reduce bone pain, fracture rates and episodes of hypercalcaemia. There is evidence that they improve the prognosis.

2. For those with more diffuse disease, general measures such as adequate hydration and use of bicarbonate for Bence-Jones proteinuria are important to prevent renal failure. Intravenous contrast material must be used cautiously and only with excellent hydration. Allopurinol may protect renal function from urate nephropathy related to treatment. Treat hypercalcaemia and bacterial infection. Avoid live vaccines. Erythropoietin may improve the anaemia.

3. Chemotherapy is indicated for patients with stage II or III disease and for those with stage I disease if they are symptomatic or have rising myeloma protein levels or progressive lytic bone lesions. Treatment is begun with high-dose steroids in combination with thalidomide or lenalidomide (reduce tumour necrosis factor alpha). An alternative is bortezomib, a proteosome inhibitor.

4. Alkylating agents should be avoided if the patient may be a candidate for bone marrow transplant. Such drugs may prevent stem cell harvesting by damaging these cells. Melphalan and prednisone were standard treatment; other alkylating agents (e.g. cyclophosphamide) are probably equally effective for patients unsuitable for bone marrow transplant. Resistance to one alkylating agent is often, but not always, associated with resistance to the others. Typically treatment is given intermittently. A week's course is repeated four weeks later for up to two years. The patient's progress must be monitored with regular protein EPG studies.

5. Relapse is treated for suitable patients with autologous stem cell bone marrow transplant.

6. Secondary acute leukaemia is being seen increasingly, related to alkylating agent therapy. Autologous bone marrow transplantation is the treatment of choice for these patients if they are less than 60 years old. The mortality rate is about 15% per year. Causes of death include infection, renal failure, leukaemia, concomitant illnesses and progressive myeloma.

Differential diagnosis

Monoclonal gammopathy of undetermined significance

A smaller monoclonal peak (<30 g/L), less than 10% plasma cells in the bone marrow and absence of lytic bone lesions suggest this diagnosis. Urinary light chains are absent. Infection, renal failure and anaemia are not increased. No therapy is required.

Waldenström's macroglobulinaemia

The EPG has a peak consisting of monoclonal IgM. These patients are generally older than those with myeloma. The hyperviscosity syndrome is often present; symptoms and signs include lassitude, confusion, bleeding, anaemia, infection, lymphadenopathy and splenomegaly, dilated retinal veins and perivenous haemorrhages, and (rarely) renal failure. Lymphadenopathy and splenomegaly do not usually occur in patients with myeloma. Lytic bone destruction and hypercalcaemia are rare. Ten per cent of the macroglobulins are cryoglobulins. An underlying lymphoproliferative disorder may be present. Treatment with plasmapheresis is effective in removing IgM paraprotein. Prednisone, fludarabine and chlorambucil are useful. Rituximab (anti-CD20 monoclonal antibody) and thalidomide have also been used successfully. Median survival is four years.

Localised myeloma
Only one plasma cell tumour is present. Solitary plasmacytomas often occur in the nasopharynx or paranasal sinuses. The major complications of myeloma are absent. Only 50% of cases show a monoclonal peak. Local radiotherapy is the usual treatment.

POEMS syndrome
This is an atypical form of myeloma. The features include:

Polyneuropathy
Organomegaly
Endocrinopathy
Monoclonal gammopathy (osteosclerotic myeloma, or IgA or IgG M proteins with lambda light chains)
Skin changes

There is a progressive sensorimotor polyneuropathy associated with myeloma-like bone lesions. Unlike multiple myeloma, over half the patients have hepatomegaly and lymphadenopathy and some have splenomegaly. Male impotence and gynaecomastia and female amenorrhoea occur as a result of hyperprolactinaemia. A few patients have hypothyroidism and one-third have type 2 diabetes. Skin changes include clubbing, hypertrichosis, thickening and increased pigmentation.

There are often high levels of the cytokines, IL-1, IL-6 and tumour necrosis factor.

Treatment of the myeloma component in the usual way often helps the other manifestations. Local bone lesions often respond to radiotherapy.

Bone marrow (haematopoietic cell) transplantation

Bone marrow transplantation is being performed for an increasing number of indications. Patients are chronically ill and often available for examinations. Two groups of patients are treated in this way: those with a malignant condition (see Table 8.21), who have their bone marrow destroyed by irradiation or chemotherapy given in marrow-toxic doses to treat a malignancy; and those with a defective bone marrow that is destroyed and then replaced (see Table 8.22). Autologous transplants (when the patient's own marrow or stem cells are stored and then reinfused) are now more common than allogenic transplants (when another person is used as the donor of marrow or stem cells).

TABLE 8.21 Malignant indications for bone marrow transplant		
Condition	**Autologous**	**Allogenic**
Acute leukaemia	Yes	Yes
Chronic myeloid leukaemia	Yes	Yes
Lymphoma	Yes	Yes
Hodgkin's disease	Yes	Yes
Carcinoma of the breast	Yes	No
Carcinoma of the testis	Yes	No
Multiple myeloma	Yes	Yes
Wilm's tumour	Yes	No

TABLE 8.22 Non-malignant indications for bone marrow transplant		
Condition	Autologous	Allogenic
Aplastic anaemia	No	Yes
Sickle cell disease	No	Yes
Thalassaemia	No	Yes
Gaucher's disease	No	Yes
Severe combined immunodeficiency	No	Yes
Fanconi's anaemia	No	Yes

The history

1. Ask what the indication for the transplant was.
2. Find out whether there has been a problem leading to the current admission to hospital (if the patient is an inpatient).
3. Ask whether other treatment has been tried unsuccessfully. (For example, bone marrow transplant is often the treatment of choice for relapse after treatment for leukaemia or lymphoma.)
4. Find out whether the bone marrow transplant was autologous or allogenic. How was the marrow ablated before transplant (radiotherapy, chemotherapy, or both) and, if the transplant was autologous, how were the stem cells harvested (from peripheral blood or by bone marrow aspiration)?
5. If the transplant was allogenic, does the patient know the donor? Only about 30% of people have an HLA-compatible relative. For the rest, a volunteer unrelated donor is used. HLA antigens are inherited together and rarely cross over. The patient may know how close the match was.
6. Ask how long the patient was in hospital after transplantation. (Engraftment is usually quicker and complications fewer after autologous transplant.) Ask specifically about problems with infection in the early period and how complications were managed.
7. Find out what effects this complicated illness and treatment have had on the patient's life and ability to work. Ask about family and financial problems. Young patients are likely to have been made sterile by the treatment. Total body irradiation and the use of alkylating agents are more likely to cause permanent sterility than other treatments. Women more often regain fertility than men. Ask tactfully whether the patient is aware of this.
8. Ask how effective the treatment has been. Does the patient feel better or worse than before and what medium- and long-term prognosis has he or she been given?
9. Ask whether there have been specific transplant-associated problems. Ask specifically about the symptoms and signs of graft versus host disease (GVHD) and the other complications of allogenic transplantation (see Table 8.23).
10. Ask about the patient's current medications.

The examination

Examine for persisting or recurrent signs of the condition for which the bone marrow transplant was performed.

1. Examine for signs of GVHD. These include skin changes similar to those of scleroderma, dry eyes and mouth (sicca syndrome), alopecia and bronchiolitis obliterans (signs of airflow obstruction).

TABLE 8.23 Complications of allogenic bone marrow transplant

Early complications	Late complications
Induction-related	*Treatment-related*
• Mucositis	• Gonadal toxicity
• Cystitis	• Cataracts
• Interstitial pneumonitis (usually CMV infection)	• Neurological
• Renal impairment	Chronic GVHD
Graft failure	Infection
Infection	Relapse of treated condition
Immunodeficiency	Second malignancy
Acute GVHD	Immunodeficiency
Veno-occlusive disease of the liver (hepatomegaly, ascites, jaundice)	

2. Examine for hepatic enlargement and ascites (veno-occlusive disease of the liver). Feel all the lymph node groups (e.g. enlarged as a result of a second malignancy, such as ALL or melanoma) and examine the eyes (e.g. secondary glioblastoma).
3. Look for signs of infection in the lungs and for herpes zoster.
4. Examine the hips (aseptic osteonecrosis).
5. Patients who have had radiotherapy may show evidence of hypothyroidism.

Management

Detailed discussion about methods of transplantation will not be required.

1. Management after transplant begins with supportive treatment to prevent infection and bleeding before engraftment occurs. Platelet and blood transfusions may be required and the patient is usually kept isolated. Transfused products are irradiated to prevent GVHD from transfused lymphocytes. Most patients receive colony-stimulating factors to speed recovery. Platelet recovery is usually the slowest and tends to determine the time of discharge from hospital.
2. Patients who have had an allogenic transplant are at risk of GVHD. This risk is reduced if the HLA match is a good one (only one locus is mismatched). Prophylaxis against GVHD with some combination of prednisone, methotrexate and cyclosporin is usual. The donor marrow may be treated to remove T cells to reduce the incidence of GVHD, but this increases the risk of graft rejection. The risk of GVHD is also increased by previous exposure to blood products and by previous pregnancy.
3. Acute GVHD can occur even when the major HLA antigens match. It occurs by definition in the first three months after transplant and is characterised by diarrhoea, skin rash and liver function test changes. Severe acute GVHD (generalised erythroderma or desquamation) reduces survival and requires aggressive treatment. It is usually treated with high doses of prednisone, antithymocyte globulin and monoclonal antibodies to T cells. Some centres use prophylactic treatment after transplant with methotrexate and tacrolimus or cyclosporin. Remember that the presence of some GVHD reduces the risk of tumour recurrence as a result of graft versus tumour activity.
4. Chronic GVHD develops after three months and affects up to half of transplant recipients. Patients develop an autoimmune-like illness with sicca syndrome, arthritis, cholestasis and bronchiolitis obliterans. It is treated with immunosuppression. It is rare for it to persist for more than three years.

5. Infection can be a problem at various times after transplant. Bacterial infection is most common during the early period before the neutrophil count reaches normal levels. It is treated with isolation and appropriate antibiotics. Fungal infection can become a problem within a week of transplant but usually resolves once engraftment has occurred. *Pneumocystis jirovecci* infection and cytomegalovirus (CMV) infection can occur within a week of transplant but are uncommon after three months. Interstitial pneumonitis occurs in up to 10% of patients. This is usually the result of CMV infection and is treated with supporting measures and ganciclovir. CMV-negative recipients should receive only CMV-negative blood products, and CMV-positive patients should receive prophylactic ganciclovir. Prophylactic treatment with fluconazole, cotrimoxazole and ganciclovir is often used to prevent these problems.

6. Graft rejection is usually a result of the activity of functional host lymphocytes and is most common in patients who have not had their marrow ablated (e.g. those with aplastic anaemia).

7. Recurrence of leukaemia may be treated with infusion of more donor T cells, although this increases GVHD.

8. Veno-occlusive disease of the liver occurs in up to 50% of patients. Most recover, but in severe cases treatment with tissue plasminogen activator may be indicated.

9. Overall, autologous bone marrow transplant is associated with similar but less severe complications. GVHD, however, does not occur.

10. The prognosis varies with the indication for the treatment (see Table 8.24). In general, malignant conditions have a better prognosis when treated with bone marrow transplant as a primary or secondary therapy than when it is used only after all else has failed. Patients with non-malignant conditions can often be very successfully treated with bone marrow transplant. For example, aplastic anaemia patients can expect up to 90% disease-free survival. Opinions differ about the use of bone marrow transplant as initial treatment for these patients.

11. Remember that, as with any complicated and life-threatening illness, pay great attention to the patient's ability to cope and the availability of support at home; these are important matters you must be able to discuss.

TABLE 8.24 Survival of bone marrow transplant patients

Condition	Five-year survival rate
Acute myeloid leukaemia	50%
Acute lymphatic leukaemia	50%
Chronic myeloid leukaemia (CML), chronic phase	70%
CML accelerated	40%
CML blast crisis	15%
Chronic lymphocytic leukaemia (CLL)	50%
Hodgkin's disease	50%
Non-Hodgkin's lymphoma	40%
Aplastic anaemia	90%
Severe combined immunodeficiency	90%
Thalassaemia	90%

Chapter 9

The rheumatological long case

It's better to be dead, or even perfectly well, than
to suffer from the wrong affliction.
Ogden Nash (1902–71)

Rheumatoid arthritis

This is a very common long case in which the diagnosis is usually straightforward and
the patient has many physical signs. The peak incidence of the onset of rheumatoid
arthritis is in the fourth decade of life and it is three times as common in women as in
men. There may be a family history and there is an association with human leucocyte
antigen [HLA]-DR4 (70%).

The history

1. Ask when the diagnosis was made—the onset of rheumatoid arthritis in
   patients over the age of 60 is associated with a worse prognosis for those who
   are rheumatoid factor positive.
2. Ask about the presenting features—most patients present with vague generalised
   symptoms, such as fatigue, anorexia and non-specific musculoskeletal pains; a
   minority present with obvious oligoarticular arthritis; and a few present with
   severe constitutional symptoms and acute arthritis. Morning stiffness lasting
   for more than an hour is very characteristic of inflammatory arthritis but not
   of osteoarthritis.
3. Ask about the initial treatment.
4. Ask about the disease progression and what joints have been involved. The
   lumbar spine is never involved and the distal interphalangeal joints are only
   rarely affected.
5. Enquire about the alterations in treatment over time and any complications
   encountered.
6. Ask about the non-articular features of the disease:
   (a) skin—Raynaud's phenomenon, leg ulcers
   (b) eyes—dry eyes (and mouth; Sjögren's syndrome), scleritis, episcleritis
       or scleromalacia perforans, cataracts (caused by steroids); iritis does not
       occur
   (c) sore throat, hoarseness or neck pain—suspect cricoaryteroid joint disease;
       recurrent headaches at the base of the skull or arm tingling from C1–2
       subluxation (obtain a lateral flexion cervical spine X-ray)
   (d) lungs—dyspnoea owing to diffuse interstitial fibrosis or pleural effusion,
       pain as a result of pleuritis

175

(e) heart—chest pain owing to pericarditis, valve disease (from rheumatoid nodules), increased atherosclerosis

(f) renal—drug use, amyloid (all rare)

(g) nervous system—peripheral neuropathy, mononeuritis multiplex, cord compression (owing to cervical spine involvement [C1–2 subluxation] or rheumatoid nodules), entrapment neuropathy (particularly carpal tunnel syndrome)

(h) blood—anaemic symptoms owing to chronic disease, iron deficiency (from blood loss), folate deficiency (diet), Felty's syndrome (rheumatoid arthritis with leucopenia and splenomegaly, and non-healing leg ulcers)

(i) systemic—fever, weight loss, fatigue

(j) vasculitic—digital arteritis, ulcers, mononeuritis multiplex, pyoderma gangrenosum.

7. Ask about drug complications:

(a) aspirin (e.g. pain or nausea, gastric erosions or peptic ulcers causing bleeding, tinnitus)

(b) NSAIDs (e.g. ulceration, renal impairment, increased cardiac risk)

(c) methotrexate is often used and has a number of side effects that need to be monitored (including hepatic and pulmonary toxicity, low white cell count and thrombocytopenia); the patient should know not to drink alcohol while taking methotrexate; an alternative drug is leflunomide (diarrhoea, alopecia, liver toxicity)

(d) penicillamine (e.g. nephrotic syndrome, thrombocytopenia, rashes, mouth ulcers, alteration in taste and, rarely, systemic lupus erythematosus [SLE], polymyositis, myasthenia gravis, Goodpasture's syndrome or pulmonary infiltration)

(e) cyclosporin—monitor renal function and blood pressure

(f) hydroxychloroquine (e.g. nausea, pigmentation, bull's eye retinopathy—need regular ophthalmological review)

(g) sulfasalazine (e.g. rash, nausea, haematological abnormalities, abnormal liver function tests, reversible oligospecima)

(h) anti-tumour necrosis factor (TNF) monoclonal antibody (e.g. increased risk of infections including reactivation of TB, positive ANA, lymphoma and demyelination)

(i) steroids.

8. Ask about the major current problem—such as decreasing hand function, paraesthesiae, severe pain etc.

9. Find out about the current activity of the disease. This can be assessed historically by asking about the number of joints that have recently been involved with active synovitis, the severity and duration of early morning stiffness (very important), functional ability, changes in weight and the degree of systemic ill-health. A severe course is more likely if there is the early appearance of rheumatoid nodules, an insidious onset and constitutional symptoms.

10. Enquire about past medical history, especially regarding peptic ulceration, drug reactions or renal disease.

11. Enquire about social background—ability to cope at home, ability to climb steps, independence in daily activities, ability to perform fine activities, the work environment, availability of support services.

12. Ask about a family history of rheumatoid arthritis.

The examination (see Table 9.1)

TABLE 9.1 Rheumatoid arthritis	
1. GENERAL INSPECTION Cushingoid appearance Weight **2. HANDS (examine all joints)** **3. ARMS** Entrapment neuropathy (e.g. carpal tunnel) Subcutaneous nodules Elbow joint Shoulder joint Axillary nodes **4. FACE** Eyes—dry eyes (Sjögren's)—scleritis, episcleritis Scleromalacia perforans—anaemia Cataract (steroids, chloroquine) Fundi—hyperviscosity Face—parotids (Sjögren's) Mouth—dryness, ulcers, dental caries, temporomandibular joint (crepitus) **5. NECK** Cervical spine Cervical nodes	**6. CHEST** Heart—pericarditis, valve lesions Lungs—effusion, fibrosis, infarction, infection, nodules (and Caplan's syndrome) Tuberculosis (steroids) **7. ABDOMEN** Splenomegaly (e.g. Felty's syndrome) Epigastric tenderness (drugs) Inguinal nodes **8. HIPS** **9. KNEES** **10. LOWER LIMBS** Ulceration (vasculitis) Calf swelling (ruptured synovial cyst) Peripheral neuropathy Mononeuritis multiplex Cord compression **11. FEET** **12. OTHER** Urine: protein, blood (drugs, vasculitis, infection, amyloidosis) Rectal examination (blood)

A thorough general examination is important. In addition to assessing for synovitis in *every* joint, look particularly at the following:

1. general appearance—steroid complications, weight; remember that the pain arises mostly from the joint capsule and that acutely inflamed joints are held in the flexed position to increase the volume of the capsule and reduce pain
2. the hands—including vasculitis and hand function; the wrist joints are almost always affected
3. arms—the elbow and shoulder joints, rheumatoid nodules and axillary node enlargement
4. the face—the eyes for Sjögren's syndrome, scleritis, episcleritis, scleromalacia perforans, cataracts, anaemia and signs of hyperviscosity in the fundi; enlarged parotid glands (Sjögren's syndrome); the mouth (dryness, dental caries, ulcers); listen for a hoarse voice and palpate the temporomandibular joints (crepitus). *Note*: rheumatoid arthritis does not cause iritis
5. the neck—for signs of cervical spine involvement
6. the chest—the heart for pericarditis, conduction defects, aortic and mitral regurgitation; and the lungs for pleural effusion, fibrosis, nodules, infarction and Caplan's syndrome
7. the abdomen—for splenomegaly and epigastric tenderness
8. the hips and knees
9. the lower legs—for ulcers, calf swelling (ruptured Baker's cyst), neuropathy, mononeuritis multiplex and signs of cord compression
10. the feet

11. the peripheral nervous system for peripheral neuropathy or mononeuritis multiplex (caused by vasculitis)
12. the skin, for cutaneous vasculitis (ischaemic ulcers on the legs or brown discoloured areas in the nail beds; *note*—exclude psoriasis)
13. urine analysis for protein and blood; and rectal examination for blood (if there is a history suggestive of NSAID complications).

Differential diagnosis

Consider the differential diagnosis of a deforming symmetrical chronic poly-arthropathy:
1. rheumatoid arthritis
2. psoriatic arthropathy and other seronegative spondyloarthropathies
3. chronic tophaceous gout (rarely symmetrical)
4. primary generalised osteoarthritis.
   Remember that the causes of arthritis plus nodules include:
1. rheumatoid arthritis (seropositive)
2. SLE—rare
3. rheumatic fever (Jaccoud's arthritis)—very rare
4. amyloid arthropathy (most usually in association with multiple myeloma).
   Note: Gouty tophi and xanthoma may sometimes be confused.

Investigations

To support the diagnosis (remembering that this is primarily a clinical diagnosis; see Table 9.2), investigations include:
1. **serological tests**
   (a) rheumatoid factor—70% of patients are seropositive; patients may at first be seronegative and seroconvert later. (*Note:* Most patients are rheumatoid factor positive if they have nodules or associated vasculitis; remember that more than 10% of well people over the age of 65 have rheumatoid factor and that it is commonly found in association with infections and other inflammatory conditions, in relatives of patients with rheumatoid arthritis and transiently after some vaccinations.)
   (b) anti-citrullinated cyclic peptide (anti-CCP)—this is more specific (97%); it is associated with a more severe disease course and erosive disease.

TABLE 9.2 Criteria for the diagnosis of rheumatoid arthritis*

1. Morning stiffness ≥1 hour for ≥6 weeks

2. Arthritis of three or more joint areas (soft-tissue swelling or fluid for ≥6 weeks of PIP, MCP, wrist, elbow, knee, ankle, MTP joints)

3. Arthritis of hand joints ≥6 weeks (*not* DIP joint)

4. Symmetrical arthritis ≥6 weeks (for joints defined in 2)

5. Rheumatoid nodules

6. Serum rheumatoid factor

7. X-ray changes of rheumatoid arthritis

*The presence of more than four of the seven criteria is diagnostic.

DIP = distal interphalangeal; MCP = metacarpophalangeal; MTP = metatarsophalangeal; PIP = proximal interphalangeal.

2. **X-ray films of involved joints**—changes to look for are:
   (a) soft-tissue swelling
   (b) joint space narrowing
   (c) juxta-articular osteoporosis
   (d) joint erosions.
   Investigations used to assess the activity of the disease include:
1. ESR or CRP—remember that the differential diagnosis of a raised ESR in rheumatoid arthritis includes:
   (a) active disease
   (b) amyloidosis
   (c) infection
   (d) Sjögren's syndrome
2. haemoglobin measurement—the severity of normochromic anaemia usually correlates with activity
3. anti-CCP, and rheumatoid factor titres
4. the presence of progressive erosions on serial X-ray films.

Treatment

1. Remember that treatment is palliative rather than curative and the limitations and problems of treatment should be made clear to the patient from the start. The principles of treatment include:
   - education
   - physiotherapy, including exercise and splinting of the joints to prevent deformity
   - occupational therapy
   - drug treatment aimed at reducing pain and inflammation (with aspirin, other NSAIDs or COX-2 inhibitors) and at preventing progression of the disease. The gastrointestinal toxicity of the traditional NSAIDs (i.e. peptic ulceration) is reduced by the COX-2 inhibitors; however, all can cause dyspepsia and renal disease (e.g. acute interstitial nephritis) and worsen renal function in patients with diabetic or atherosclerotic kidney disease; all NSAIDs are probably associated with an increased risk of myocardial infarction. If there is aspirin allergy, sodium salicylate is an alternative.
2. The use of slow-acting or disease-modifying, antirheumatic drugs (DMARDs) is now recommended early on for patients with active progressive disease, especially if there is evidence of joint destruction (see Table 9.3). These drugs include methotrexate, sulfasalazine, hydroxychloroquine, cyclosporin, leflunomide, azathioprine, penicillamine and gold (oral or injected). These medications have a slow onset of action (weeks for methotrexate to months for gold). There is evidence that they can lead to healing of bone erosions. Monitoring should include full blood count, urine testing for proteinuria and specific tests for

TABLE 9.3 Risk factors for destructive disease
1. High titre rheumatoid factor or positive anti-CCP
2. Constitutional symptoms
3. Insidious onset
4. Erosions early on X-ray
5. Rheumatoid nodules early
6. HLA DR-4

certain drugs, such as liver function tests for methotrexate, or ophthalmological examination and assessment of visual fields for hydroxychloroquine.

3. Methotrexate can be given orally or intramuscularly, usually 10–25 mg weekly, but starting with a low dose. It is usually better tolerated than the other DMARDs and is often the drug of first choice and given early in the course of the disease to decrease inflammation and sometimes the development of synovitis. Methotrexate may sometimes cause an increase in the number of rheumatoid nodules. It can be given alone or in combination with hydroxychloroquine and sulfasalazine. To decrease the risk of side effects of methotrexate, especially mouth ulcers, folic acid is given daily. Safety monitoring includes full blood count and liver function tests. Adverse reactions include rash, abnormal liver function tests (transaminases), leucopenia, thrombocytopenia and interstitial lung disease. It should not be given to patients with glucose-6-phosphate dehydrogenase deficiency.

4. Alternative agents in use include leflunomide (a pyrimidine antagonist that inhibits the proliferation of T cells) and cytokine-targeted monoclonal antibodies (anti-TNF, interleukin [IL]-1-receptor antagonists). The antibodies are either chimeric (infliximab) or completely humanised (adalimumab). Anti-TNF antibodies have been shown to be effective treatment when used in combination with methotrexate. These agents may be directed against TNF (infliximab, adalimumab) or against the TNF receptor (etanercept). They are given as subcutaneous injections or as an infusion (infliximab). Anti-TNF is effective in controlling symptoms and has been shown to reduce disease progression and the development of erosions. It increases susceptibility to serious infections (especially reactivation of TB) and there is an increased risk of lymphoma. These drugs are very expensive, but there is increasing evidence that their early use has dramatic effects on the prognosis of this disease. Other regimens include the use of cyclosporin in combination with methotrexate.

5. Parenteral gold therapy is also disease-modifying; it should always be given with a test dose first (5–10 mg), then 50 mg weekly until 1000 mg is reached, then decrease the frequency of the injections over several months to 50 mg once a month. Oral gold may be less effective. Gold is now used much less often, having been superseded by the above regimens. Monitor regularly for proteinuria and bone marrow depression (leucopenia or thrombocytopenia), which are indicators for the cessation of therapy.

6. d-penicillamine use is restricted by complications of renal toxicity and bone marrow depression; it is not often used now.

7. Local steroid injections are helpful for acute involvement of a joint and may give prolonged relief from pain and swelling and improve function. The main indications for steroid use are:
   - vasculitic complications of rheumatoid arthritis (where high doses are needed)
   - severe progressive disease, until suppressive treatment with another slow-acting antirheumatic drug becomes effective
   - chronic low-dose treatment, which may be justifiable in the elderly.

8. Surgery may be very effective treatment for severely diseased joints. Hip, shoulder and knee replacements are the most successful operations. Arthroplasty and relief of contractures can be of value, especially in the hands.

   The prognosis of this chronic, but often intermittent disease varies. Only a small minority have no permanent joint problems 10 years after diagnosis, and half have a disability that interferes with work by this time. The greater the number of involved joints at the outset and the more abnormal the inflammatory markers, the worse the prognosis. Life-expectancy is reduced by up to seven years as a result of the increased risk of gastrointestinal bleeding, the increased risk of infection and a threefold increased risk of atherosclerosis.

Systemic lupus erythematosus

This multisystem disorder occurs usually in patients between 20 and 40 years of age. Women are more often affected than men (8:1) and there is an increased incidence in families (monozygotic twins have a 50% concordance). There are associations with HLA-DR2, with HLA-DR3, and with homozygous deficiencies of the early components of complement. It presents diagnostic as well as long-term management problems. The diagnosis requires at least four of the 11 published criteria either currently or in the past (see Table 9.4.)

TABLE 9.4 American Rheumatism Association criteria for SLE

1. Malar rash—sparing the nasolabial folds

2. Discoid rash

3. Photosensitivity rash

4. Oral ulcers

5. Arthritis—non-erosive and affecting two or more peripheral joints

6. Serositis—pleurisy or pericarditis, with audible rub, effusion or ECG changes

7. Renal disorder—persistent proteinuria > 0.5g/day or cellular casts

8. Neurological disorder—seizures or psychosis not related to drugs or metabolic abnormalities

9. Haematological disorder—haemolytic anaemia, leucopenia, lymphopenia, thrombocytopenia

10. Immunological disorder—anti-DNA antibodies in abnormal titre, or anti-Sm antibody, or positive anti-phospholipid antibodies

11. Antinuclear antibody disorder—abnormal ANA titre

Note: Four or more manifestations of the 11 must be present serially or simultaneously

---

The history

1. Ask about the presenting symptoms (see Table 9.4):
   (a) general symptoms—malaise (100% of patients), weight loss (60%), nausea and vomiting (50%), thrombosis of veins or arteries (15%)
   (b) musculoskeletal symptoms (95%)—arthralgia, arthritis (typically symmetrical and non-erosive), myalgia and myositis
   (c) dermatological symptoms (85%)—skin rash, alopecia, oral and nasal ulcers
   (d) fever (77%)
   (e) neuropsychiatric symptoms (60%)—delirium, dementia, convulsions, chorea, neuropathy, loss of vision (optic neuritis), stroke, headache, symptoms resembling multiple sclerosis, anxiety and depression
   (f) renal tract symptoms (50%)—haematuria, oedema, renal failure (just about any type of glomerulonephritis)
   (g) respiratory tract symptoms (45%)—pleurisy
   (h) cardiovascular symptoms (40%)—pericarditis, myocarditis, valvular lesions, premature coronary artery disease (increased atherosclerosis)
   (i) haematological symptoms (50%)—lymphadenopathy, anaemia
   (j) gastrointestinal symptoms (30%)—nausea, diarrhoea, pseudo bowel obstruction, perforation

(k) thrombophlebitis, recurrent abortions or fetal death in utero (suggests antiphospholipid syndrome)

(l) sicca symptoms (secondary to Sjögren's syndrome)

(m) reduced activities of daily living and ability to work as a result of the effect of this chronic and relapsing disease on the patient's life.

2. Ask about any drug history (e.g. procainamide, hydralazine) (see Table 9.5). Remember, newer antiarrhythmic and antihypertensive drugs have made classical drug-induced lupus less common and typically the symptoms resolve rapidly with cessation of the drug; autoantibody levels (anti-histone) diminish slowly. Anti-TNF drugs can also cause a lupus-like syndrome with a positive ANA and anti-double-stranded DNA; minocycline and hydralazine do this too, but with these drugs ANCA (antineutrophil cytoplasmic antibody) is positive as well.

3. Ask about any treatment given and any complications of treatment.

4. Ask about problems during pregnancy and use of contraception.

5. Enquire about the family history.

6. Enquire about the patient's understanding of the implications of this chronic and incurable disease and its prognosis.

TABLE 9.5 Drugs inducing SLE

1. Procainamide (most patients are ANA-positive within 1 year; 15–20% develop SLE)

2. Hydralazine (most patients are ANA-positive within 1 year; 5–10% develop SLE)

3. Isoniazid*

4. Methyldopa*

5. Penicillamine*

6. Chlorpromazine*

7. Anticonvulsants,* particularly phenytoin (not sodium valproate)

Note: There is an increased incidence of drug-induced lupus in slow acetylators who will develop a positive ANA and clinical manifestations sooner than rapid acetylators. Drug-induced lupus is more common in the elderly because of the more frequent use of drugs in this group. There is usually no renal or nervous system disease, no antibody to dsDNA, and improvement *may* occur if the drug is withdrawn.

*Rarely cause overt SLE, but ANA is commonly positive.

The examination (see Table 9.6)

1. Inspect the patient for weight loss and Cushingoid appearance (because of steroid treatment) and assess the patient's general mental state.

2. Examine all the skin for a discoid erythematous raised rash, a photosenstivity rash and a classical malar rash. Remember that discoid lupus erythematosus (DLE) occurs in 20% of SLE patients. This disfiguring skin disease leads to permanent hair loss with telangiectasia, scaling, circular erythematous lesions and follicular plugging. There is often destruction of skin appendages. DLE can occur without other features of SLE.

3. Look at the hands for vasculitis, which can produce nail-fold infarcts and ischaemia or gangrene, and rash (e.g. photosensitivity, diffuse maculopapular rash).

4. Look for Raynaud's phenomenon and arthropathy (fusiform swelling of the PIP joints or synovitis, possibly in a rheumatoid arthritis distribution—10% develop swan neck deformity and ulnar deviation of the fingers).

5. Look at the forearms for livedo reticularis and purpura as a result of vasculitis or thrombocytopenia. Test for proximal myopathy caused by actual disease or secondary to steroid treatment.

TABLE 9.6 Systemic lupus erythematosus

1. GENERAL INSPECTION
Cushingoid
Weight
Mental state
	5. CHEST
	Cardiovascular system—endocarditis
	Respiratory system—pleural effusion,
	    pleurisy, pulmonary fibrosis, collapse
	    or infection

2. HANDS Vasculitis Rash Arthropathy (symmetric polyarthritis)	**6. ABDOMEN** Hepatosplenomegaly Tenderness
3. ARMS Livedo reticularis Purpura Proximal myopathy (SLE, steroids)	**7. HIPS** Aseptic necrosis
	8. LEGS Feet—small joint synovitis Rash Proximal myopathy Cerebellar ataxia Neuropathy (uncommon) Hemiplegia Mononeuritis multiplex
4. HEAD Alopecia, lupus hairs Eyes—scleritis, cytoid lesions etc. Mouth—ulcers (painless), infection Rash (e.g. butterfly)—spares nasolabial folds Cranial nerve lesions Cervical adenopathy	**9. OTHER** Urine analysis (proteinuria) Blood pressure (hypertension) Temperature chart

6. Inspect the head. Look for alopecia. Lupus hairs are characteristic: they occur above the forehead and are short, broken hairs that grow back quickly after hair loss (except in patients with DLE).

7. Look at the eyes for keratoconjunctivitis sicca and for pale conjunctivae owing to anaemia, and look at the fundi for cytoid lesions (hard exudates secondary to vasculitis).

8. Look in the mouth for ulcers and infection. Note any facial rash (butterfly photosensitivity rash [30%], discoid lupus or diffuse maculopapular rashes). Feel the cervical and axillary nodes.

9. Examine the chest. In the cardiovascular system, note signs of pericarditis or murmurs (Libman-Sacks endocarditis is very uncommon).

10. In the respiratory system, note signs of pleural effusion, pleuritis, interstitial lung disease or atelectasis.

11. Examine the abdomen for splenomegaly (usually mild) and hepatomegaly. Feel for abdominal tenderness.

12. Examine the hips for signs of aseptic necrosis.

13. Examine for proximal weakness in the legs, cerebellar ataxia, hemiplegia and transverse myelitis. Assess mental status (cognitive changes, even psychosis).

14. Also examine for neuropathy (mainly sensory) and mononeuritis multiplex, as well as thrombophlebitis and leg ulceration.

15. Look at the urine analysis for evidence of renal disease (haematuria and proteinuria).

16. Take the blood pressure (it may be elevated in renal disease). Also look at the temperature chart for fever, indicating active disease or secondary infection.

TABLE 9.7 Antibodies associated with connective tissue diseases

Disease	Antibodies associated
Systemic lupus erythematosus	Anti-single-stranded DNA—not specific (useless!) Anti-dsDNA (70%)—high titres are specific Anti-Sm (30%)—specific for lupus Anti-RNP (30% in low titre)—high titre in MCTD Anti-Ro-SS-A (30%)—associated with primary Sjögren's syndrome, congenital heart block; can cause nephritis Anti-SS-B (15%)—associated with Sjögren's syndrome Antihistone (drug-induced SLE usually from hydralazine, or procainamide; 95%) Antiphospholipid (50%)—include anticardiolipin and lupus anticoagulant Antierythrocyte (60%)—occasionally causes anaemia Anti-platelet Antilymphocyte (70%)—possible leucopenia
Scleroderma and CREST	Anticentromere (CREST: 70%; scleroderma: 10%) Antinucleolar, anti-Scl-70 (scleroderma: 30%) Anti-RNP, anti-SS-A (scleroderma occasionally in low titre) Antinuclear antigen (90%)
Sjögren's syndrome	Anti-SS-A (70%), anti-SS-B (60%)
Mixed connective tissue disease (MCTD)	Anti-RNP (100%)
Polymyositis and dermatomyositis	Anti-Jo-1 (polymyositis: 30%; dermatomyositis: 30%) Anti-Mi2 (10% dermatomyositis) Anti-SRP (aggressive disease)

CREST = calcinosis cutis; Raynaud's phenomenon; (o)esophageal involvement; sclerodactyly; telangiectasia; RNP = ribonucleoprotein; Sm = smith; SRP = signal recognition protein.

Investigations

1. Diagnosis depends on a combination of the symptoms, signs and laboratory test results (see Tables 9.4, 9.5 and 9.7). Almost all cases are ANA-positive, which is very sensitive but not specific (if ANA-negative, check SSA/SSB). Very specific tests for SLE are anti-dsDNA (including titre, 100% specific) and anti-Sm (positive virtually only in SLE).

2. Patients who do not fit the criteria may have another connective tissue disease. Mixed connective tissue disease (MCTD) is suggested by the overlapping clinical features of scleroderma, polymyositis and SLE and the presence of characteristic antibodies to nuclear ribonucleoprotein (nRNP), which is one of the extractable nuclear antigens. Anti-nRNP is present in high titre and produces a speckled pattern on fluorescent antibody testing in patients with MCTD. When these patients are followed for many years, they may start to resemble patients with progressive systemic sclerosis or SLE, or may continue with a relatively undifferentiated connective tissue disease.

3. MRI scans and lumbar puncture (increased protein and mononuclear cells) may be indicated if central nervous system lupus is suspected. Central nervous system symptoms often correlate poorly with serological measures of the activity of the disease. Do not miss bacterial meningitis in SLE.

4. Haematological tests:

(a) Anaemia—normochromic, normocytic and related to the chronic inflammatory processes—is very common. Immune haemolytic anaemia is less common and the Coombs' test then gives a positive result.

(b) The ESR tends to be elevated but the CRP is often normal, except during episodes of serositis.

(c) Leucopenia (especially lymphopenia) occurs in over half the patients and may be caused by antibody directed against leucocytes.

(d) The lupus anticoagulant and anticardiolipin antibodies, or both, are found in about 10% of cases. Characteristically, there is a prolonged partial thromboplastin time with kaolin (PTTK), which is not corrected by the addition of normal plasma. It is associated with thrombosis rather than bleeding.

(e) Thrombocytopenia occurs in 15% of cases and is associated with anti-platelet antibodies.

5. Immunological tests:

(a) The characteristic abnormalities are the presence of autoantibodies (see Table 9.7). ANAs are present in 99% of cases and are usually detectable from the time of onset of symptoms. The antigens involved include single- and double-stranded DNA, SS-A and SS-B, and Sm antigen (an acidic nuclear protein). Many antibodies persist even when the disease is quiescent. Antibodies to dsDNA and Sm are the most specific for SLE and are therefore the most useful diagnostically. The latter, however, is not very sensitive.

(b) Complement abnormalities are usual during exacerbations of the disease, with a reduction in total haemolytic complement (CH50) and in the components of the classical pathway (C3 and C4). The combination of a low CH50 and normal C3 suggests an inherited deficiency of complement components and is strongly associated with SLE. The finding of high levels of anti-dsDNA and lower complement levels is usually associated with active disease and especially renal involvement.

(c) Positive rheumatoid factor occurs in 10% of cases at low titre. Skin biopsy in SLE can be helpful; positive immunofluorescence of the basement membrane in involved skin occurs in 95% of patients.

Treatment

Current work suggests that appropriate treatment to suppress exacerbations of SLE will prolong life. Many patients have mild disease without life-threatening complications. The prognosis of SLE is generally good. There is a 75% 10-year survival rate; the major causes of death are infections, renal failure, lymphoma and myocardial infarction.

1. Arthralgias, myalgia and fever respond to rest and NSAIDs.

2. Exposure to sunlight should be avoided and sunscreen used.

3. Hydroxychloroquine is useful in the management of arthritis and skin rash. Annual retinal and visual field examinations must be performed in patients on this drug because of the cumulative risk of retinal toxicity.

4. Raynaud's phenomenon may respond to calcium channel antagonists.

5. Steroids are indicated for central nervous system involvement, pericarditis, myocarditis, pleurisy, severe haemolytic anaemia and thrombocytopenia. Use of high initial doses with gradual reduction once improvement occurs is the proper method of treatment.

6. Hypercoagulability (thrombotic episodes and antiphospholipid antibodies) should be treated with warfarin for life, with a target INR of 2.5–3.

7. Management of renal disease is difficult. Renal biopsy usually shows abnormalities, but often only mild changes. Virtually any type of glomulonephritis may occur. Renal biopsy is indicated early if there is any clinical or biochemical

evidence of renal disease or if the urine sediment is abnormal. Four main groups of biopsy abnormalities can be identified:
- mesangial proliferation
- focal glomerulonephritis
- diffuse proliferation
- membranous proliferation.

Mesangial proliferation has the best prognosis—disease is unlikely to progress. Diffuse proliferative glomerulonephritis has the worst prognosis and aggressive treatment (e.g. high-dose pulse steroids plus cyclophosphamide) is recommended. Membranous proliferation has a low rate of response to treatment. SLE is not a contraindication to dialysis or renal transplant in those patients who develop renal failure, but there is a higher than average risk of graft failure.

8. Calcium and vitamin D supplements should be offered to protect against osteoporosis. Bisphosphonates should be considered if long-term steroid treatment is likely.
9. Azathioprine is indicated as a steroid-sparing agent. Cyclophosphamide is a more toxic alternative. Intermittent pulses of cyclophosphamide may be helpful. These agents are particularly indicated in active glomerulonephritis.
10. Mycophenalate and a number of new biological agents are being tested in clinical trials. Autologous stem cell transplant is also an experimental treatment.
11. Remember that postpartum exacerbations of lupus may occur. Spontaneous abortions are common in women with antiphospholipid antibodies. Treatment with anticoagulation (heparin plus low-dose aspirin—never prescribe warfarin) may be effective in reducing the risk of abortion. Steroids may be used in pregnancy because, except for dexamethasone, these do not cross the placenta. Women with the anti-Ro (SSA/SSB) antibody may have babies with permanent complete heart block and transient erythematous rashes.

Systemic vasculitis

Patients with a systemic vasculitic illness will often be used for the long-case examination because of the complex nature of these illnesses and the frequent need for hospitalisation. The fact that these illnesses tend to affect multiple body systems across numerous specialties is ideal to test candidates' general approach to internal medicine. The majority of cases seen in the examination will have a vasculitis such as Wegener's granulomatosis, giant cell arteritis or polyarteritis nodosa. Occasionally, less common adult vasculitides, such as Churg-Strauss syndrome or microscopic polyarteritis, will be encountered.

The long-case examination for the patient with systemic vasculitis requires the candidate to take a careful history and examine the patient in a thorough general manner, as well as look for specific abnormalities in each disease. Candidates will be expected to have a good knowledge of the various investigative tools available to diagnose vasculitis. The course of treatment will invariably be discussed in this type of case, particularly the side effects of long-term medications and likely prognosis.

The history

In most cases, the onset of a systemic vasculitic illness is subacute rather than acute. The patient has often seen several practitioners before a diagnosis is made. The history will be critical in determining the diagnosis if the patient has a systemic vasculitis and presents a diagnostic problem, or indeed if there are significant management issues.

1. First, ask about the systemic features that would suggest a vasculitic illness: fatigue, malaise, fever, myalgia and arthralgia will be very frequent in these

patients. Ask about vasculitic skin rash, which would normally be in the form of palpable purpura. Ask about the pattern of joint involvement.

2. Next ask about a history of renal disease, particularly hypertension or renal failure, and any gastrointestinal symptoms.

3. **Wegener's granulomatosis** (small or medium-sized vessels, venules and capillaries causing a pulmonary–renal syndrome): the upper and lower respiratory tract are almost invariably involved and frequent symptoms include:
   • nasal congestion
   • rhinorrhoea
   • bloody nasal discharge
   • cough (which is initially a dry cough, but may evolve into haemoptysis)
   • breathlessness.

4. **Giant cell arteritis:** patients are generally in the sixth, seventh or eighth decade of life. About 20% of patients with polymyalgia rheumatica develop giant cell arteritis. The usual specific symptoms are:
   • severe bitemporal headache
   • less commonly, visual disturbance (e.g. diplopia) or visual loss
   • jaw claudication, or occasionally tongue claudication.
   Other focal neurological symptoms can also occur.

5. **Polyarteritis nodosa** (medium-sized arteries): the specific symptoms depend on which arteries are involved—coronary arteries, mesenteric arteries or renal arteries. Suspect this possibility if there are multiple systems involved (e.g. foot drop with chest and abdominal pain). Ask about risk factors for hepatitis B (one-third of cases).

6. **Churg-Strauss vasculitis** (small vessels causing a pulmonary–renal syndrome): patients almost invariably have asthma first, then a peripheral eosinophilia. Ask about a previous history of:
   • asthma
   • allergic rhinitis, nasal polyps
   • eczema
   • cough and breathlessness
   • peripheral nervous system disease, either in the form of symmetrical peripheral neuropathy or mononeuritis multiplex.

7. **Microscopic polyarteritis** (small vessels causing a pulmonary–renal syndrome): the major problem is usually with renal impairment and lung disease, which may not have any specific symptoms. Systemic symptoms of vasculitis are generally very prominent.

8. **Mixed essential cryoglobulinaemia** (small vessels due to rheumatoid factor bound to IgG): patients present with:
   • palpable purpura of the extremities
   • Raynaud's disease
   • arthritis
   • neuropathy.
   Hepatitis C is common.

The examination

1. The patient with systemic vasculitis usually looks unwell. Check for fever, sinus tachycardia, pallor and signs of recent weight loss.

2. Look for livedo reticularis (a net-like pattern). The differential diagnosis includes cholesterol atheroembolism after a vascular procedure, antiphospolipid syndrome and vasculitis. Other mimics of vasculitis include atrial myxoma, bacterial endocarditis and thrombotic thrombocytopenic purpura (TTP).

3. Other physical signs will be more specific to the actual underlying illness:
   - **Wegener's granulomatosis:** look for the classical collapse of the nasal septum (a saddle-shaped nose, which also occurs in relapsing polychondritis). There may be evidence of tachypnoea and crackles throughout the lung field. Fluid overload may occur in the setting of worsening renal failure.
   - **Giant cell arteritis:** tender and indurated temporal arteries will often be present. There may be abnormal eye signs if there is retinal involvement. Focal neurological signs should be sought.
   - **Polyarteritis nodosa:** there may be evidence of painful skin nodules in rare cases, as well as palpable purpura and livedo reticularis. Look for mononeuritis multiplex.
   - **Churg-Strauss vasculitis:** look for signs of allergic disease, such as swollen nasal turbinates, nasal polyps and evidence of bronchospasm. Examine the peripheral nervous system carefully, looking for single nerve lesions or symmetrical peripheral neuropathy generally affecting the lower limbs.
   - **Microscopic polyarteritis:** urinalysis is the key—look for any evidence of proteinuria or haematuria.
   - **Mixed essential cryoglobulinaemia:** look for Raynaud's disease, palpable purpura and peripheral neuropathy. Assess for signs of liver disease (hepatitis C).

Investigations

Investigations will be critical in determining the diagnosis in systemic vasculitis.

1. In most cases a biopsy of affected tissue is the most reliable way of making the diagnosis; other investigations will raise the suspicion that vasculitis is the problem and direct the clinician to a suitable biopsy site.
2. It will often be necessary to exclude systemic infection, malignancy or generalised autoimmune disease.
3. In vasculitis, the ESR is invariably raised, often at levels of >70 mm/h. There is frequently a normochromic normocytic anaemia and there may be neutrophilia. The platelet count may be elevated.
4. Renal function will often be impaired in Wegener's granulomatosis, polyarteritis nodosa and microscopic polyarteritis.
5. Abnormal liver function tests, particularly elevated transaminase levels, may be found in Wegener's granulomatosis and in polyarteritis nodosa. Liver function abnormalities are also reported in giant cell arteritis.
6. Urine abnormalities will often be found in the form of urinary casts and the presence of dysmorphic red blood cells in the urine, particularly in Wegener's granulomatosis, microscopic polyarteritis and polyarteritis nodosa.
7. The chest X-ray will often show a bilateral diffuse interstitial abnormality in Wegener's granulomatosis (see Fig 15.22) and a peripheral fluffy, patchy infiltrative pattern in Churg-Strauss vasculitis.
8. **Wegener's granulomatosis:** the critical investigation is the cytoplasmic (c) antineutrophil cytoplasmic antibody (c-ANCA). This will be present in a vast majority of cases of Wegener's granulomatosis. Further testing of this antibody will reveal the presence of anti-pr3 antibodies. The presence of a typical clinical syndrome with a positive c-ANCA and pr3 antibodies is virtually diagnostic of Wegener's granulomatosis. The need for a tissue biopsy may be avoided if these tests are positive. Occasionally, patients with upper airways disease only will not have a positive c-ANCA test.
9. **Giant cell arteritis:** diagnosis depends on a positive tissue sample. Don't delay starting steroids to make a definite diagnosis (the biopsy can be done within two weeks of starting steroids). Temporal artery biopsy should reveal the

diagnosis as long as a generous biopsy is taken by the surgeon, but the artery on the other side may need to be sampled in some cases.

10. **Polyarteritis nodosa:** tissue samples are often not available. Many organs may be involved (see Table 9.8). If symptoms or signs point this way, a biopsy of nerve, muscle or testis may be diagnostic; renal biopsy is not helpful. Angiography is sometimes helpful in this illness, particularly of the mesenteric arteries, but possibly also of the coronary arteries. Bead-like aneurysmal dilation of the arteries is suggestive of polyarteritis.

11. **Churg-Strauss vasculitis:** 50% of patients will have a positive perinuclear (p) ANCA test. The other important diagnostic tool is the tissue biopsy, which will reveal intense eosinophilia. Sural nerve biopsy will sometimes be required in the setting of neuropathy and this will show vasculitis.

12. **Microscopic polyarteritis:** this is characterised by a positive p-ANCA result. This antibody is directed against myeloperoxidase. Renal biopsy is usually necessary to establish the diagnosis.

13. p-ANCA is rare in other inflammatory diseases, but common in patients with vasculitis (c-ANCA is specific for Wegener). ANCA titres do not correspond with the clinical severity of the patient's illness and they may be only markers of disease. Remember that p-ANCA tests may be positive (but MPO negative) in other conditions including inflammatory bowel disease, autoimmune hepatitis and primary sclerosing cholangitis, as well as in health (5%).

TABLE 9.8 Clinical findings in patients with polyarteritis nodosa

Site	Clinical problem	Incidence
Muscles and joints	Myalgia, arthritis	65%
Kidneys	Hypertension, renal impairment	60%
Gut	Nausea, vomiting, abdominal pain, bowel, liver or pancreatic infarcts	45%
Peripheral nervous system	Mononeuritis multiplex, peripheral neuropathy	50%
Central nervous system	Strokes and seizures	25%
Skin	Purpura, infarcts, Raynaud's phenomenon	40%
Heart	Cardiac failure, infarction, pericarditis	35%
Genitourinary	Ovarian, testicular pain or infarction	20%

Treatment

Systemic vasculitis will generally require aggressive immunosuppressive medication. Failure to suppress the vasculitis aggressively can result in permanent injury, progressive deterioration and death.

1. **Wegener's granulomatosis (deadly if untreated):** high-dose corticosteroids and daily oral cyclophosphamide should be instituted. Trimethoprim sulfamethoxazole is adjunctive therapy. Biological agents are being investigated for treatment of Wegener's. Rituximab shows the most promise, but should not be used at this stage unless other agents have failed.

2. **Giant cell arteritis:** high-dose oral corticosteroids are required, typically for one to two years.

3. **Polyarteritis nodosa:** the untreated five-year survival rate is less than 20%. A combination of high-dose prednisone and cyclophosphamide will usually be very effective (90% long-term remission). Treatment may often be discontinued after remission is obtained and the long-term prognosis is very good. Interferon

alpha, or the antiviral drug vidarabine, may help to induce remission if there is associated hepatitis B infection.

4. **Churg-Strauss vasculitis:** the eosinophilic vasculitis of the Churg-Strauss syndrome is generally very steroid responsive, but occasionally other cytotoxic agents need to be used. Steroids alone have been shown to increase the five-year survival rate from 25% to 50%.

5. **Microscopic polyarteritis:** corticosteroids combined with immunosuppressive agents are usually required, with renal support in patients who develop renal failure.

6. The duration of treatment for all of these vasculitic illnesses needs to be individualised. Patients with giant cell arteritis can come off treatment after about two years, but some have disease for several years. Most of the other diseases will require maintenance therapy.

7. Patients often suffer the effects of long-term steroid therapy and immuno-suppression, such as osteoporosis, hypertension, diabetes and accelerated vascular disease. Prevention should be aggressively pursued. Infection (e.g. *Pneumocystis* pneumonia) is common in this group and can be serious or fatal.

8. Patients on cyclophosphamide need careful monitoring of their blood count and careful counselling to ensure adequate fluid intake and avoid haemorrhagic cystitis. They also deserve an annual urinalysis for haematuria once therapy is ceased; haematuria may indicate the development of bladder cancer.

Antiphospholipid antibody syndrome

Antiphospholipid syndrome is a disease that not infrequently requires patients to be admitted to hospital for its various complications. It therefore may crop up as a long case in the examination. The disease can be either primary or secondary. The secondary form is usually a complication of other autoimmune conditions, the most common of which is SLE. The main antibody in this disease is directed against the phospholipid-beta$_2$-glycoprotein 1 complex, on which it exerts a procoagulant effect. It has also been described in HIV infection.

The history

Patients with antiphospholipid syndrome commonly suffer thrombosis (see Table 9.9).

TABLE 9.9 Clinical manifestations of the antiphospholipid antibody syndrome
1. Cardiac—myocardial infarction, valvular heart disease, pulmonary hypertension
2. Haematological—haemolytic anaemia, thrombocytopenia, migraine, epilepsy, transverse myelopathy
3. Renal—renal vein thrombosis
4. Endocrine—Addison's disease (adrenal vein thrombosis)
5. Neurological—cerebral ischaemia (stroke, multi-infarct dementia)
6. Gastrointestinal—bowel ischaemia
7. Obstetric—recurrent abortions, intrauterine growth retardation
8. Dermatological—livedo reticularis, ulcers

1. Ask about venous thromboses. The most common site is the deep lower limb or pelvic veins, but the axillary veins can be involved.

2. Ask about arterial thromboses. Stroke and myocardial infarction are the most common arterial complications.

3. Enquire about a history of recurrent first-trimester and later abortion. Anti-phospholipid syndrome is far more common in females and otherwise unexplained first-trimester abortions are very characteristic of this disease. Other obstetric complications include intrauterine growth retardation and an increased tendency for hypertension in pregnancy.
4. Ask about bleeding problems associated with thrombocytopenia, skin changes (especially livedo reticularis), central nervous system complications such as migraine and chorea, and eclampsia or pre-eclampsia with the HELLP syndrome:
    Haemolysis, Elevated Liver enzymes, Low Platelets
5. Ask about features of the underlying disorder, such as SLE, which suggest the patient has a secondary form of antiphospholipid syndrome.

The examination
Unless the patient has an active thrombosis there are unlikely to be any abnormal physical signs. Look especially for:
1. signs of any associated autoimmune diseases, particularly skin rashes and joint abnormalities in SLE, and dry eyes and mouth in Sjögren's syndrome
2. livedo reticularis rash on the lower limbs
3. heart murmurs from sterile valve vegetations.

Investigations (see also p 149)
1. The detection of IgG anticardiolipin antibodies is diagnostic for the antiphospholipid syndrome if the antibodies are in high titre and found in the correct clinical context. IgM anticardiolipin antibodies may be detected, although these are less specific.
2. The lupus inhibitor is a related antibody (both are antibodies to phospholipid) that confers an even greater risk of thrombosis and pregnancy complications. The lupus inhibitor is also associated with a prolonged activated partial thromboplastin time (APTT) not corrected in a mixing study.
3. Antibodies to beta$_2$-glycoprotein-1 (B2-GP-1) in high titre may be present in the appropriate clinical setting.
4. In any patient with antiphospholipid syndrome, it is worth checking the ANA and other autoimmune serology as indicated. The platelet count should also be measured. The venereal disease research laboratory (VDRL) test may be falsely positive.
5. X-rays of the hands may show calcinosis in scleroderma patients (see Fig 9.1).

Treatment
1. Any patient with thrombotic complications of the antiphospholipid syndrome should be considered for treatment with anticoagulants for life (consider whether the benefits exceed the risks for individual patients).
2. The patient with anticardiolipin antibodies, but no clinical abnormalities, presents a difficult clinical situation. There are no data to support routine anticoagulation in this situation, but clearly there is a risk of arterial thrombosis.
3. The patient who has had obstetric problems in the past but no history of thrombosis also presents a dilemma for clinicians. The literature supports the use of anticoagulation therapy only in those with anticardiolipin antibodies or lupus inhibitor in whom a thrombotic complication has previously occurred.
4. Women who have suffered recurrent abortion will require treatment during pregnancy. Low-molecular-weight heparin would normally be used throughout the pregnancy, with the addition of low-dose aspirin. There is no good evidence that corticosteroids improve survival of the fetus.

Figure 9.1 X-ray of the hands showing marked calcinosis (arrows).
Figure reproduced courtesy of The Canberra Hospital.

Systemic sclerosis (scleroderma)

This is a progressive disease of multiple organs. Although a rare disease, it crops up commonly in examinations. It is more common in women (3:1). The five-year survival at diagnosis is only 70%.

The history

1. Ask about symptoms:
   (a) dermatological symptoms—Raynaud's phenomenon (commonly the first symptom), tight skin, disability from sclerodactyly
   (b) arthritis—arthropathy in a rheumatoid distribution, carpal tunnel symptoms
   (c) gastrointestinal symptoms—dysphagia, heartburn (oesophagitis), diarrhoea (malabsorption)
   (d) renal tract symptoms—hypertension, chronic kidney disease
   (e) respiratory symptoms—symptoms of interstitial lung disease, pleurisy, known diagnosis of pulmonary hypertension
   (f) cardiac symptoms—symptoms of pericarditis, palpitations (arrhythmias), symptoms of cardiac failure (dilated cardiomyopathy)

(g) other symptoms—erectile dysfunction, hypothyroidism, history of non-melanoma skin cancer.

2. Graft versus host disease can mimic scleroderma. Also ask about a history of exposure to polyvinyl chloride (PVC), l-tryptophan (eosinophilic myalgia syndrome) and drugs (e.g. bleomycin, pentazocine). Nephrogenic systemic fibrosis can occur in dialysis patients exposed to gadolinium during an MRI. Also ask about drugs likely to aggravate Raynaud's phenomenon (e.g. beta-blockers); a possible association with silicone breast implants seems to have been negated.

3. Ask about treatment received (e.g. d-penicillamine) and side effects thereof.

4. Enquire about degree of disability—function at home, ability to work, financial security.

Scleroderma may be classified as limited or diffuse. Limited disease means involvement of the skin up to the elbows (and may include the face) without chest, abdominal or internal organ involvement, except for the oesophagus. These patients are usually anticentromere positive.

In CREST (typically a more limited form of scleroderma, usually with oesophageal involvement, which causes dysphagia), sclerodactyly is usually limited to the distal extremities and/or face. The signs are:

Calcinosis (calcific deposits in subcutaneous tissue at the ends of the fingers) (see Fig 9.1)
Raynaud's phenomenon (resulting in loss of tissue pulp at the ends of the fingers)
(o) Esophageal involvement
Sclerodactyly (tightening of the skin on the fingers)
Telangiectasia

Progressive pulmonary fibrosis (ILD) is more common in patients with diffuse disease, but pulmonary hypertension is six times more common in patients with limited disease; it tends to occur late in the course of the disease. Patients with rapidly progressing dyspnoea are more likely to have pulmonary hypertension than ILD.

Localised scleroderma is called *morphea*. It presents as single or multiple plaques of skin induration.

The examination (see Table 9.10)

1. Make a general inspection for weight loss (owing to malabsorption or dysphagia).

2. Look at the hands. Look for the signs of limited scleroderma. These include sclerodactyly (tightening of the skin of the fingers) with extension up to the elbow, telangiectasia, finger tapering, pitting scars, signs of calcinosis (calcific deposits in subcutaneous tissue at the ends of the fingers) and the effects of Raynaud's phenomenon (loss of tissue pulp at the ends of the fingers). Nail-fold capillaroscopy is useful, but few have the skill. The presence of dilated tortuous vessels (giant loops) almost always indicates an underlying connective tissue disorder of some sort. Assess hand function.

3. Look at the arms for skin changes and assess proximal weakness (myositis).

4. Examine the head. Note any alopecia. Look at the face for 'salt-and-pepper' pigmentation, loss of wrinkling, 'bird-like' or 'mouse-like' facies (because of puckering of the mouth) and telangiectasia. Check for any difficulty in closing the eyes, for dryness of the eyes (Sjögren's syndrome) and pale conjunctivae (anaemia). Check for any difficulty opening the mouth wide and for dryness and puckering of the mouth.

TABLE 9.10 Systemic sclerosis

1. GENERAL APPEARANCE
'Bird-like' facies
Weight loss (malabsorption)
Anaemia (malabsorption, bleeding from a watermelon stomach)

2. HANDS
CREST—calcinosis, atrophy of distal tissue pulp (Raynaud's), sclerodactyly, telangiectasia
Dilated capillary loops
Small joint arthropathy and tendon crepitus
Fixed flexion deformity
Hand function

3. ARMS
Oedema (early) or skin thickening and tightening
Pigmentation
Vitiligo
Hair loss
Proximal myopathy

4. HEAD
Alopecia
Eyes—loss of eyebrows, anaemia, dryness (Sjögren's), difficulty with closing
Mouth—dryness, puckered, difficulty with opening

Pigmentation
Telangiectasia

5. DYSPHAGIA
Ask patient about swallowing

6. CHEST
Tight skin ('Roman breast plate')
Heart—cor pulmonale, pericardial effusion, pericarditis, failure, arrhythmias, pulmonary hypertension, ischaemia
Lungs—fibrosis, reflux pneumonitis, chest infections, lung carcinoma, vasculitis

7. LEGS
Skin lesions
Vasculitis
Small joint arthropathy
Patellar crepitus

8. OTHER
Blood pressure (hypertension in renal involvement)
Urine analysis (proteinuria)
Temperature chart (infection)
Stool examination (steatorrhoea)
Cancer elsewhere (non-melanoma skin cancer)

5. Look at the chest for the 'Roman breast plate' effect as a result of skin tightening.
6. Examine the cardiovascular system for pericarditis, arrhythmias, cor pulmonale and cardiac failure (owing to myocardial fibrosis).
7. Examine the respiratory system for interstitial lung disease, reflux pneumonitis, infection, lung carcinoma and vasculitis.
8. Look for jaundice and xanthelasma (primary biliary cirrhosis occurs rarely with CREST). Scratch marks may be visible from pruritis.
9. Look at the legs for vasculitis and ulceration.
10. Take the blood pressure.
11. Check the urine analysis and temperature charts.

Investigations

1. The ESR may be raised. Anaemia may be present owing to chronic disease, iron deficiency (secondary to bleeding from oesophagitis), folate or vitamin B$_{12}$ deficiency (secondary to malabsorption), or a microangiopathic haemolytic anaemia, which is usually associated with renal disease.
2. Hypergammaglobulinaemia (particularly IgG) is present in 50% of cases. Rheumatoid factor is present in 25% and ANA is found in most cases. Anti-Scl-70 is positive in a minority with diffuse scleroderma. Anticentromere antibody is particularly associated with CREST (up to 70%) (see Table 9.7).
3. Investigations for malabsorption and dysphagia may be necessary.

4. Assess visceral involvement with chest X-ray films, respiratory function tests, high-resolution CT of the chest, gastroscopy or oesophageal manometry, depending on the clinical presentation.

Treatment

This debilitating chronic disease will expose the patient to the need for recurrent investigations and adjustments to treatment. These matters need careful explanation from the outset. Prognosis is worse in men and those with renal or late-onset disease. Patients with skin and gut involvement, but without other organ disease, have the best prognosis.

1. Symptomatic treatment includes avoiding vasospasm (by avoiding smoking, beta-blockers and cold weather). Aggressive treatment of reflux with proton pump inhibitors is important to prevent the formation of oesophageal strictures. Nifedipine, phenoxybenzamine, prazosin or methyldopa may help Raynaud's phenomenon. The prostacyclin analogue iloprost showed promise for Raynaud's phenomenon in scleroderma.
2. Artificial tears are useful for dry eyes and NSAIDs may help with joint symptoms.
3. Treat malabsorption (particularly bacterial overgrowth, with antibiotics).
4. d-penicillamine (an immunosuppressant drug that also interferes with collagen cross-linking) may be helpful for skin disease and may improve survival. It has been usual to start treatment with a low dose. Randomised studies have shown no advantage of higher doses. The drug has a number of severe side effects (see Table 9.11). Monthly full blood counts are usually recommended.
5. Cyclophosphamide is used if there is lung involvement and may improve other complications of the disease, especially if used early. Treatment is usually given for nine months.
6. Pericarditis, inflammatory myopathy and early interstitial lung disease may respond to steroids.
7. The endothelin receptor antagonist, bosentan, has been approved for the treatment of pulmonary artery hypertension associated with scleroderma for patients with WHO class III or IV symptoms.
8. Aggressive treatment of hypertension to prevent renal failure is vital—ACE inhibitors are the drug class of choice. An ACE inhibitor is often given to patients even with abnormal renal function to prevent hypertensive renal crises. Dialysis is not contraindicated.
9. Many other drugs have been tried for patients with scleroderma, including angiotensin receptor blockers, selective serotonin reuptake inhibitors, serotonin antagonists, topical nitrates and platelet inhibitors. There are no controlled trials showing that treatment can reverse the course of the disease.

TABLE 9.11 Side effects of d-penicillamine	
Severe	**More minor**
Glomerulonephritis and nephrotic syndrome	Alteration of taste
Myasthenia gravis	Skin rashes
Thrombocytopenia	Fever
Leucopenia	Nausea
Aplastic anaemia	Anorexia

Chapter 10

The endocrine long case

I would like to see the day when somebody would be appointed surgeon somewhere who had no hands, for the operative part is the least part of the work.

Harvey Cushing (1869–1939)

Osteoporosis (and osteomalacia)

Osteoporosis is increasingly encountered in the long-case examination. The patient is often a postmenopausal woman or is taking corticosteroids for an acute or chronic inflammatory illness. Osteoporosis will commonly form part of another medical problem. Osteoporotic fractures can affect 30% of postmenopausal women over their lifetime. Many older women have undergone screening bone densitometry and may be aware that they have asymptomatic osteoporosis. Patients who have had a hip fracture or who have evidence of an endocrine disorder, malabsorption, liver disease, Crohn's disease or bone marrow disease, or who are taking certain medications, should have the possibility of osteoporosis considered while they are being evaluated (see Table 10.1).

The history

1. Ask about a history of fractures, particularly fractures of the wrist (risk increases from age 55), hip (risk increases from age 70), humerus and ribs, and vertebral compression fractures (especially T12), which may have occurred with minimal stress (risk increases from age 55). Acute back pain that subsides over weeks or months and then recurs may be caused by compression fractures.
2. If the patient has had a hip fracture, ask about any secondary complications, including pulmonary thromboembolism and nosocomial infections.
3. Ask about symptoms of bone pain, which may be diffuse, and proximal muscle weakness. These features may occur with osteomalacia (characterised by defective bone mineralisation in adults).
4. Ask about risk factors for osteoporosis (see Table 10.2). Determine the menstrual history and age of onset of menopause. Enquire about symptoms of thyroid excess or thyroid hormone replacement (thyroxine). Determine whether there are symptoms or a history of anaemia (e.g. coeliac disease).
5. Ask about toe pain and proximal weakness (osteomalacia, usually due to vitamin D deficiency—then you must exclude malabsorption).
6. Ask whether the patient has had skeletal X-ray examinations. Note that X-rays are insensitive for bone loss, because a substantial reduction of bone mass must occur before changes will be visible on the X-rays.

TABLE 10.1 Major secondary causes of osteoporosis

1. Endocrine diseases
   (a) Hyperthyroidism
   (b) Hyperparathyroidism
   (c) Cushing's syndrome
   (d) Growth hormone deficiency
   (e) Hyperprolactinaemia
   (f) Hypogonadism
2. Gastrointestinal diseases
   (a) Malabsorption syndromes (e.g. coeliac disease, Crohn's disease, gastric bypass)
   (b) Chronic cholestasis (e.g. primary biliary cirrhosis)
3. Malnutrition
   (a) Anorexia nervosa
   (b) Scurvy
   (c) Alcoholism
4. Bone marrow disorders
   (a) Multiple myeloma
   (b) Disseminated carcinoma
   (c) Lymphoma
   (d) Leukaemias
5. Connective tissue diseases
   (a) Marfan's syndrome, Ehlers-Danlos syndrome
   (b) Osteogenesis imperfecta
   (c) Rheumatoid arthritis
6. Drugs
   (a) Chronic heparin therapy
   (b) Steroids
   (c) Thyroxine over-replacement
   (d) Lithium
   (e) Phenytoin
   (f) Cyclosporin

7. Take a careful drug history. Medications that cause osteoporosis include alcohol, heparin, steroids, thyroxine over-replacement, anticonvulsants (by affecting vitamin D metabolism), and cyclosporin.
8. Enquire about a poor diet (a low-fat diet often limits calcium intake) or inadequate sunlight exposure if the patient is a nursing-home resident, or has a history of renal disease or phenytoin use (all risk factors for osteomalacia). Ask about the patient's exercise history, as physical activity throughout life preserves bone mass. Cigarette smoking reduces skeletal mass.
9. Determine any risk factors for falls: a greater risk of falls increases the risk of fracture at any level of osteoporosis.
10. Determine the social impact of the disease (e.g. immobility, pain, fear of falling).

TABLE 10.2 Causes of osteomalacia

1. Unavailability of vitamin D:

   (a) vitamin D malabsorption (e.g. coeliac disease, pancreatic insufficiency, cirrhosis)

   (b) abnormal vitamin D metabolism (e.g. chronic renal failure, pseudohypoparathyroidism)

   (c) decreased vitamin D bioavailability (e.g. inadequate sunlight, nephrotic syndrome, peritoneal dialysis)

2. Phosphate unavailability caused by phosphate-binding antacids, hereditary hypophosphataemia, tumour-induced osteomalacia (e.g. fibrous dysplasia of bone) and Fanconi's syndrome type 1 or 2

3. Normal anion gap metabolic acidosis (e.g. distal renal tubular acidosis [type I] with hypokalaemia and hypercalciuria, often caused by autoimmune disease such as Sjögren's syndrome or SLE)

The examination

There are usually no signs of osteoporosis unless a recent fracture has occurred.

1. Examine for bone tenderness and proximal weakness (osteomalacia). Look for bowing of the legs (rickets).
2. Look for signs of thyroid disease and Cushing's syndrome.
3. Thoracic kyphosis may be a sign of vertebral fractures.
4. Assess weight and general nutritional status.

Investigations

1. Bone densitometry using dual-energy X-ray absorptiometry (DEXA) of the lumbar spine and/or proximal femur remains the test of choice for evaluation of bone mineral density (BMD; see Table 10.3). *Osteopenia* is used to refer to a bone mineral density between 1 and 2.5 standard deviations below peak bone mass; *osteoporosis* refers to a bone mineral density of more than 2.5 standard deviations below peak bone mass. The measurement is often given as a T score. This is the number of standard deviations by which the measured bone density falls below the average for a young normal person of the same sex. Thus, a T score of less than –2.5 defines osteoporosis.

TABLE 10.3 Indications for bone mineral density assay

- Fracture occurring after minimal trauma

- All women ≥65 years and men ≥70 years (but guidelines vary)

- Monitoring of known low BMD after at least one year

- Monitoring of bone loss after prolonged steroid use or as a result of hypogonadism

- Monitoring of bone loss in primary hyperthyroidism, chronic liver disease, chronic renal disease, Crohn's disease, known malabsorption and rheumatoid arthritis

- Measurement of BMD 12 months after change in treatment for known low BMD

2. Review the serum calcium and alkaline phosphatase results. In osteoporosis, serum calcium and alkaline phosphatase levels should be normal. Alkaline phosphatase is usually elevated in all forms of osteomalacia. Check 25-OH vitamin D levels (not 1,25-OH vitamin D) if there are any risk factors for osteomalacia. If there is vitamin D deficiency, then serum 25-OH vitamin D levels are usually low (e.g. vitamin D malabsorption, chronic liver disease, lack of exposure to sunlight—especially common in nursing-home patients).

Assessment of calcium, parathyroid hormone and vitamin D levels will usually distinguish the most important causes of osteomalacia and allow specific diagnostic tests to be appropriately directed (see Table 10.4). A sustained elevation of alkaline phosphatase should lead to consideration of osteomalacia, as well as Paget's disease and metastatic malignancy to bone.

3. A full blood count and ESR estimation should be ordered to look for evidence of myeloproliferative disease, and renal and liver function tests should be ordered to exclude renal or hepatic disease.

4. Thyroid stimulating hormone should be measured to rule out thyrotoxicosis.

5. If osteoporosis is unexpectedly severe, then an EPG should be considered to rule out multiple myeloma. In men, a serum testosterone level is worthwhile.

TABLE 10.4 Tests in bone disease

Disease	Calcium	Phosphate	25-OH vitamin D	Parathyroid hormone	Alkaline phosphatase (bone)
Osteoporosis	N	N	N	N	N
Osteomalacia or rickets owing to malabsorption or dietary lack	Low–N	Low–N	Decreased	Increased–N	Increased
Osteomalacia with renal bone disease	Variable	N–increased	Variable	Increased–N	Increased
Familial hypophosphataemic rickets	N	Decreased	N	N	Increased
Primary hyperparathyroidism	Increased	Decreased–N	N	Increased–high N	Increased
Paget's disease	N	N	N	N	Increased
N = normal.					

6. Ask to review any skeletal X-rays.
   • In osteoporosis of the spine, there is characteristic loss of trabecular bone in the vertebral body, including accentuation of the vertebral endplates. The vertebral trabeculae become more prominent with the loss of horizontal trabeculae. Also look for collapse, anterior wedging and the codfish deformity (from expansion of the intervertebral disc; see Fig 10.1).
   • In osteomalacia, X-rays may show some decrease in bone density with coarsening of trabeculae and blurring of the margins. A specific abnormality is Looser's zones (pseudo fractures) in the long bone shafts; these are ribbon-like zones of rarefaction. Other characteristic abnormalities may include a triangular (trefoil) pelvis and biconcave collapsed vertebrae. If there is secondary hyperparathyroidism present with osteomalacia, then bone cysts, erosion of the distal ends of the clavicles and subperiosteal resorption in the phalanges may be seen.

7. In difficult cases, an iliac crest bone biopsy with double tetracycline labelling can help distinguish osteoporosis from osteomalacia.

Figure 10.1 X-ray of the lumbar spine showing loss of bone density (1), codfish deformity (2) and anterior wedging (3).
Figure reproduced courtesy of The Canberra Hospital.

8. Consider undertaking tests for secondary causes of osteoporosis if the clinical picture suggests this may be helpful.

Treatment
Established osteoporosis is currently not reversible with medical therapy. Early intervention can prevent progression of osteoporosis and is of value. Secondary causes of osteoporosis should be identified and corrected if present.

1. **Calcium.** Because calcium absorption decreases with age, calcium therapy has a modest benefit in both early and late postmenopausal women. Consumption of 1200–1500 mg of calcium daily in adults over the age of 65 is advisable.

2. **Vitamin D supplementation.** Moderate or severe vitamin D deficiency (serum 25-OH D < 25 nmol/L) should be treated with high-dose supplements of vitamin D of 3000–5000 IU/day for six to 12 weeks and then 1000 IU/day from then on. Elderly women in nursing homes who have inadequate intake should receive supplementation of vitamin D 800 IU/day and calcium 1200 mg/day. This has been shown to reduce non-vertebral fracture risk.

3. **Generally recommend ceasing smoking, avoiding excess alcohol consumption.** Institute fall prevention measures and prescribe regular weight-bearing exercise. Consider a hip protector.

4. **Bisphosphonates (risendronate and alendronate).** These drugs increase bone mineral density in postmenopausal women and have been shown to reduce the risk of fracture for postmenopausal women with osteoporosis by 50%. Patients unable to tolerate oral bisphosphonates can be given the drug as an infusion once every three months or, with some of the newer agents, once a year. The oral drugs can cause oesophageal ulceration that presents with odynophagia, usually within one to two months of commencing therapy. Osteonecrosis of the jaw is another serious possible side effect, which is more likely to occur with intravenous formulations in the presence of previous dental infections. These drugs are now indicated for patients older than 70 who have a BMD T score of −3 or less and for those who have had a fracture after minimal trauma.

   Strontium ranelate is an alternative drug for people who are unable to take bisphosphonates. Its effectiveness for preventing hip fractures has not been established, but there is evidence for its use in protecting against vertebral and rib fractures. It should be taken at bedtime at least two hours after eating.

5. **Oestrogen.** Hormone replacement therapy will prevent loss of cortical and trabecular bone in postmenopausal women. Therapy is probably more effective if started earlier in menopause as bone loss is most rapid then. Because oestrogen increases the risk of endometrial carcinoma, combination with progesterone is important unless a hysterectomy has been performed. A past history of endometrial cancer is a contraindication. There is an increased risk of breast cancer, as well as DVT and pulmonary embolism. Cardiovascular risk is also increased and hence its use in postmenopausal women has declined.

6. **Selective oestrogen receptor modulators.** Raloxifene, closely related to tamoxifen, reduces the risk of spine fractures. It increases the risk of DVT, but lowers the risk of breast cancer (and is not associated with an increased risk of endometrial cancer). Tamoxifen is a mixed oestrogen receptor antagonist and agonist that prevents bone loss. It increases the risk of endometrial cancer.

7. **Parathyroid hormone peptide.** This drug is very effective for osteoporosis but very expensive.

8. **Calcitonin.** There have been inconsistent results with calcitonin and any effect is smaller than with other therapies. The drug can be given subcutaneously or intranasally. Administration can cause nausea, flushing and inflammation.

9. **Men with osteoporosis.** In men who have osteoporosis and androgen deficiency, androgen replacement should be given unless there is a history of prostatic carcinoma. If there is secondary hypogonadism, human chorionic gonadotrophin or pulsatile gonadotrophin-releasing hormone may be worthwhile. Bisphosphonates and teriparatide (PTH) are efficacious in men; the role of raloxifene is not clear.

10. **Steroid-induced osteoporosis.** This is very important because, if prednisone is considered likely to be needed for a number of months or longer, then measures to prevent bone loss are important from the time steroids are begun, particularly in postmenopausal women or when high doses are needed. Co-administration of bisphosphonates is of value here. Calcium and 25-OH vitamin D in combination have also been shown to be effective. These are the only drugs that have been shown to reduce fracture risk for patients on steroids. Other general measures such as cessation of smoking and a regular exercise regimen are probably important and should be recommended to the patient.

11. **Surgical treatment of fractures.** This is often required. Frail elderly patients with other medical problems require careful assessment of anaesthetic risk.

Vertebral fractures may cause severe pain that requires potent analgesics. Bed rest should be as brief as possible. Injection of bone cement into the vertebral body (vertebroplasty) is a new treatment that may relieve pain and possibly has other benefits.

Hypercalcaemia

Hypercalcaemia is a common medical problem and therefore can appear in a long case. It is most likely to be a diagnostic problem. Most patients (90%) have hyperparathyroidism or malignancy (see Table 10.5). The asymptomatic patient usually has hyperparathyroidism. A malignant condition that is advanced enough to cause hypercalcaemia is likely to have caused other symptoms.

TABLE 10.5 Causes of hypercalcaemia
1. Primary hyperparathyroidism (from a solitary adenoma, or rarely multiple endocrine neoplasia)
2. Malignancy (e.g. metastatic breast cancer, lung or renal cancer releasing humoral mediators, haematological malignancies)
3. Increased vitamin D (excess ingestion, granulomatous disease) (increased 25-OH vitamin D)
4. Increased bone turnover (e.g. hyperthyroidism, thiazide diuretics, vitamin A intoxication)
5. Renal failure (CKD, secondary hyperparathyroidism)
6. Familial hypocalciuric hypercalcaemia
7. Other (e.g. lithium: increases parathyroid hormone)
CKD = chronic kidney disease.

The history

1. If the patient tells you that he or she has high calcium levels, enquire about the non-specific symptomatic manifestations. These include tiredness, weakness and episodes of confusion. Enquire about anorexia and constipation, as well as nausea and vomiting; acute abdominal pain from acute pancreatitis may have occurred. Enquire about polyuria and polydipsia. Ask about a history of hypertension or a slow heart rate.
2. Enquire about a history of peptic ulcer or renal colic ('stones, moans, bones and abdominal groans' from primary hyperparathyroidism). Ask about joint pain from pseudogout (chondrocalcinosis in primary hyperparathyroidism). Enquire about a past history of hypertension (hyperparathyroidism).
3. Ask the patient whether he or she was known to have a neck mass in the past or has had an operation to remove the parathyroid gland. In most cases a single adenomatous gland is found but they can be multiple. Surgical parathyroidectomy is the definitive treatment for primary hyperparathyroidism. Most neck masses will be coincidental thyroid nodules rather than a benign or malignant parathyroid tumour.
4. Ask whether the patient has had an eye examination and whether calcium was seen (band keratopathy). Also ask whether X-rays of the bones have been taken. In hyperparathyroidism, X-rays of the hand may show subperiosteal reabsorption with a moth-eaten appearance on the radial sides of the phalanges and in the distal phalangeal tufts (osteitis fibrosa cystica), as well as in the distal clavicles.
5. Determine whether there is any past history of malignant disease, including diseases that metastasise to bone (e.g. carcinoma or myeloma) or haematological disease such as lymphoma (ectopic vitamin D production).

6. Ask about drugs, including thiazide diuretics, lithium and ingestion of calcium or vitamin D.

7. Enquire about known renal failure, a cause of secondary hyperparathyroidism because of resistance to parathyroid hormone and growth of the size of the glands. These enlarged glands then produce partly non-suppressible parathyroid hormone and hypercalcaemia.

8. Ask about symptoms of thyrotoxicosis or phaeochromocytoma. Ask about recent immobilisation.

9. Check whether there is a family history of high serum calcium levels, such as familial hypocalciuric hypercalcaemia (autosomal dominant). Classically a patient with this condition has had hypercalcaemia since a relatively young age, with only a slight elevation in the serum parathyroid hormone level at most, and with a personal or family history of unsuccessful neck exploration; it does not require any therapy. A family history of hypercalcaemia may also occur with the multiple endocrine neoplasia syndromes, MEN1 and MEN2A. These are both autosomal dominant conditions. These patients may have symptoms related to the other features of their MEN syndrome (e.g. peptic ulceration from the Zollinger-Ellison syndrome owing to excess gastrin secretion).

10. Many patients are asymptomatic and had hypercalcaemia detected on a routine set of biochemical tests. Hyperparathyroidism has been recognised much more commonly since automated biochemical analyses have become routine.

The examination

1. Look for any evidence of a neck scar from parathyroid surgery, as well as forearm scars from re-implantation of the parathyroid gland from the neck.

2. Evaluate the patient for evidence of malignancy, including lymphadenopathy or organomegaly.

3. Look for evidence of renal failure.

4. Carefully evaluate the respiratory system for any evidence of sarcoidosis, as well as tuberculosis or histoplasmosis.

5. Take the pulse for bradycardia, a result of a high serum calcium level. Measure the blood pressure for evidence of phaeochromocytoma.

6. Examine for signs of thyrotoxicosis.

7. Look for pigmentation from Addison's disease.

8. Examine for proximal weakness and signs of pseudogout in the joints.

9. Examine the cornea for band keratopathy (calcification horizontally across the centre of the cornea).

Investigations

1. Look at the total serum calcium level. Remember that apparently high calcium levels can be the result of haemoconcentration while the blood is being collected. Correct for hypoalbuminaemia: add 0.02 mmol/L to the serum calcium concentration for every 1 g/L by which the serum albumin level is less than 40 g/L. The calcium level at which symptoms occur varies, but most patients have symptoms when the corrected calcium level reaches 3 mmol/L. Higher levels are associated with tissue calcification and the risk of renal failure, especially if the phosphate level is normal or increased by renal impairment. Once the calcium level approaches 4 mmol/L, unconsciousness and cardiac arrest can occur.

2. Measure the parathyroid hormone (PTH) level. If elevated, primary hyperparathyroidism is the most likely diagnosis (the PTH can be inappropriately in the high normal range in 10%; the phosphorous should be low). If the patient is taking lithium or thiazide, the test should be repeated after discontinuing drug

treatment, because these drugs may influence both calcium and parathyroid hormone secretion.

3. In a young otherwise asymptomatic person with a marginal elevation of parathyroid hormone, a 24-hour urine calcium examination should be asked for to exclude familial hypocalciuric hypercalcaemia (FHH). Alternatively, collect a fasting morning spot urine and measure the urine calcium/creatinine clearance ratio (<0.01 in FHH). This autosomal dominant condition is caused by faulty calcium sensing by the parathyroid glands and renal tubules.

4. If there is a low or undetectable parathyroid hormone level, consider the possibility of granulomatous disease, including sarcoidosis, tuberculosis, berylliosis, leprosy and lymphoma. An increased level of 25-OH vitamin D supports this possibility.

5. Ask to review the chest X-ray. Investigations to look for malignancy if suspected may then be required (e.g. protein electrophoresis, CT scan etc.).

Treatment

There is evidence that asymptomatic patients with hyperparathyroidism who are not treated have increased bone loss compared with controls. Significant increases in fracture risk (especially of the wrist and spine) have been demonstrated.

1. If the diagnosis is hyperparathyroidism and the patient is symptomatic, has renal stones or has a reduced bone density, surgical parathyroidectomy is usually indicated. If the patient is asymptomatic, then treatment is more controversial, but younger patients (<50 years) with higher serum or 24-hour urine calcium levels will usually be offered surgery. Preoperative localisation is not required for the skilled surgeon, but if there is a need for a repeat procedure this can be evaluated using ultrasonography, CT or technetium-99m sestamibi scanning.

2. Note whether there has been hypocalcaemia after surgery. If there is no residual parathyroid tissue left, lifelong vitamin D therapy is necessary or, alternatively, autotransplantation of parathyroid tissue into the forearm may be offered.

3. In malignant hypercalcaemia, the underlying tumour should be treated. Steroids are often effective in lowering the serum calcium level. With granulomatous disease, steroids are also effective in lowering the calcium level (but avoid if infection is the cause); chloroquine may be useful in patients who cannot tolerate steroids. Lithium treatment may need to be stopped. Hypercalcaemia does not necessarily mean lithium toxicity.

4. Familial hypocalciuric hypercalcaemia rarely causes symptoms and should not be treated with parathyroidectomy. Consider screening all first-degree relatives.

5. In an emergency, rehydration with intravenous saline and frusemide is indicated for hypercalcaemia. Parenteral calcitonin lowers calcium levels only transiently. The use of intravenous bisphosphonates is very effective.

Paget's disease of the bone (osteitis deformans)

This is usually a disease of the elderly but it may occur in younger patients. In populations from western or southern Europe up to 10% of people over the age of 85 are affected. The condition is characterised by excessive resorption of bone and increased formation of new bone in an irregular 'mosaic' pattern. Bone turnover may be increased 20 times early in the course of the disease. The aetiology is unknown but may be caused by a persistent paramyxovirus infection of osteoclasts. There are reports of familial occurrence (15% have a family history) and of autosomal dominant inheritance. The condition is rare in Asian populations. It presents as a management problem.

The history

1. Ask about symptoms that led to the diagnosis:
   (a) isolated elevation of alkaline phosphatase on routine blood testing
   (b) an incidental finding on an X-ray
   (c) bone pain
   (d) secondary osteoarthritis
   (e) change in height or hat size
   (f) progressive bone deformity or pathological fracture; gait abnormalities associated with change in length of a long bone
   (g) neurological symptoms—hearing loss, neurological gait disturbance (suggestive of basilar invagination with long tract signs, or cerebellar involvement or spinal cord compression), cranial nerve symptoms, headache
   (h) symptoms of congestive cardiac failure
   (i) symptoms of renal colic (as there is an increased incidence of calcium nephrolithiasis in this disease, especially during the resorptive phase)
   (j) gout, secondary to increased bone turnover
   (k) sarcoma of bone (very rare—less than 1% of cases, occasionally multicentric)
   (l) symptoms of hypercalcaemia—thirst, polyuria, nausea, coma (a rare occurrence even in immobilised patients, or alternatively caused by coexisting primary hyperparathyroidism, which is common)
   (m) pathological fractures, especially of the convex side of weight-bearing bones; can be multiple.
2. Enquire about articular pain, which may be caused by secondary osteoarthritis in joints adjacent to sites of Pagetic involvement, and true bone pain. Secondary osteoarthritis is characterised by pain and stiffness, which improves with joint movement; alternatively it may initially be exacerbated by weight-bearing and relieved by rest. True bone pain is more often constant or gnawing and is worse at night. A sudden exacerbation of bone pain may indicate a pathological fracture or the development of an osteosarcoma.
3. Ask about treatment, its effectiveness and side effects.
4. Enquire about disability at home and work. Remember, though, that most patients are asymptomatic.

The examination (see Table 10.6)

1. Inspect generally for short stature and obvious deformity.
2. Look at the face. Measure the skull diameter (>55 cm may be abnormal). Look for prominent skull veins, feel for bony warmth (actually caused by vasodilatation in the skin) and auscultate for systolic bruits. Examine the fundi for angioid streaks (see p 326) and for papilloedema or optic atrophy, which are rare. Also assess visual acuity and visual fields.
3. Test to see if hearing is decreased as a result of ossicle involvement or eighth nerve compression. Remember, *all* the other cranial nerves may rarely be affected owing to overgrowth of foramina or basilar invagination, so examine them carefully.
4. Look at the neck for basilar invagination. These patients have a short neck and low hairline, the head is held in extension and neck movements are decreased.
5. Assess the jugular venous pressure and examine the heart for signs of cardiac failure owing to a hyperdynamic circulation.
6. Examine the back. Note any deformity, especially kyphosis. Tap for tenderness. Feel for warmth. Auscultate for systolic bruits over the vertebral bodies.

TABLE 10.6 Paget's disease	
1. GENERAL INSPECTION Short stature Limb deformity Obvious osteosarcoma (bony swelling) **2. FACE** Skull diameter (measure) Auscultate skull (bruits) Fundi—angioid streaks, optic atrophy Hearing (ossicle or VIII nerve involvement) Other cranial nerves (foramina overgrowth or basilar invagination) **3. NECK** Short neck (basilar invagination) Jugular venous pressure—cardiac failure (high output) **4. BACK** Deformity	Tenderness Warmth Bruits **5. LEGS** Bowing femur, tibia Tenderness, warmth, swelling bones Hip examination (movements) Knee examination **6. GAIT** **7. NEUROLOGICAL ASSESSMENT OF LIMBS** (spinal cord compression, basilar invagination) **8. OTHER** Urine (blood) Height (measure)

7. Look at the legs for anterior bowing of the tibia and lateral bowing of the femur. Feel for warmth. Note any changes of osteoarthritis in the hips and knees. There may be limitation of hip movements—especially abduction, which suggests protrusio acetabulae—and fixed flexion deformity of the knees. Be careful, as the bones may be tender.

8. Sarcomas (a feared, but rare complication) should be looked for, particularly in the femur, humerus and skull; they usually present as tender, localised swellings. They can be multiple.

9. A full neurological examination is necessary for spinal cord compression and basilar invagination, which may even cause quadriparesis. If the patient is mobile, do not forget to assess walking for any disability (p 374). Cerebellar signs may also rarely occur with basilar invagination.

10. Check the urine analysis (for blood, as renal stone incidence is increased) and measure the patient's height (for serial follow-up).

Investigations

These are indicated in symptomatic patients requiring treatment and in asymptomatic subjects to determine the extent of skeletal involvement. Paget's disease is occasionally confused with osteoblastic bone secondaries (e.g. from prostate, Hodgkin's disease) or fibrous dysplasia.

1. Testing for hypercalcaemia may be worthwhile for any patient who is immobilised.

2. The serum alkaline phosphatase level is an indicator of disease activity, as is the urinary hydroxyproline level. Other biochemical markers of bone turnover will also be increased (e.g. osteocalcin, urine or serum cross-links of collagen).

3. Radiologically the bones most often involved are the pelvis, femur, skull and tibia (see Fig 10.2). Look for bony enlargement, increased density, an irregular widened cortex and cortical infractions (incomplete pseudofractures) on the convex side of the bowed long bones. The early lytic phase of the disease, presenting with a flame-shaped osteolytic wedge advancing along the bones, is often overlooked. Secondary arthritic changes may occur (e.g. hips). Bone scanning is more sensitive than an X-ray in assessing the extent of disease.

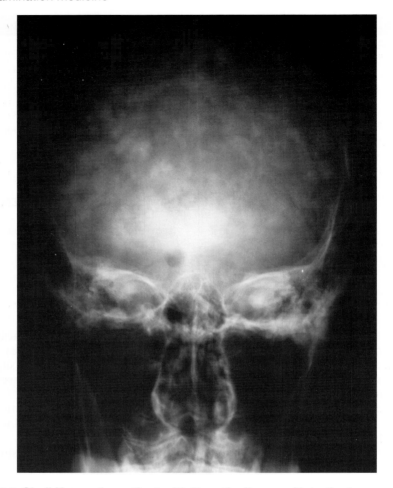

Figure 10.2 Skull X-ray of a patient with Paget's disease. Note the bony enlargement of the cranium.
Figure reproduced courtesy of The Canberra Hospital.

CT scanning or MRI may be useful in the investigation of an atypical lesion, especially if sarcoma is suspected.

Treatment

The indications for treatment are bone pain, progressive deformity or complications such as neural compression or high-output cardiac failure, and as a prelude to orthopaedic surgery. Treatment of patients with Pagetic involvement of weight-bearing bones may be indicated to attempt to prevent deformity and pathological fracture. Proof of benefit is not available, however.

1. Simple analgesics (paracetamol) or NSAIDs, including COX-2 inhibitors, should be used first to control pain. Orthopaedic procedures such as total hip replacement may be indicated.
2. A number of drugs are available that reduce bone resorption.
   (a) An oral bisphosphonate (e.g. alendronate) is usually the first-line treatment. These drugs are effective at reducing hydroxyproline excretion and often relieve symptoms, but may exacerbate bone pain initially. They also impair bone mineralisation and may cause osteomalacia. However, bone

turnover is reduced and new bone is usually more normal in structure. The bisphosphonates should be given in combination with calcium supplements and vitamin D. Ulcerating oesophagitis causing dysphagia is an important side effect. The bisphosphonates are not generally indicated for asymptomatic patients. Intravenous infusions of the potent bisphosphonate pamidronate may produce prolonged suppression of Pagetic activity and may normalise bone turnover in patients with mild disease without adverse effects on bone mineralisation or bone formation.

(b) Calcitonin of salmon or human origin, given subcutaneously, often improves bone pain and may be useful in the treatment of neurological complications. Although side effects (nausea, flushing and diarrhoea) are common and may limit treatment in up to 20% of patients, it is still regarded as a first-line therapy. Resistance to salmon calcitonin after one to two years may indicate the development of neutralising antibodies. Serum alkaline phosphatase levels and urinary hydroxyproline levels are useful guides to the effect of treatment; a 50% reduction in either test value indicates a good response to treatment.

(c) Mithramycin, given intravenously, can be very effective. It is reserved for occasions when rapid remission is required (e.g. spinal cord compression). There may be significant increases in bone lysis and predisposition to fractures with this drug, as well as bone marrow depression.

3. Surgery, including osteotomy for misshapen femurs, may be useful. It is important for the patient to avoid immobilisation in the postoperative period because of the risk of hypercalcaemia.

4. The appearance of osteosarcoma (see Fig 10.3) is associated with a poor prognosis. Preoperative chemotherapy followed by amputation—the current treatment for spontaneously occurring tumours—is being evaluated.

Acromegaly

Although an uncommon condition, acromegaly is a chronic illness and common as a long or a short case (see p 325).

The history

The patient will probably know the diagnosis, although if the condition has been suspected only recently investigations may still be underway. The patient may be in hospital for these tests because of a complication of the condition or, perhaps more likely, has been brought in for the clinical examinations.

1. Find out when the diagnosis was made and how long ago; in retrospect, the patient may have had symptoms for years. The average time taken to make the diagnosis is more than 10 years.

2. Ask why the diagnosis was suspected. The onset of abnormalities is usually very gradual. The common features of the condition are listed in Table 10.7. Ask what changes the patient has been aware of and whether these have improved with treatment. Bony and acral changes are irreversible and early diagnosis is worthwhile.

3. Ask about the associations and complications of the condition. The mortality rate for untreated acromegaly is about twice that of the age-matched population, mostly as a result of an increased risk of cardiovascular disease. There is also an increase in the incidence of colonic polyps and carcinoma of the colon.

4. There is now a recognised association with obstructive sleep apnoea and questions should be asked about snoring, daytime sleepiness and other relevant symptoms. The reason for the association is the enlargement of the tongue and swelling of the upper airway.

Figure 10.3 MRI of the lower leg of a patient with Paget's disease. A large osteosarcoma of the tibia can be seen (arrow).
Figure reproduced courtesy of The Canberra Hospital.

TABLE 10.7 Symptoms and signs in acromegaly
Acral enlargement*
Enlarged jaw and facial features*
Sweating*
Soft-tissue enlargement*
Headache*
Peripheral neuropathy
Paraesthesiae
Carpal tunnel syndrome
Skin tags and colon polyps
Symptoms of sleep apnoea
Impotence and hypogonadism
Muscle weakness
Galactorrhoea
Diabetes mellitus
*In >50% of patients.

5. Ask if the patient knows what investigations have been performed (see investigations below).
6. Ask about current and past treatment and how helpful this has been. Pituitary surgery and radiotherapy have a number of complications.
7. As with any chronic illness, the effect of acromegaly on the patient's life may be severe. Ask about occupation and ability to work.

The examination
See page 325.

Investigations
1. The preferred test is measurement of insulin-like growth factor I (IGF-I). Unlike growth hormone (GH), the level of IGF-I does not fluctuate and the absolute level reliably reflects the average GH level. There is physiological elevation of the level in pregnancy and during puberty, but otherwise elevation is very specific for acromegaly. The diagnosis can be confirmed with a glucose tolerance test, where GH suppression (normal to <2 mU/L) is measured in response to a glucose load. Failure of suppression is characteristic of acromegaly, but the test is non-specific and may be abnormal in renal impairment, thyrotoxicosis and diabetes.
2. In 25% of acromegalic patients, the prolactin level is elevated and this can be associated with galactorrhoea. Other pituitary hormone levels may be low because of interference with normal pituitary function by the large mass of the tumour. Baseline pituitary function should be assessed with measurements of prolactin, cortisol, thyroxine, follicle-stimulating hormone (FSH), luteinising hormone (LH) and free alphasubunit.
3. Imaging is performed once an elevated IGF-I is confirmed. MRI scanning is the modality of choice as it provides excellent anatomical definition of the tumour (see Fig 10.4).

Treatment
The aim of treatment is to prevent excess GH production without interfering with normal pituitary function. Early diagnosis makes treatment easier and more effective, and IGF-I testing makes the diagnosis easier.

Acromegaly is cured when the IGF-I level is normal and GH is suppressed to less than 5 mU/L after an oral glucose load. However, symptomatic relief can be obtained without complete cure.

Medical treatment with long-acting somatostatin analogues is increasingly useful, both before surgery and afterwards if removal is incomplete. Overall, surgery remains the treatment of first choice.

Medical treatment
1. Long-acting somatostatin analogues, such as octreotide, are now available. These drugs mimic the inhibition of GH release by somatostatin. They have the advantage that they are long-acting enough to be effective when given by subcutaneous injection. The usual dose is 100 µg three times a day, but this can be increased to up to 1500 µg/day. Unlike somatostatin, these drugs do not significantly inhibit insulin secretion. Unless surgery or radiotherapy has cured the disease, octreotide must be continued indefinitely. Symptoms such as headache, arthralgia and sweating improve after a few weeks. The drugs sometimes cause a reduction in the size of the tumour, which can make surgery easier. Side effects of treatment are usually relatively mild and include discomfort at the injection site, diarrhoea, anorexia, abdominal bloating and cholelithiasis.

Figure 10.4 MRI of the brain showing a large pituitary tumour (arrow).
Figure reproduced courtesy of The Canberra Hospital.

Long-acting depot injections are now available but expensive. For this reason, they are usually reserved for patients in whom other treatment has not been completely successful or is contraindicated.

2. Bromocriptine is also available for treating acromegaly. It causes a paradoxical suppression of GH release in acromegalics, but at tolerated doses remission is not usually obtained. Side effects include nausea, anorexia and hypotension. The drug is most often used as adjunctive treatment after radiotherapy or surgery.

3. Newer dopamine agonists that are more effective than bromocriptine include cabergoline.

Surgery

1. Trans-sphenoidal pituitary surgery is effective at selectively resecting the benign adenoma and preserving pituitary function in 50–80% of surgically treated cases. If cure is defined as a return of IGF-I to the normal range, then surgical cure is less often obtained. Nevertheless, symptoms are almost always greatly relieved by surgical debulking of the tumour.

2. The perioperative mortality rate should be less than 1%.

3. Uncommon complications include cerebrospinal fluid rhinorrhoea, diabetes insipidus and stroke. Hypopituitarism follows eventually in about 10% of patients.

Radiotherapy

Radiotherapy is usually considered as a second-line treatment where surgery has not been completely effective.

1. Conventional radiotherapy delivers about 5000 cGy to the pituitary over five weeks. It works only slowly. GH levels take a year to fall by 25%. Even after 10 years few patients achieve normal IGF-I levels. Hypopituitarism is common after radiotherapy, but other side effects are rare.
2. Newer, more promising techniques use computerised MRI to deliver larger doses accurately to the gland ('stereotactic radiosurgery').

Types 1 and 2 diabetes mellitus

This is a common subject for the long case since diabetic patients are always available. A large proportion of long-case patients have type 2 diabetes, often as part of the 'metabolic syndrome'. Diabetes usually presents a management rather than a diagnostic problem. The examiners like this disease because it tests very practical management skills.

Juvenile diabetes (immune-mediated diabetes) is called type 1 and maturity-onset diabetes (non-immune-mediated diabetes) is called type 2. Most type 1 diabetes (type 1A) is associated with autoimmune destruction of islet cells, but a small proportion of these diabetics do not have these abnormalities (type 1B). The cause of diabetes in these patients is not known, but it is more common in Asian populations. Type 2 diabetes is increasingly found in obese adolescents and children. More than 90% of diabetics have type 2 disease.

Don't forget the criteria for diagnosis of diabetes mellitus—a fasting (overnight) blood sugar level of 7.0 mmol/L or higher on at least two separate occasions or, in the absence of fasting hyperglycaemia, a two-hour postprandial glucose level of 11.1 mmol/L or higher. Fasting blood glucose levels between 6.1 and 7.0 mmol/L are considered to represent impaired fasting glucose levels. There is evidence that complications of diabetes may occur in some populations when the fasting glucose level is over 6.1 mmol/L.

The history

1. Ask about the age at which diabetes was diagnosed and its manner of presentation—thirst, polyuria and polydipsia, weight loss, infection, ketoacidosis, asymptomatic glycosuria. Remember the rare causes of glucose intolerance (see Table 10.8).
2. Ask about the treatment initiated at diagnosis and major changes that have occurred over time (insulin is required for survival in type 1 diabetes, which usually has an onset below age 30 years; in type 2 diabetes, control typically becomes more difficult with time).
3. Ask about the diet prescribed (see Table 10.9). The previous strict dietary rules using exchanges and portions have largely been abandoned, but some patients may still use them (one exchange = 15 g of carbohydrate = 60 calories = 250 kilojoules [kJs] [but the definition does vary]; e.g. for an average-sized male, three exchanges for each main meal and two exchanges for morning and afternoon tea and supper are required to provide an even carbohydrate distribution—50% of the diet). Ask whether the patient knows about the glycaemic index (GI) factor.
4. Ask whether oral hypoglycaemic drugs have been used or are being taken.
5. Ask about insulin treatment—how much and when taken. The usual dose is 0.5 units/kg/day, with 40% of the dose comprising a long-acting insulin. Also ask where the insulin is injected and by whom, and find out the type of insulin syringe used (e.g. a pen injector).

TABLE 10.8 Causes of glucose intolerance

1. Diabetes mellitus
2. Counter-regulatory hormone excess (rare)

   Acromegaly

   Cushing's syndrome

   Phaeochromocytoma

   Glucagonoma (associated with necrolytic erythema)
3. Pregnancy
4. Drugs

   Steroids or oral contraceptives

   Streptozotocin

   Thiazide diuretics (temporary and mild, secondary to hypokalaemia)

   Phenytoin, diazoxide (insulin secretion inhibited)
5. Pancreatic disease

   Chronic pancreatitis or carcinoma

   Haemochromatosis (decreased insulin production with or without increased insulin resistance)
6. Chronic liver disease (insulin resistance)
7. Syndromes:
   - Lipoatrophic diabetes (generalised lipoatrophy, hepatomegaly, hirsutism, hyperpigmentation, hyperlipidaemia)
   - Type A syndrome (usually young women with acanthosis nigricans and polycystic ovary disease)
   - Type B syndrome (acanthosis nigricans and autoimmune disease)

TABLE 10.9 Dietary recommendations for type 1 and type 2 diabetes

Protein 10–20% kJ/day

Saturated fat <10% kJ/day

Polyunsaturated fat 10% kJ/day

Carbohydrate (50–55%) and monounsaturated fats for the rest

Artificial sweeteners as required

Fibre 30 g/day

Minimise cholesterol intake (<300 mg/day)

6. Ask about the progress of the disease:
   (a) assessment of control adequacy—does the patient test the urine or (more likely and desirable) use a home blood glucose monitoring meter? Which glucose reagent strip is used and which meter? (Remember that different meters require different reagent strips.) Enquire how often the test is done, the usual results, at what time of day the test is performed (pre- or postprandial or both) and whether the dose is adjusted at other times (e.g. gastrointestinal upset). Ask about recent glycosylated haemoglobin (HbA_{1c}) results. Ask about symptoms of poor control:

    (i) hyperglycaemia—polyuria, thirst, weight loss, intermittent blurring of vision, hospital admissions with ketoacidosis (type 1 diabetes only)

    (ii) hypoglycaemia/hypoglycaemia awareness—ask the patient to describe the symptoms and how they are managed; ask specifically about morning headaches, morning lethargy and night sweats (symptoms suggestive of nocturnal hypoglycaemia), weight gain and seizures; ask about the time of day in relation to food, alcohol, exercise and insulin injection

  (b) involvement of other systems:

    (i) vascular system—ischaemic heart disease, intermittent claudication, cerebrovascular disease

    (ii) nervous system—peripheral neuropathy, autonomic neuropathy (causing erectile dysfunction, fainting, nocturnal diarrhoea) (see Table 15.43), amyotrophy

    (iii) eyes—regular visits to an ophthalmologist or retinal photography at the diabetes clinic and treatment received (ask especially about laser treatment)

    (iv) renal system—dysuria, nocturia, oedema, hypertension; is the patient taking an ACE inhibitor or AR blocker for renal protection; has there been proteinuria?

    (v) skin—boils, vaginitis and balanitis, *Candida*, necrobiosis lipoidica.

7. Ask about drug history—steroids, thiazides, oral contraceptives, beta-blockers.

8. Ask about associated other diseases—history of pancreatitis, Cushing's syndrome, acromegaly.

9. Enquire about social background—type of work, living conditions (living alone or with family), coping with giving insulin (associated blindness etc.), eating habits, financial situation, driving (type of licence held).

10. Ask about variations in weight and a regular exercise program. Have diet and exercise led to a fall in weight since the diabetes was diagnosed?

11. Ask about cardiovascular risk factors, including family history, serum cholesterol level, smoking and hypertension, and drug and non-drug attempts at control of these factors (except family history).

12. Enquire about family history of diabetes and obstetric history (e.g. big babies, stillbirths), and other risk factors for type 2 diabetes (see Table 10.10).

13. Ask whether the patient has an 'action plan' for hypoglycaemic symptoms and what this involves.

TABLE 10.10 Risk factors for type 2 diabetes

Family history (first-degree relatives)
Age over 45
Overweight (BMI >27 kg/m^2)
Race (Australian Aboriginals—at risk with BMI >22 kg/m^2; Pacific Islander)
Previous abnormal fasting glucose (6.1–7.0 mmol/L)
Gestational diabetes
Hypertension
Polycystic ovaries

The examination

Detailed examination is essential, looking specifically for complications of the disease. In particular, don't forget to look at the retina. Inspect the feet and assess for peripheral neuropathy. Test the urine. If the patient is obese, assess BMI and waist circumference.

Management

The general aim is to regulate diet, exercise and insulin so as to allow the patient to lead a normal life while avoiding short- and long-term complications.

In adults with type 1 diabetes, multiple injection regimens are preferred because the improved control prevents or retards the progression of complications.

The newly diagnosed diabetic

The major management decision here is whether insulin is required. In some cases this will be obvious (e.g. for the type 1 patient with ketoacidosis), but for many elderly obese diabetics the position is not so clear. If insulin is not indicated at presentation, attempt to gain control first by weight loss and diet, followed by oral hypoglycaemic agents.

1. **Weight loss.** Weight loss to achieve ideal body weight increases insulin sensitivity. Abdominal obesity (waist–hip ratio >0.9 for women and >0.8 for men) increases the risk of metabolic complications. Realise that there is some disagreement about the ideal diet, but achieving ideal weight is essential.
2. **Diet.** The recommended diet (see Table 10.9) should be tailored to the patient's requirements and activities. For example, kilojoule recommendations for a 20-year-old man undertaking normal activities are 175 kJ/kg of body weight and for a 75-year-old man are 140 kJ/kg. Distribution of carbohydrate should be worked out on an individual basis. Fat intake should be kept to ≤30% of kilojoules for patients who are not overweight and considerably less for obese patients. The distribution of kilojoules is more important for insulin-requiring patients, who should usually have about 20% for breakfast, 35% for lunch, 30% for dinner and 15% for supper. Patients who use short-acting insulin before each meal may be able to vary the insulin dose to suit the meal. The diet should include high-fibre foods and monounsaturated fats. Polyunsaturated fats can raise triglyceride levels but monounsaturates tend to reduce them. Patients with nephropathy may be advised to restrict protein intake, usually to about 10% of kilojoule intake.
3. **Oral hypoglycaemic agents.** The use of oral hypoglycaemic agents is generally accepted.
   (a) Metformin is the only available biguanide and is regarded as the agent of choice in the obese patient with type 2 diabetes. Side effects of biguanides include:
      (i) diarrhoea, anorexia, nausea and occasionally vomiting
      (ii) vitamin B_{12} malabsorption
      (iii) lactic acidosis (the risk is increased in the elderly and in patients with cardiovascular, liver and renal disease); the drug is contraindicated in heart failure
      (iv) interaction with radiocontrast materials; the drug should be stopped on the day of a procedure requiring contrast and for 48 hours afterwards.
      Metformin rarely causes hypoglycaemia and there is a synergistic effect when it is used in combination with sulfonylureas.
   (b) Sulfonylureas include first-generation drugs (e.g. chlorpropamide and tolbutamide) and second-generation drugs (e.g. gliclazide, used for obese

patients; glipizide, used for thin patients; and glibenclamide). Second-generation drugs are as effective as the first-generation ones and are associated with fewer drug interactions. The mechanism of action of sulfonylureas is to increase insulin action peripherally and to increase insulin secretion. Side effects of sulfonylureas include:

(i) possibly an increase in the cardiovascular death rate—this fear seems not to have been well founded, as the UKPDS (see below) did not find any increase in cardiovascular mortality for patients on these drugs

(ii) prolonged hypoglycaemia—this is greatest with glibenclamide, which is therefore not recommended for those over the age of 60; gliclazide and glipizide are as effective and are safer

(iii) weight gain (owing to increase in appetite and mild hypoglycaemia)

(iv) bone marrow depression

(v) cholestatic jaundice

(vi) skin rash

(vii) alcohol intolerance, causing flushing

(viii) water retention and hyponatraemia (syndrome of inappropriate antidiuretic hormone).

The effectiveness of the sulfonylureas is variable and rates of secondary failure vary between agents. Primary failure occurs in 40% of cases and secondary failure in 3–30%; only 20–30% of patients continue with satisfactory control. Substitution of one drug for another may be worth trying before abandoning oral hypoglycaemic therapy.

(c) Thiazolidinediones (TZDs) are a newer class of oral hypoglycaemic drugs. They reduce insulin resistance, blood sugar levels and triglycerides. Pioglitazone and rosiglitazone are available in Australia: their use is restricted to patients whose HbA$_{1c}$ is over 7% during the preceding three months and who are on maximum tolerated doses of metformin and a sulfonylurea. Patients on insulin must also be on metformin and have a raised HbA$_{1c}$. Liver function tests must be performed every two months for the first year and the drug stopped if the alanine aminotransferase (ALT) level rises above 2.5 times normal. The drugs are associated with small rises in HDL and LDL cholesterol and with peripheral oedema. They are contraindicated for patients with class III or IV heart failure.

(d) Acarbose inhibits intestinal alpha-glucosidase, slowing polysaccharide degradation and absorption. It is a useful agent taken before meals with other treatment. Side effects include flatulence, diarrhoea and abdominal pain, but there is no major toxicity.

(e) Other agents include amylin analogues (suppress glucagon, and used in conjunction with insulin), incretin mimetics (stimulate insulin release and suppress glucagon; injection only) and dipeptidyl-peptidase 4 inhibitors (reduce inactivation of natural incretin).

Insulin therapy

1. Insulin requirements initially are generally between 0.4 and 1.0 U/kg/day. An anorectic agent should be considered when requirements exceed 1.5 U/kg/day. Insulin therapy is often begun on an outpatient basis and under these circumstances small doses (e.g. 0.25 U/kg/day), sufficient to prevent ketosis, are used with a view to avoiding hypoglycaemia.

(a) Possible insulin regimens include: the basic bolus regimens, using a short-acting insulin at mealtimes (actrapid or humulin R) with an intermediate- or long-acting insulin at suppertime (isophane, lente or ultralente insulin); twice-daily double mix, using a combination of short- and intermediate-acting insulin (premixed ratios—short:intermediate 15:85, 20:80, 30:70 and 50:50—are commercially available, or the patient may mix insulins in a syringe); and in patients with type 2 diabetes, a combination of oral hypoglycaemic agents at mealtimes with an intermediate- or long-acting insulin at supper.

(b) Continuous subcutaneous insulin infusion is a treatment option, but infusion devices remain beyond the means of most patients with diabetes and may be associated with an increased risk of morbidity and mortality related to hypoglycaemia. The administration of intraperitoneal insulin via the dialysate can be useful in the management of patients on continuous ambulatory peritoneal dialysis (CAPD), and continuous intraperitoneal infusion has been attempted in some centres.

(c) Human insulin has replaced the highly purified (monocomponent) insulins but bovine insulin is still available. When a patient is changed from bovine to human insulin, the insulin dosage should be reduced by about 20% because of differences in insulin kinetics. Many patients report altered symptoms of hypoglycaemia and a more rapid onset of symptoms after changing to human insulin. Aim for euglycaemia: ideally the glucose level should be between 3.5 and 7.0 mmol/L throughout the day and night.

2. Insulin resistance is defined as a requirement of more than 200 units per day. Causes of insulin resistance are:
   (a) obesity (decreased receptor number)
   (b) insulin antibodies (uncommon, and an indication for a more purified insulin)
   (c) circulating antagonist hormones—growth hormone (e.g. in puberty), cortisol, thyroxine, glucagon
   (d) association with acanthosis nigricans (e.g. receptor abnormalities, lipodystrophies). Remember, injecting into a lipoatrophied site may cause poor control because of unpredictable absorption.

3. Insulin allergy has been uncommon since the widespread introduction of human insulins, but they can cause immediate local reactions (e.g. pruritus, local pain) or delayed reactions (e.g. swelling). Urticaria and anaphylaxis can also occur. Treatment in mild cases is with antihistamines and local steroids, but in severe cases desensitisation is important. Insulin allergy is more common in patients who stop and start insulin therapy.

4. Fasting hyperglycaemia is a major management problem. The 'Somogyi effect' refers to rebound morning hyperglycaemia following nocturnal hypoglycaemia, which is thought to be caused by the release of counter-regulatory hormones. This is now, however, a matter of considerable debate. The treatment is to reduce the evening insulin dose. The 'dawn' phenomenon is early morning hyperglycaemia in the *absence* of nocturnal hypoglycaemia; the treatment is to increase the insulin coverage without inducing hypoglycaemia.

5. Causes of hypoglycaemia in a previously stable diabetic on insulin therapy are:
   (a) decreased food intake, increased exercise or weight loss
   (b) injection errors
   (c) diabetic renal disease
   (d) rare causes—high level of insulin antibodies, malabsorption, hypothyroidism, autoimmune adrenal insufficiency, panhypopituitarism or an insulinoma.

6. Haemoglobin A_{1c} gives an indication of control over the preceding three months: aim for a level of 7% or less, although the numbers may be distorted by one or two high blood sugar levels. Spurious readings may occur in renal failure, iron deficiency, haemoglobinopathies and pregnancy.

Diabetes education

Because diabetes is a lifelong disease, detailed education by the team looking after the patient is important. Regular follow-up is essential.

1. Blood glucose monitoring with a glucose meter is essential for all patients who can manage it—initially, testing several times a day before and two hours after meals, and before bed, may be necessary; later, in stable diabetes, twice-daily may be enough.

2. Exercise promotes glucose utilisation; in the well-controlled diabetic it is important to reduce the dose of regular insulin before exercise or supplement with glucose. (*Note:* Exercise in the poorly controlled diabetic may precipitate ketoacidosis because of increased release of counter-regulatory hormones.)

Management of chronic complications

Complications are probably a result of damage caused by glycosylated proteins. Convincing evidence that tight control prevents or reverses complications is now available. Following the Diabetes Control and Complications Trial published in 1994 and the more recent United Kingdom Prognosis in Diabetes Study (UKPDS), clinicians now agree that rigorous control of blood sugar levels and aggressive control of blood pressure and other cardiovascular risk factors is essential. These measures are probably more effective in the early stages of the disease.

1. The blood pressure can be managed with any antihypertensive but the use of an ACE inhibitor or AR blocker is strongly indicated when proteinuria has been detected, and is often used routinely. The goal blood pressure is less than 130/80 mmHg.

2. Lipid control with the statins is being assessed in a number of trials. The high cardiovascular risk of these patients suggests that aggressive lipid-lowering with one of these drugs will be of value. Remember to control other risk factors, such as smoking (for retinopathy and vascular disease) and alcohol intake (for neuropathy and hypertriglyceridaemia). Aspirin prophylaxis in patients with risk factors or patients over age 40 is no longer generally indicated.

3. Ideally, all patients should be assessed every two years by an ophthalmologist. Less sophisticated fundoscopy may miss early diabetic retinopathy (see Table 15.43). Retinal cameras can now be used at the clinic to take clear retinal photographs, which can be repeated often and 'read' by an ophthalmologist. Retinopathy almost always precedes diabetic nephropathy.

4. Diabetic nephropathy is a common cause of chronic renal failure and results from arteriolar disease or glomerulosclerosis (classic Kimmelstiel-Wilson lesion or, more commonly, diffuse intercapillary glomerulosclerosis). The evolution of diabetic nephropathy has been well studied and can be divided into the following stages:

(a) glomerular hyperfiltration
(b) microalbuminuria
(c) dipstick proteinuria
(d) proteinuria in the nephrotic range
(e) end-stage renal failure.

5. Microalbuminuria is defined as a urinary albumin excretion of 20 to 200 μg/minute (measured using sensitive immunoassays) on more than two occasions in the absence of urinary tract infection and intercurrent illness. The albumin-to-creatinine ratio may be a more sensitive way of assessing the presence of significant proteinuria. Regular screening for microalbuminuria is now considered an important component of good diabetes management. The microalbuminuria stage is probably reversible with a combination of ACE inhibitor therapy, strict metabolic control and possibly dietary protein restriction.

6. Once proteinuria develops, progression to end-stage renal failure appears inevitable over a period of about five to 10 years. The rate of progression may be modified by:
   (a) control of hypertension—ACE inhibitors are the agents of choice, but it is important to be aware of the risk of hyperkalaemia as a result of hyporeninaemic hypoaldosteronism and deteriorating renal function in patients with renovascular disease
   (b) treatment of urinary tract infections
   (c) dietary protein restriction
   (d) possibly improving glucose control.
       ACE inhibition is indicated as soon as proteinuria is detected. ARBs are an alternative for those intolerant of ACE inhibitors. ACE-I and ARB combination treatment may reduce proteinuria further, but has little additive effect on blood pressure and is associated with an increased risk of acute renal failure. There is an increased incidence of papillary necrosis with urinary tract infection.

7. The best form of management for end-stage chronic renal failure in a diabetic is peritoneal dialysis and early renal transplantation. Remember that diabetics with chronic renal failure almost invariably also have retinopathy, which may be worsened by haemodialysis.

8. For those with severe systemic complications or end-stage renal disease, whole-organ pancreas (with or without kidney) transplantation is a promising therapeutic option. A number of successful kidney/pancreas transplants have been performed. Patients are generally euglycaemic without hypoglycaemic treatment. This is the treatment of choice for diabetics with renal failure.

The pregnant diabetic

Remember that blood sugar levels are normally lower in pregnancy. A woman with no diabetic history should be screened for gestational diabetes in the 24th–28th week. A 50-g glucose load is given and the blood sugar is measured one hour later. The normal result is <7.0 mmol/L. Between 7.0 and 7.8 mmol/L is borderline (repeat) and ≥7.8 mmol/L means that a formal 75-g glucose tolerance test is required: a fasting level of ≥5.3 mmol/L and a two-hour level of ≥8.6 mmol/L indicates gestational diabetes mellitus.

1. Insulin requirements vary during pregnancy owing to the effects of human placental lactogen (HPL). In the first trimester, insulin requirements usually remain unchanged or may decrease, but in the second trimester some increase in insulin requirements occurs owing to rising HPL levels. By the third trimester insulin requirements are usually at least 50% higher than before pregnancy, but after delivery there is a dramatic decrease in insulin requirements.

2. Blood glucose control should be improved as much as possible before conception in a diabetic woman wanting to undertake pregnancy. Haemoglobin A_{1c} should be normalised, as strict metabolic control at the time of conception has been shown to prevent the otherwise increased incidence of congenital malformations in the offspring of diabetic mothers. The complications of poor control seen in the infant are:
   (a) congenital malformations such as spina bifida (incidence about 6%, double the normal rate)
   (b) macrosomia
   (c) intrauterine fetal death in the later stages of pregnancy
   (d) hypoglycaemia after delivery
   (e) complications related to immaturity (e.g. respiratory distress syndrome, hypocalcaemia, jaundice).

3. Use of home blood glucose monitoring, with testing of both pre- and postprandial glucose levels, is essential. Strict glucose control must be maintained during labour and delivery. Paediatric services and a neonatal intensive care unit should be available. Remember that statins, ACE inhibitors and ARBs *must* be ceased in pregnancy.

Chapter 11

The renal long case

> When the patient dies the kidneys may go to the
> pathologist, but while he lives the urine is ours.
>
> *Thomas Addis (1881–1949)*

Chronic kidney disease (chronic renal failure)

Chronic kidney disease (CKD) by itself is not a particularly common subject for the long case. However, it is a difficult and important topic and kidney disease is often present in that very common long case, the obese diabetic with hypertension and vascular disease. Keep in mind the current CKD classification (see Table 11.1). The patient will usually know that he or she has renal disease. Methodical questioning to establish the diagnosis, cause, management and complications is necessary.

TABLE 11.1 Stages of chronic kidney disease

Stage	Description	GFR (mL/minute)
0	Increased risk for chronic kidney disease (e.g. diabetes, hypertension)	>90
1	Kidney damage but normal GFR	>90
2	Kidney damage and mild GFR reduction	60–89
3	Moderate reduction in GFR	30–59
4	Severe reduction in GFR	15–29
5	Kidney failure	<15
GFR = glomerular filtration rate.		

The history

Questions regarding symptoms, diagnosis and aetiology

1. The earliest symptoms of renal failure include nocturia, lethargy and loss of appetite. The first episode of overt renal failure may have been precipitated by a further insult, such as use of NSAIDs, radiocontrast injections, infection, ACE inhibitors or AR blockers (if bilateral renal artery stenosis), dehydration or anaemia.
2. **Glomerulonephritis (see Tables 11.2 and 11.3).** Determine whether there is a history of proteinuria, haematuria, oliguria, oedema, sore throat, sepsis, rash,

haemoptysis or renal biopsy. Ascertain treatment details (e.g. antihypertensives, immunosuppressives, anti-platelet therapy, dialysis).

3. **Analgesic nephropathy.** Ask about the number, type and duration of analgesics consumed, urinary tract infections, hypertension, haematuria, gastrointestinal blood loss, nocturia, renal colic (sloughed papillae, stones), transitional cell cancer and anaemia. This cause of renal failure is now very uncommon following the withdrawal of compound analgesics containing aspirin and phenacetin.

4. **Polycystic kidneys.** Ask about family history, how the disease was diagnosed, haematuria, polyuria, loin pain, hypertension, renal calculi, headache, subarachnoid haemorrhages and visual disturbance (intracranial aneurysm). Also ask about deafness and a history of persistent haematuria (hereditary nephritis—Alport's syndrome).

5. **Reflux nephropathy.** Ask about childhood renal infections, cystoscopy, operations, treatment (e.g. regular antibiotics) and enuresis.

6. **Diabetic nephropathy.** Ask about other complications and therapy. An ACE inhibitor or AR blocker is preferred for all cases with diabetic nephropathy.

7. **Hypertensive nephropathy.** Ask how the disease was diagnosed, duration and control of hypertension, treatment and compliance with medication, angiography, family history.

8. **Connective tissue disease.** Think especially of systemic lupus erythematosus and scleroderma.

9. Find out whether the patient is aware of the long-term prognosis. If he or she is not on dialysis yet, has this been discussed? Is the patient likely to be eligible for dialysis or the transplant list?

10. Ask when the underlying condition was diagnosed and how it is being treated. The progression to end-stage kidney disease may be rapid or very prolonged.

TABLE 11.2 The nephrotic syndrome

Clinical features

1. Proteinuria (>3.5 g/24 h)

2. Hypoalbuminaemia (serum albumin <30 g/L)

3. Oedema

4. Hyperlipidaemia (increased LDL and cholesterol levels)

Causes

1. Primary (80%)

   Idiopathic membranous glomerulonephropathy is the most common cause in adults over 40 years of age. Other primary causes include focal glomerular sclerosis, membranoproliferative glomerulonephritis and minimal change nephropathy

2. Secondary

   Systemic disease—SLE, diabetes mellitus, Hodgkin's disease (minimal change), solid tumours (membranous), amyloid, multiple myeloma

   Infection—hepatitis B (membranous), HIV (collapsing focal sclerosis), infective endocarditis

   Drugs—gold, d-penicillamine, probenecid, non-steroidal anti-inflammatory drugs, heroin

Note: Renal vein thrombosis is a complication and rarely a cause of the nephrotic syndrome.

TABLE 11.3 Classification of glomerulonephritis

Primary

Diffuse

1. Minimal change

2. Membranous

3. Proliferative

   Post-streptococcal (and after other infections)

   Mesangiocapillary

   Crescentic

   Mesangioproliferative

Focal

1. IgA nephropathy

2. Focal glomerulosclerosis

Glomerulonephritis as part of a systemic disease

1. Systemic lupus erythematosus

2. Wegener's granulomatosis

3. Polyarteritis nodosa (PAN)

4. Goodpasture's syndrome

5. Henoch-Schönlein purpura

6. Infective endocarditis

7. Cryoglobulinaemia ± hepatitis C

8. Myeloma

9. Diabetes mellitus

10. Haemolytic uraemic syndrome

Questions regarding management

1. **Conservative management.**

   (a) Ask about follow-up, medications, diet, salt and water allowance, investigations performed (particularly renal biopsy) and whether erythropoietin has been given subcutaneously in an attempt to elevate the haemoglobin.

   (b) Has the patient been advised to restrict protein intake? There is controversy about the value of protein restriction in delaying end-stage renal failure. There is some evidence that restriction to 40–59 g/day may be helpful. Patients with nephrotic syndrome should be much less restricted. The concern about protein restriction is that it leads to more rapid loss of muscle mass without much delay in end-stage renal failure.

   (c) What effect have the disease and the dietary and other restrictions had on the patient's quality of life and his or her family?

2. **Dialysis (see Table 11.4).** Ask about haemodialysis or peritoneal dialysis, including where performed, how often, how many hours per week, relief of symptoms with treatment and subsequent complications. Also ask about shunts, other operations (e.g. renal tract operations, parathyroidectomy) and medications taken.

---

3. **Transplant work-up and management.** Ask when and how many, whether living relative or cadaver, postoperative course, improvement, symptoms since transplantation, medications, follow-up and long-term complications (e.g. neoplasia, steroid complications).
4. **Bladder management for reflux or neurogenic bladder.**
5. **Social arrangements and ADLs.** Ask about employment, the family's ability to cope, travel, sexual function and financial situation.

TABLE 11.4 Dialysis

Peritoneal dialysis (CAPD or APD)	
Advantages	Simple, reliable and safe (from a cardiovascular point of view). Removes large fluid volumes. Allows greater freedom of diet and fluid intake. Preferable for diabetics.
Disadvantages	Peritonitis, exit-site infections (around catheter). Protein loss (7–10 g/day usually; 30–40 g/day with peritonitis). Basal atelectasis. Abdominal hernias. Does not control uraemia in hypercatabolic patients. Hyperglycaemia. Catheter displacement. 'Peritoneal membrane failure'. Perforation of bladder and bowel (rare). Hydrothorax (rare).
Haemodialysis	
Advantages	Takes approximately 18 hours per week (5 hours three times/week, plus set-up time). No protein loss. Large volumes can be ultrafiltrated.
Disadvantages	Circulatory access problems (thrombosis, infection of vascular access). Heparin may increase bleeding. Increased cardiovascular instability. Anaemia. Osteodystrophy. Dialysis dementia (aluminium).

Note: Mortality from dialysis is caused by myocardial infarction (60%) or sepsis (20%) in most cases. Acquired cystic disease in native kidneys may occur; <5% are malignant. Arthropathy and carpal tunnel syndrome may occur in long-term dialysis patients owing to amyloid (beta$_2$-microglobulin) deposition.

APD = automated peritoneal dialysis (exchanges done at night); CAPD = chronic ambulatory peritoneal dialysis.

Questions regarding complications
1. **Conservatively treated patients.** Ask about symptoms of anaemia, bone disease, secondary gout or pseudo gout, pericarditis, hypertension, cardiac failure, peripheral neuropathy, pruritus, peptic ulcers, impaired cognitive function and poor nutrition. Have the doses of renally excreted drugs given for other conditions been reduced? Remember that although most drugs that require a loading dose are begun at their usual dose (and then continued at a reduced maintenance dose), digoxin, which has an altered volume distribution, must have its loading dose reduced.
2. **Dialysis patients.** Ask about shunt blockage and access problems, infection, pericarditis, peritonitis etc.
3. **Transplant patients.** For patients with recent transplants ask about graft pain or swelling (failure of graft function, rejection), infection, urine leaks and steroid side effects. For those with long-term renal grafts, ask about serum creatinine levels, proteinuria, recurrent glomerulonephritis (dense deposit disease), avascular necrosis, skin cancer and reflux nephropathy. Find out about compliance with drugs and whether the patient knows about rejection episodes and treatment (e.g. with muromonab–CD3).

The examination *(see Table 11.5)*

TABLE 11.5 Chronic kidney disease (renal failure)	
1. GENERAL INSPECTION Mental state Hyperventilation (acidosis), hiccups Sallow complexion Hydration Fever	Bladder Liver Lymph nodes Ascites Bruits Rectal (prostatomegaly, bleeding)
2. HANDS Nails—Terry's nails, brown lines Vascular shunts Asterixis Neuropathy	**7. LEGS** Oedema—nephrotic syndrome, cardiac failure etc. Bruising Pigmentation Scratch marks Gout Neuropathy Vascular access
3. ARMS Bruising Pigmentation Scratch marks Urea frost (whole crystal deposits— terminal uraemia) Myopathy	
	8. BACK Tenderness Oedema Spina bifida scar
4. FACE Eyes—anaemia, jaundice, band keratopathy Mouth—dryness, fetor Rash (vasculitis etc.) Facial hair—cyclosporin Saddle nose (Wegener's granulomatosis)	**9. URINE ANALYSIS** Specific gravity, pH Glucose—diabetes Blood—'nephritis', infection, stone etc. Protein—'nephritis' etc.
	10. URINE SEDIMENT Red cells Casts
5. CHEST Heart—pericarditis, failure Lungs—infection	**11. OTHER** Blood pressure—lying and standing Fundoscopy—hypertensive and diabetic changes etc.
6. ABDOMEN Scars—dialysis, operations Kidneys—transplant kidney, renal mass Tenckhoff catheter, exit-site infection	

A complete physical examination is always essential. Look particularly for the following.

1. General appearance—mental state, hyperventilation, Kussmaul's breathing, hiccupping and the state of hydration.
2. Hands—nails for white transverse opaque bands or lines in hypoalbuminaemia; a brown arc near the ends of the nails (Terry's nails) in renal failure. Also palmar crease pallor, vasculitis, vascular shunts at the wrist, asterixis and peripheral neuropathy.
3. Arms—bruising, pigmentation, scratch marks, subcutaneous calcification, myopathy, fistulae and skin cancers, especially squamous cell carcinomas.
4. Face—eyes for jaundice, anaemia and band keratopathy (caused by hyper-calcaemia); mouth (dry, fetor); rash (e.g. SLE); and a cushingoid appearance.
5. Chest—pericardial rub, cardiac failure, lung infection, pleural effusion and venous hum (shunt).
6. Abdomen—palpable kidney, scars (owing to dialysis or transplants), renal

artery bruit (a systolic bruit, or occasionally a systolic–diastolic bruit in the upper abdomen, suggests possible renal artery stenosis), bladder enlargement, rectal examination (for prostatomegaly, urethral mass and signs of blood loss), nodes (lymphoma, cytomegalovirus or other infections if the patient is immunosuppressed), ascites (dialysis or other causes), and femoral bruits and pulses.

7. Urine—for blood, protein, specific gravity, pH, glucose, urine microscopy and examination of the urinary sediment for casts.

8. Legs—oedema, bruising, pigmentation, scratch marks, peripheral neuropathy, vascular access (for shunts) and myopathy.

9. Back—bone tenderness and sacral oedema.

10. Blood pressure lying and standing. Fundoscopy.

Investigations

1. Determine renal function:
   (a) glomerular filtration rate (GFR)—creatinine clearance (creatinine clearance levels of <10 mL/min are considered indications for dialysis) and plasma creatinine/urea level; the GFR is routinely calculated by laboratories and the patient may know these results
   (b) tubular function—plasma electrolyte levels, urine specific gravity and pH, glycosuria, serum phosphate and uric acid, aminoaciduria, serum calcium and plasma albumin levels
   (c) urine analysis and urinary protein excretion (protein-to-creatinine ratio)
   (d) others if necessary—diethylenetriamine penta-acetate scan for renal artery stenosis or urinary tract obstruction.

2. Determine renal structure:
   (a) ultrasound—renal size and symmetry, signs of obstruction; small kidneys suggest chronic disease
   (b) plain X-ray film of the abdomen (KUB—kidneys, ureters, bladder)
   (c) intravenous pyelogram (IVP) under good hydration (but avoid in patients with diabetes mellitus or myeloma, or when the creatinine level is >150 mmol/L—it has largely been replaced by less invasive tests)
   (d) CT scan (same restrictions as for IVP if contrast is to be used; the use of oral N-acetylcysteine before and after the use of contrast material and more importantly hydration with IV fluids does offer some renal protection)
   (e) cystoscopy and retrograde pyelography
   (f) other—renal artery Doppler study, renal angiography.

3. Consider investigations aimed towards the likely underlying disease process— renal biopsy; measurement of antinuclear antibody; hepatitis B surface antigen; hepatitis C; HIV; complement; immune complexes; immunoelectrophoresis; micturating cystogram; urine cytology.

4. Consider investigations aimed at assessing the widespread effects of renal failure—blood count; serum ferritin and iron saturation level; midstream urine examination; calcium, phosphate and alkaline phosphatase levels; parathyroid hormone level; nerve conduction studies; arterial Doppler studies.

5. Decide whether there are features that favour chronic over acute kidney disease: nocturia, polyuria, longstanding hypertension, renal osteodystrophy, peripheral neuropathy, anaemia, hyperphosphataemia and hyperuricaemia. The differentiation of acute and chronic renal failure is also aided by determining kidney size. They are usually small in chronic kidney disease, but the exceptions to this rule include:
   • diabetic nephropathy (early)
   • polycystic kidneys

- obstructive uropathy
- acute renal vein thrombosis
- amyloidosis
- rarely other infiltrative diseases (e.g. lymphoma), which can all produce chronic renal failure but maintain normal kidney size.

  In general, however, kidneys enlarge or maintain normal size in acute renal failure and are small in chronic renal failure.

6. Look for anaemia and the presence of burr cells in the peripheral blood film, which are usually indicative of chronic kidney disease but may occur in acute renal failure (e.g. in SLE), thrombotic thrombocytopenic purpura and the haemolytic uraemic syndrome.

7. Always ask about previous urine analyses, such as insurance examinations, in which proteinuria may have been detected and followed up, thus giving a clue about chronic glomerulonephritis.

Treatment

This most chronic disease (see Table 11.6) has profound affects on the patient and his or her relatives. The association between the patient and the renal physician and nursing staff becomes a very intense one, often lasting many years. It is important to ask detailed questions about the way the patient copes with the condition, whether work and travel are possible, and what the patient feels about the long-term prospects. Also ask whether a dialysis patient has considered accepting a kidney from a live donor.

TABLE 11.6 Complications and treatment of chronic renal failure
Anaemia
Causes include erythropoietin deficiency, poor nutrition (especially folate deficiency), blood loss, haemolysis, bone marrow depression, chronic disease and aluminium toxicity.
Treatment should include prophylactic folate supplements for dialysis patients. Erythropoietin is very effective for the chronic anaemia of renal failure and can normalise the haematocrit. Erythropoietin is commonly used in conjunction with intravenous iron supplements (as oral iron is poorly absorbed in end-stage renal disease).
Bone disease
Maintenance of normal calcium and phosphate levels is the key to preventing the problem. Treatment with calcium carbonate or sevelamer (to bind phosphate in the gut), vitamin D analogues and low calcium concentration in dialysis fluids is necessary.

1. Osteomalacia—diagnosis by:
   (a) X-ray films (decreased density, Looser's zones)
   (b) low calcium, phosphate and vitamin D levels
   (c) high serum alkaline phosphatase level

2. Tertiary hyperparathyroidism—diagnosis by:
   (a) X-ray film (microcysts on radial side of the middle phalanx, erosion of the clavicular ends, 'Rugger jersey' spine (see Fig 11.1), telescoped terminal phalanges, metastatic calcification of vessels)
   (b) high phosphate and parathyroid hormone levels, and a high calcium level

3. Osteoporosis
4. Osteosclerosis

(Continues)

TABLE 11.6 Complications and treatment of chronic renal failure (Continued)
Bone disease (continued)
5. Aluminium-induced bone disease
6. Dynamic bone disease (reduced bone formation) is the most common type of bone disease in dialysis patients due to over-suppression by phosphate binders; note PTH is low
Peripheral neuropathy
This is now uncommon in patients receiving adequate dialysis. It is more often a result of diabetes than of renal failure itself. Combined pancreatic islet and renal transplant may help.
Hypertension
This needs careful monitoring and control of salt and fluid balance as well as judicious use of antihypertensive drugs (an ACE inhibitor or ARB slows disease progression).
Infection
These patients are at risk of infection because of the kidney disease itself, the immunosuppressive drugs given to treat glomerulonephritis and their need for frequent intravenous vascular access.
Acidosis
This is often treated with dialysis and carefully monitored. Sodium bicarbonate often helps.
Hyperkalaemia
This should be treated with a low-potassium diet and ion-exchanging resins if necessary. Dialysis is very effective.

1. Treat reversible causes of deterioration. These include:
   (a) hypertension
   (b) urinary tract infection
   (c) urinary tract obstruction
   (d) dehydration
   (e) cardiac failure
   (f) drug use (e.g. radiocontrast, NSAIDs, aminoglycosides, cyclosporin)
   (g) hypercalcaemia
   (h) hyperuricaemia with urate obstruction
   (i) hypothyroidism or rarely hypoadrenalism.
2. Monitor and control the blood pressure very carefully. Treat lipids.
3. Carefully attend to salt and water balance and acidosis.
4. Normalise the calcium and phosphate levels with diet, phosphate binders or calcitriol.
5. Restrict dietary protein. Although this may delay slightly the need for dialysis, it leads to wasting and protein malnutrition. It is no longer universally recommended.
6. Assess and treat sexual dysfunction.
7. Dialyse when indicated (see below).
8. Consider transplantation.

The absolute indications for dialysis are (see Table 11.4):
1. uraemic symptoms despite conservative management (GFR <15 mL/min)
2. volume overload despite salt and water restriction and diuretic use
3. hyperkalaemia unresponsive to conservative measures

Figure 11.1 Spine X-ray of a patient with chronic kidney disease showing alternating dense and radiolucent bands—'Rugger jersey spine'.
Figure reproduced courtesy of The Canberra Hospital.

4. progressive deterioration of renal function (dialyse before symptoms develop)
5. acute renal failure (dialyse early).

   Note: Dialysis may be started earlier to avoid these complications.

Renal transplantation

Renal transplantation is now a widely accepted, commonly performed treatment for end-stage renal failure. Patients unfortunately continue to have a number of chronic problems that may bring them into hospital and make them available for examinations. Cadaveric transplantation is generally more common than the use of matched family donors. Specific contraindications to renal transplantation include recent malignancy, an untreatable focus of infection and severe external disease.

The prognosis continues to improve and the introduction of cyclosporin and other immunosuppressives has made a substantial difference to survival rates. The one-year graft survival rate is now more than 90% in experienced centres. The selection of patients for transplant is difficult. Shortages of donor organs mean that transplant is not offered to elderly patients, those with other serious illnesses or those with unrevascularised coronary artery disease.

The history

1. Ask the patient about the cause of the original renal failure (p 223). Find out how long the transplant has been in situ and whether this is the patient's first transplant. Ask whether the kidney came from a relative or was a cadaveric graft.

2. The patient should be well informed about previous rejection episodes and how these have been managed. Find out whether this is the reason for the current admission. Clinically, rejection may be marked by fever, swelling and tenderness over the graft. The patient should be aware of all these signs. There is also often a reduction in urine volume. A rise in creatinine level is usual. Ask about recent graft biopsies, which may have been necessary to assess rejection, recurrence of disease or drug toxicity.

3. Find out what immunosuppressive drugs the patient is taking and in what doses. He or she should know whether changes in doses have been required recently because of problems with any of the drugs.

4. Ask about specific complications of immunosuppression.
   (a) Cyclosporin can result in significant side effects. The drug can be associated with an increase in hirsutism, tremor, gout, renal impairment, increased liver function tests (especially bilirubin), hypertension, hyperkalaemia, hypomagnesaemia, gingival hypertrophy and rarely haematological malignancy.
   (b) Ask about ischaemic heart disease and peripheral vascular disease, infections and malignancy, as the incidence of these conditions remains higher than in the general population.

The examination

1. Look particularly at the skin for squamous and basal cell carcinomas.

2. Note any signs of Cushing's syndrome and hirsutism (e.g. cyclosporin).

3. Examine the abdomen carefully, noting the position and site of the allograft and whether it has any tenderness or bruits.

4. Look for old vascular access sites for haemodialysis and decide whether there will be problems finding sites for access for further dialysis if this is required.

5. Examine the lungs for signs of infection and the mouth for *Candida*. Inspect the gums. Note gouty tophi. Look at the temperature chart.

Investigations

1. It is important to obtain the serum creatinine level and, if possible, establish whether the serum creatinine level has been rising or falling since the time of transplantation. A slightly elevated creatinine level is considered acceptable in patients on cyclosporin treatment as this drug interferes with renal function.

2. The electrolyte levels and liver function test results are important. Cyclosporin can cause hepatotoxicity and renal impairment, as can cytomegalovirus infection of the liver.

3. A white cell count should be obtained to look for leucocytosis (infection or steroids) and leucopenia (e.g. excessive doses of azathioprine). The azathioprine dose is usually adjusted according to the neutrophil count. The haemoglobin is usually normal in patients with a successful transplant and good function.

4. The results of blood cultures should be sought if there has been any suggestion of recent infection. Urinary tract infection must also be considered and early urine microscopy is helpful.

5. Exclude prerenal and postrenal disease. A renal scan and ultrasound with measurement by Doppler is useful for estimating renal artery blood flow.

Management

1. The majority of patients receiving chronic dialysis are candidates for renal transplantation. The donor's kidneys must be ABO-compatible. Typing by human leucocyte antigens (HLA) -A, -B and -DR improves graft survival. Three HLA antigens are inherited from each parent. A complete match is for six antigens. The graft survival rate for these patients is 50% at 20 years. The long-term graft survival rate declines with a decrease in the number of matches. The recipient is usually screened for antibodies to class 1 antigens (HLA-A and -B) before receiving the transplant, as their presence is associated with hyperacute rejection.

2. Management problems include acute tubular necrosis, infection, cyclosporin nephrotoxicity (acute vasoconstriction, haemolytic uraemic syndrome or dose-related nephrotoxicity) and rejection episodes.

3. Rejection is prevented by the use of steroids, azathioprine (or mycophenolate) and cyclosporin. Acute rejection episodes are treated with three pulse doses of 0.5–1 g intravenous methylprednisolone or monoclonal antibody (e.g. muromonab–CD3) if the episode is resistant to steroids. Azathioprine is given in doses of 1.5–3 mg/kg/day; it is metabolised by the liver so its dose does not need to be varied according to renal function, but the dose is usually adjusted according to the neutrophil count. The use of allopurinol should be avoided because it interferes with azathioprine excretion and increases bone marrow toxicity. Prednisone is given in maintenance doses of approximately 7.5–10 mg daily after about six months. A gradually rising creatinine level may be a sign of cyclosporin toxicity (which, if caused by interstitial fibrosis, is not reversible) or of chronic rejection. This is a difficult clinical problem, but graft biopsy can be used to decide whether the cyclosporin should be stopped or immunosuppression increased.

4. Opportunistic infections typically occur a month or more post transplant. *Toxoplasma*, *Nocardia* and *Aspergillus* are now less common with current immunosuppressive protocols; viral infections (especially CMV) dominate. Infection must be aggressively diagnosed (e.g. by blood cultures and lung biopsy) and treated. When infections are life-threatening, immunosuppressive treatment, apart from prednisone, should be suspended.

5. The major cause of graft loss is chronic rejection.

6. Recurrence of glomerulonephritis in the transplanted kidney occasionally occurs and is most common with focal glomerulosclerosis. IgA nephropathy, Goodpasture's syndrome and membranoproliferative glomerulonephritis (especially type II) can also recur.

Chapter 12

The neurological long case

> The brain is a wonderful organ. It starts working the moment you get up in the morning and does not stop until you get into the office.
>
> *Robert Frost (1874–1963)*

Multiple sclerosis

This is a common chronic disease. Patients suffering from multiple sclerosis (MS) are readily available for the clinical examinations. They are mostly very well informed about, and interested in, their disease. MS usually begins in early adult life and is more common in women (2:1).

The history

Diagnosis requires at least two neurological events separated in time and place within the central nervous system (CNS). MS is primarily a clinical diagnosis.

1. Ask about the presenting symptoms (listed here in approximate order of importance):
   (a) episodes of spastic paraparesis, hemiparesis or tetraparesis (may present as gradually progressive disease in late-onset MS)
   (b) episodes of limb paraesthesiae (owing to posterior column, medial lemniscus or internal capsule involvement)
   (c) episodes of visual disturbance—loss of acuity, pain on eye movement, loss of central visual field (optic neuritis)
   (d) episodes of ataxia (owing to cerebellar or posterior column involvement)
   (e) band sensations around trunk or limbs
   (f) less common symptoms, such as vertigo, symptoms of cranial nerve disorders (e.g. tic douloureux), urinary urgency, incontinence of faeces, impotence, depression, euphoria, dementia, seizures, bulbar dysfunction (pseudobulbar palsy).
2. Ask about precipitating factors, such as heat (hot baths etc.), infection, fever, pregnancy and exercise.
3. Ask about family history: MS is seven times more common in immediate relatives (sibling risk is 5%).
4. Ask about social disability—sexual function, ability to work, financial problems.
5. Ask about place of birth: MS is more common in subjects who spent their childhood in temperate latitudes than in tropical regions. Smoking is also a risk factor.
6. Find out what treatments have been tried and with what success and side effects.

Various unproven treatments are often tried by patients with this incurable disease. Ask whether any of these have been used.

The examination

1. The signs can be very variable. Look particularly for signs of spastic paraparesis and posterior column sensory loss, as well as cerebellar signs.
2. Examine the cranial nerves. Look carefully for loss of visual acuity, optic atrophy, papillitis and scotomata (usually central). Internuclear ophthalmoplegia is an important sign and is almost diagnostic in a young adult. It can also occur in patients with SLE or Sjögren's syndrome who may have disease confined to the CNS, or with brain stem tumours or infarcts. Internuclear ophthalmoplegia is weakness of adduction in one eye as a result of damage to the ipsilateral medial longitudinal fasciculus; there is nystagmus in the abducting eye. In MS, internuclear ophthalmoplegia is often bilateral. Other cranial nerves may rarely be affected by lesions within the brain stem (III, IV, V, VI, VII, pseudobulbar palsy). Charcot's triad consists of nystagmus, intention tremor and scanning speech, but occurs in only 10% of patients.
3. Look for Lhermitte's sign (an electric shock-like sensation in the limbs or trunk following neck flexion). This can also be caused by other disorders of the cervical spine, such as subacute combined degeneration of the cord, cervical spondylosis, cervical cord tumour, foramen magnum tumours, nitrous oxide abuse and mantle irradiation.
4. Rarely, Devic's disease, usually seen in children or young adults, is present (bilateral optic neuritis and transverse myelitis occurring within a few weeks of one another) and may be a variant of MS.

Investigations

The differential diagnosis of multiple CNS lesions includes SLE, Sjögren's syndrome, Behçet's disease, acute disseminated encephalomyelitis, meningovascular syphilis, paraneoplastic effects of carcinoma, sarcoidosis, Lyme disease and multiple emboli from any source. It is important to distinguish MS affecting predominantly the spinal cord from other diseases—especially subacute combined degeneration of the cord (more common in the older population) and spinal cord compression presenting with root pain and persistent levels of sensory loss.

MS is essentially a clinical diagnosis, but the following tests may be helpful:

1. MRI is the imaging modality of choice. Typical changes are present in the great majority of patients with MS. Gadolinium contrast studies show leakage into the brain from blood vessels for up to months after the formation of a new lesion. T2-weighted images will show persisting changes probably owing to a combination of oedema, gliosis and inflammation. The extent of these abnormalities does not correlate well with the clinical picture, but T1-weighted images may show hypodense areas whose extent does correspond to the patient's symptoms. These probably represent irreversible damage and axonal loss. CT scan may reveal low-density, sometimes contrast-enhancing, plaques in white matter (subcortical or periventricular, but only in 10–50% of cases). CT scanning is no longer in routine use for diagnosis of MS.
2. Cerebrospinal fluid in chronic MS contains oligoclonal IgG bands (70%) and an altered IgG:albumin ratio. Myelin basic protein may be elevated in acute demyelination. There are usually fewer than 50 white cells per millilitre in the cerebrospinal fluid, but acute severe demyelination may result in a cell count exceeding 100/mL.
3. Visual-evoked responses are delayed in 80% of established cases and indicate previous optic neuritis (important if there is only one other clinically detectable

lesion present). Auditory-evoked responses and somatosensory-evoked responses may be abnormal, but are not usually diagnostic

4. Antimyelin antibodies are of uncertain value.

A definite diagnosis is not possible without the presence of two or more CNS episodes, usually separated in time and place. The first may be a clinical abnormality and the second detected by MRI or visual-evoked responses. These include objective CNS changes usually involving long tract signs and symptoms: pyramidal, cerebellar, optic nerve, posterior columns and medial longitudinal fasciculus. Gradual progression of symptoms may be used to make the diagnosis if typical cerebrospinal fluid abnormalities are present. The MRI should show four distinct areas of abnormality at least 3 mm in diameter. There should be no other explanation for the symptoms (see above).

Treatment

There are two aspects to treatment of these patients: (1) supportive and symptomatic treatment and (2) attempts to alter the disease progression. In addition, there are many support groups and organisations for patients with MS. These often give sensible advice to these distressed people and should be recommended to patients. It is most important, however, that the diagnosis is secure before patients are labelled with this condition with its numerous long-term implications.

1. The course of the disease:
   (a) *Relapsing–remitting MS:* relapses with or without complete recovery, but stable between episodes. Offer disease-modifying therapy.
   (b) *Secondary progressive MS:* about half of the patients with relapsing–remitting MS develop secondary progressive MS within 10 years. They experience gradual progression of their symptoms without distinct episodes.
   (c) *Primary progressive MS:* these patients (10%) have increasing symptoms without distinct episodes from the start.
   (d) *Progressive relapsing MS:* in these patients there is gradual worsening with episodes of deterioration occurring later in the course of the illness.
2. General support is essential. During exacerbations, bed rest with meticulous nursing is vital. Treatment of bladder dysfunction, severe spasticity (e.g. with baclofen), tic douloureux and facial spasm (e.g. carbamazepine and physio-therapy) is important.
3. Drug treatment:
   (a) Interferon beta 1a and interferon beta 1b have been shown to reduce the frequency of exacerbations by about one-third when used at an early stage of disease and to reduce the accumulation of CNS white matter lesions. They are more effective for the relapsing forms of the disease (see below).
   (b) Glatiramer acetate (subcutaneous) takes up to a year to provide benefit; the drug can induce non-cardiac chest pain.
   (c) Natalizumab (monoclonal antibody to alpha 4 integrin) caused progressive multifocal leucoencephalopathy and is no longer used.
   (d) Methotrexate given in weekly doses of 7.5 mg reduces the progression of disability and the MRI signs of disease activity for up to two years. Azathioprine (2–3 mg/kg/day) is sometimes used for chronic progressive disease and appears to have a modest beneficial effect. Cyclophosphamide may slow progression in patients under the age of 40. Its side effects make it difficult to use. Mitoxantrone has been used in rapidly progressive disease but causes cardiac toxicity.
   (e) Plasmapheresis and intravenous gammaglobulin may help exacerbations when steroids fail.

At 15 years after the first episode, 80% of patients have significant symptoms that prevent them from working and require help with normal activities. If the initial episode is limited to a single abnormality and the MRI is normal, only 10% will go on to develop a second episode over the following 10 years. If the MRI is abnormal, up to 80% will experience further episodes.

Myasthenia gravis

This disease presents both diagnostic and management problems. Peak incidence in women is in the third decade of life, but in men it is in the seventh decade. Overall it is more common in women (2:1). Exacerbations and remissions (incomplete) are common.

The history

1. Ask about symptoms at presentation:
   (a) ocular—diplopia (90%), drooping eyelids
   (b) bulbar—choking (weakness of pharyngeal muscles), dysarthria, difficulty (especially fatigue) when chewing or swallowing
   (c) limb girdle—proximal muscle weakness; there is fatigue on exertion and prompt partial recovery on resting.
2. Ask about a history of difficult anaesthesia (owing to prolonged weakness after muscle relaxation) and past episodes of pneumonia (as a result of bulbar and respiratory weakness).
3. Determine how the diagnosis was made, including whether electrodiagnostic studies were done and whether the patient had blood tests for acetylcholine receptor antibodies.
4. Ask about a history of thymectomy.
5. Enquire about other treatment—including drug dose and when the last dose was taken, plasma exchange or immunosuppressive therapy.
6. Ask about drug use, which may interfere with neuromuscular transmission (see below).
7. Ask about other organ-specific autoimmune disease associations (SLE, rheumatoid arthritis).
8. Enquire about the social history.

The examination

1. Examine for muscle fatigue, particularly the elevators of the eyelids and the oculomotor muscles (tested by sustained upward gaze), bulbar muscles (tested by counting or reading aloud) and the proximal limb girdles (tested by holding the arms above the head).
2. Look for the Peek sign (orbicularis oculi weakness—close the eyelids: within 30 seconds in myasthenia they will begin to separate and you will see the lower sclera).
3. Asking the patient to smile may produce a snarling expression. Speech on prolonged speaking may sound dysarthric or nasal because of weakness of the palate.
4. Weakness of neck flexion may be prominent.
5. Look for a thymectomy scar.
6. Reflexes are preserved, there is no sensory loss and muscle atrophy is usually minimal.

Investigations

Tests for myasthenia gravis include the following:
1. **Acetylcholine receptor antibodies (anti-AChR)**—these occur in 80–90% of cases, with false-positive results being rare (but the frequency of positive tests

is lower in pure ocular and inactive myasthenia gravis). The titre is not directly related to disease severity. Antistriated muscle antibody is detectable in 90% of patients with a thymoma but is also common in elderly patients without a thymoma; muscle specific kinase antibodies (MuSK) are present in 40% of 'seronegative' (ACh antibody negative) patients.

2. **Electromyogram (EMG)**—in myasthenia gravis, repetitive stimulation at low frequencies causes an asymptotic reduction (there is progressively less reduction with each shock) in muscle action potential amplitudes if that particular muscle is affected. Needle examination of affected muscles shows motor unit potential variation and, sometimes, fibrillation potentials and myopathic change. Single-fibre EMG shows increased jitter and blocking.

3. **Thymoma investigations**—chest X-ray, thoracic CT scan or MRI.

4. **Associated conditions**—hyperthyroidism and autoimmune diseases (check thyroid function tests, rheumatoid factor and antinuclear antibodies).

5. **Respiratory function tests**—these patients may have severe respiratory impairment.

Treatment

The prognosis of myasthenia gravis is good: 50% of patients have a remission, although 5–10% die from respiratory failure.

Symptomatic

1. Anticholinesterases are the mainstay of treatment in mild cases. Pyridostigmine is the usual one prescribed. Potassium supplements and potassium-sparing diuretics (e.g. spironolactone) may give additional improvement but are rarely used these days.

2. It is important to avoid drugs that interfere with neuromuscular transmission, including streptomycin, gentamicin, quinidine and procainamide.

3. Sudden worsening of the patient's symptoms so as to be life-threatening (because of respiratory failure) is called a myasthenic crisis. It is often precipitated by infection, which must be treated aggressively with antibiotics (not aminoglycosides) and intensive respiratory support. Mechanical ventilation and a course of plasmapheresis may be required.

4. Sometimes the problem may be excessive anticholinesterase inhibitor treatment (cholinergic crisis). Temporary suspension of drug treatment and monitoring of muscle strength may be all that is required for these episodes.

Disease-suppressing

1. Steroids are indicated for generalised severe disease when anticholinesterases are inadequate. They are then needed in the long term. They may aggravate disease initially (in the first week to 10 days), so all patients should be observed closely when treatment is commenced.

2. Failed steroid treatment in patients with severe disease is an indication for immunosuppressive drug therapy (e.g. azathioprine, cyclosporin, mycophenolate). Azathioprine has been shown to be effective as a steroid-sparing agent and to reduce relapses and prolong remissions. It should not be used as initial management or on its own. There is less evidence for other treatment, however.

3. Rituximab has been tried in desperate cases. This chimeric antibody attaches to the CD20 membrane site of B lymphocytes and attracts killer T cells and antibodies that destroy the lymphocytes which make the pathological antibodies. A course of treatment is very expensive.

4. Thymectomy is advisable early for many patients with generalised myasthenia

gravis if they are ACh-antibody positive. The exceptions are elderly patients or those with an easily inducible remission. Thymomas occur in 10% of cases (and of these, 25% are malignant) and thymic hyperplasia occurs in 65%. Of such patients, after resection, 70% show improvement and 25% of those who improve undergo remission. Causes of failed response to thymectomy include incomplete removal, ectopic tissue and fulminant disease.

5. Plasmapheresis is useful in acute situations such as in myasthenic crisis, preparation for surgery or in the peripartum period. Very ill patients may need repeated treatments.

Differential diagnosis

The differential diagnosis of proximal muscle weakness is important. The ocular muscle dystrophies also need to be considered. The Lambert-Eaton syndrome is occasionally confused with myasthenia gravis. This syndrome results from presynaptic failure of release of acetylcholine, caused by small cell carcinoma of the lung (in 50% of cases) or autoimmune disease. In the Lambert-Eaton syndrome:

- there is proximal muscle weakness and pain, and power may increase on repeated effort; reflexes are reduced or absent
- the ocular and bulbar muscles are usually spared
- the EMG is helpful (high-frequency stimulation causes an increment, whereas low-frequency stimulation causes a decrement and muscle action potential amplitudes are low).

Symptoms may be reduced by 3,4-diaminopyridine (DAP: safe and effective) or guanidine; steroids and plasma-exchange therapy can also be effective. Some patients with small cell carcinoma of the lung have a neurological remission if the tumour is completely removed. Treatment with d-penicillamine may cause a mild reversible form of myasthenia.

Guillain-Barré syndrome

This disease is not uncommon in the examination, as patients may be in hospital for an extended period and present management difficulties. It is the most common acute polyneuropathy and can affect both sexes and all ages.

The history

1. Ask about the presenting symptoms of ascending motor weakness, their time course and whether they are decreasing or increasing. The patient may report difficulty breathing. Other symptoms include paraesthesiae or sensory loss (sensory neuropathy is usually minimal) and symptoms of cranial nerve palsies, particularly bulbar lesions (all cranial nerves except I, II and VIII can be affected).
2. Ask about a preceding respiratory or gastrointestinal infection (which occurs in up to 50% of cases one to three weeks beforehand). Also enquire about other precipitating events, such as surgical operation, vaccination, intercurrent malignant disease (e.g. Hodgkin's disease), SLE and HIV infection.
3. Ask about previous episodes of disease (in chronic relapsing polyneuropathy).
4. Ask about evidence of autonomic neuropathy, such as postural hypotension, labile blood pressure, difficult to control arrhythmias and, rarely, sphincter dysfunction (see Table 15.42).
5. Enquire about the social history.

The examination

1. Predominantly, distal muscle weakness without atrophy is present, although 25% have more proximal than distal weakness. The upper limbs may be more affected

than the lower limbs. Tendon reflexes are reduced or absent concomitant with the degree of weakness. Muscle tenderness is common (one-third of cases).
2. Signs of autonomic neuropathy (severe postural changes in blood pressure and cardiac arrhythmias) must be looked for.
3. Sensory loss is usually minimal but if present affects the posterior columns (vibration and proprioception) more than the spinothalamic tracts.
4. Always measure forced expiratory time.

Investigations
Guillain-Barré syndrome is a clinical diagnosis. Helpful tests include the following:
1. **immune stimulus**—identify the immune stimulus by Monospot test, cold agglutinins, tests for cytomegalovirus, HIV or *Campylobacter*
2. **cerebrospinal fluid examination**—look for a raised protein level and the relative lack of white blood cells in 90% of cases; 10% have 10–50 mononuclear cells/mL
3. **respiratory function tests (FEV$_1$, FVC)**—assess the progressive involvement of respiratory muscles; the patient can progress rapidly (even over hours) to respiratory failure requiring intubation and should be admitted to hospital, even if only mildly affected
4. **nerve conduction and EMG studies**—many nerves may have to be studied to find abnormalities because this disease is patchy, but abnormalities include slowed motor conduction, conduction blocks, increased distal motor latencies, reduced sensory action potentials and increased F wave latencies. EMG evidence of denervation takes 10 days to three weeks to appear and may indicate axonal involvement with a worse prognosis.

Treatment
Prognosis is good—most patients make a complete recovery over time (up to a year), but 2% die (usually of respiratory complications, pulmonary emboli, cardiac arrhythmias) and 10% have a major residual deficit. If the deficit does not diminish in three weeks or the patient has autonomic neuropathy, a poorer prognosis is more likely.
1. Physiotherapy is used to prevent contractures. Respiratory support in an intensive care unit is essential if the vital capacity is less than 1 L.
2. Plasmapheresis or intravenous gammaglobulin shortens the time to recovery from respiratory paralysis and hastens the return of mobility. They are equally effective and combined treatment offers no additional benefit. Treatment should be begun as soon as possible. Rapid improvement is much more likely if treatment is begun within two weeks of the first symptoms. Relapses may occur and are more common after intravenous gammaglobulin than after plasmapheresis.
3. Steroids (and ACTH) are not beneficial.

Differential diagnosis
Infections such as glandular fever, acute viral hepatitis, *Mycoplasma* pneumonia, *Campylobacter jejuni* and HIV can cause Guillain-Barré syndrome. Post influenza vaccine disease is rare. The differential diagnosis of acute ascending motor paralysis includes diphtheria, polio, polyarteritis nodosa, acute intermittent porphyria, tick or snake bites and rhabdomyolysis, arsenic poisoning and botulism. Critical illness myopathy or polyneuropathy must not be missed. Remember that diphtheria, botulism and myasthenia gravis usually begin with bulbar symptoms.

The differential diagnosis of autonomic neuropathy includes diabetes mellitus, alcoholism, acute intermittent porphyria and amyloidosis.

Transient ischaemic attacks and 'funny turns'

Patients presenting with a 'funny turn' can pose a difficult diagnostic problem as there are many possible explanations. The problem may be neurological, cardiac, endocrinological or psychiatric. A careful history and physical examination should enable the candidate to produce a sensible differential diagnosis and management plan. Treatment is usually fairly straightforward once the diagnosis is made.

The history

1. It may be possible from the history to establish whether cerebrovascular disease and, in particular, transient ischaemic attacks (TIAs) explain the funny turns.
    (a) TIAs occur suddenly; there is focal neurological loss that is maximal at onset and does not spread or intensify. By definition the symptoms must resolve within 24 hours. Specific enquiry should be made about unilateral weakness or clumsiness, difficulty understanding or expressing spoken language, altered sensation unilaterally, and partial or complete loss of vision in one eye or bilateral blindness.
    (b) Faintness, confusion, simultaneous bilateral weakness, slurred speech and spinning sensations are not localising symptoms and are less suggestive of a TIA.
2. Neurological deficits that have lasted for longer than 24 hours are consistent with the syndrome of a completed stroke.
    (a) The absence of focal symptoms in a patient with severe headache and vomiting suggests subarachnoid haemorrhage. Vomiting and focal symptoms may occur with intracerebral haemorrhage, but headache is present in less than 50% of these patients.
    (b) In ischaemic stroke, the symptoms typically begin abruptly, often during sleep, and are not usually associated with headache or vomiting.
3. Presyncope refers to a sense of impending loss of consciousness, manifest as faintness or light-headedness and often associated with sweating, nausea, anxiety and visual dimming.
    (a) Causes of this condition can include cardiac arrhythmias, postural hypotension, cough syncope and micturition syncope.
    (b) Vasovagal syncope or presyncope can often be diagnosed clinically if the history is typical: an episode begins with clamminess, sweating and nausea and often occurs in a crowded room or after something upsetting has happened.
4. Epilepsy needs to be considered in the differential diagnosis.
    (a) Partial epilepsy is usually accompanied by an aura or a warning (e.g. flashing lights, twitching of the face or a limb, unilateral tingling or numbness, buzzing noises or humming).
    (b) Primary generalised epilepsy begins with loss of consciousness; eyewitness accounts are crucial in making a diagnosis. Tongue-biting and incontinence with tonic–clonic movements suggest primary generalised epilepsy.
    (c) Remember that seizure activity may accompany cerebral hypoxia of any cause (e.g. Stokes-Adams attacks). A long period of drowsiness often follows a major seizure.
5. Vertigo is the illusion of movement of the self or the environment. The sensation may be rotational. Often nausea, vomiting, imbalance and anxiety are associated.
    (a) Causes of this condition include vestibular neuronitis, acute labyrinthitis, benign positional vertigo, Ménière's disease, vertebrobasilar insufficiency, posterior fossa neoplasms, cerebellar haemorrhage and MS.

(b) Cerebellar haemorrhage characteristically causes severe associated nausea and vomiting, and is of sudden onset.

(c) Ask whether the vertigo is related to the position of the head (e.g. made worse by turning over in bed or by looking up). This symptom suggests labyrinthine disease, most commonly benign positional vertigo.

6. Unsteadiness of gait may be secondary to a number of disorders of the peripheral or central nervous system. Drug side effects, neoplasms, cerebellar and extrapyramidal diseases can present in this way.

7. Hypoglycaemia is an important, albeit rare, cause of funny turns and must always be considered in the differential diagnosis of suspected cerebrovascular disease. It is associated with hunger, sweating, tremor and tachycardia (owing to catecholamine release), as well as neurological dysfunction. Causes of hypoglycaemia include: too much insulin or oral hypoglycaemic agent and not enough food; reactive or postprandial, usually among patients with gastric surgery; or fasting (especially among patients with hypopituitarism, adrenal insufficiency, cirrhosis, alcoholism or rarely an insulinoma).

8. There are a number of cardiac causes of funny turns or syncope.

(a) A dizzy feeling related to standing up and without any component of true vertigo suggests postural hypotension. This can be a complication of antihypertensive treatment, especially with vasodilating drugs, and occasionally occurs in patients with single-chamber ventricular pacemakers (pacemaker syndrome).

(b) Orthostatic hypotension is common in the elderly and in patients with autonomic neuropathy (e.g. secondary to diabetes mellitus).

(c) Episodes of complete heart block may complicate ischaemic heart disease or be caused by degenerative disease of the conducting system. These patients describe syncope occurring without warning. Unless they have been injured by the fall they feel normal again immediately.

(d) Ventricular and supraventricular tachyarrhythmias may cause dizziness or syncope, possibly associated with palpitations. Ventricular arrhythmias are more likely in patients with known structural heart disease (e.g. previous infarction). Remember that antiarrhythmic drugs can cause bradycardia and are associated in some cases with dangerous proarrhythmic effects.

(e) Patients with severe aortic stenosis may present with exertional syncope, which is usually associated with ischaemic-like chest pain.

9. Other conditions that need to be considered include episodes of hyperventilation or panic attacks. Patients who sigh often because of anxiety are rarely aware of any abnormality of their breathing. Their dizziness is often accompanied by a sensation of swaying. Transient global amnesia sometimes presents as a funny turn involving temporary disorientation and loss of memory.

10. Find out about risk factors and associated symptoms.

(a) If a TIA or stroke is suspected, enquire about risk factors for vascular disease (in particular, smoking, hypertension, diabetes and hyperlipidaemia).

(b) Neck pain may indicate arterial dissection.

(c) Symptoms of connective tissue disease or thrombotic episodes may be relevant.

(d) Ask for a list of all the drugs the patient has been taking. Enquire about medications that increase the risk of vascular episodes, including oral contraceptives and some peripheral vasodilator drugs that can lower blood pressure. Also ask specifically about sedatives, hypoglycaemic agents, anticonvulsants and drugs affecting cardiac conduction.

The examination

A complete examination of the neurological and cardiovascular systems is essential but must be guided by the symptoms.

1. The fundi should be carefully examined for evidence of emboli, hypertensive changes, diabetic changes and ischaemic retinopathy. Test the visual fields (e.g. left or right half visual field loss in a carotid territory stroke). Look for nystagmus.
2. Carotid bruits should be listened for, but their absence does not exclude tight carotid stenosis. Unfortunately, even if a bruit is present, this does not necessarily indicate tight common or internal carotid artery stenosis, because external carotid artery stenosis can also cause a bruit.
3. If indicated, perform the Hallpike test for benign paroxysmal positional (positioning) vertigo (BPPV).
4. Check all the pulses. Decide whether atrial fibrillation is present. Test the blood pressure lying and standing for postural hypotension. Listen for murmurs (e.g. as a result of aortic stenosis, infective endocarditis, rheumatic heart disease or a prosthetic valve). Examine for peripheral vascular disease. Note the presence of an electronic pacemaker.
5. Palpate over the temporal areas for the tenderness of giant cell arteritis.

Figure 12.1 MRI of the brain showing a metastatic cerebellar tumour (arrow).
Figure reproduced courtesy of The Canberra Hospital.

Investigations

1. In patients with a suspected, but not typical, TIA it is worthwhile checking a full blood count, ESR (elevated in temporal arteritis and in connective tissue disease), fasting plasma glucose (for evidence of diabetes or hypoglycaemia), cholesterol (for hypercholesterolaemia), urinalysis (for evidence of renovascular disease) and an ECG (for evidence of ischaemic heart disease, arrhythmia or heart block). Look for a long QT interval. Patients in sinus rhythm, but with bifascicular or trifascicular block, may be having episodes of complete heart block. Serological testing for tertiary syphilis (*Treponema pallidum* haemoglutination test [TPHA]) is rarely indicated.

2. A CT or MRI scan of the head (see Figs 12.1 and 12.2) should be performed for all patients with a TIA or stroke, as 5% of TIAs are caused by structural lesions. A CT scan is also worth performing in patients with established stroke to exclude haemorrhage, as this may alter management.

3. A carotid ultrasound should be performed in patients who have carotid territory TIAs. Suggestive features of a carotid artery TIA include monocular visual loss, unilateral sensory disturbances or weakness, or aphasia. Vertebrobasilar TIAs, on the other hand, may cause bilateral visual loss, weakness or sensory disturbance, and crossed sensory and motor loss. If a greater than 70% stenosis of the origin of the internal carotid artery on the symptomatic side is found, carotid angiography should be considered with a view to endarterectomy or angioplasty, which is of value in otherwise fit patients.

Figure 12.2 MRI of the brain showing a cerebellar infarct (arrow).
Figure reproduced courtesy of The Canberra Hospital.

4. TOE should be considered in any stroke patient with abnormalities on examination of the heart or with abnormalities on the ECG (or chest X-ray). It is also recommended when no other cause has been found for the episode. A TOE with contrast injection may reveal a patent foramen ovale. This known cause of paradoxical embolism is present in up to 30% of people. Trials are underway to establish the benefits (if any) of catheter-based closure of these when they are detected in patients with otherwise unexplained stroke, but remember that stroke is an uncommon cause of syncope.

5. Patients with atrial fibrillation should have their thyroid function checked and an echocardiogram performed to look at left ventricular size—a predictor of risk of embolic events.

6. In relatively young patients with a TIA (<50 years of age), careful attention to the possibility of a connective tissue disease is worthwhile. Check an antinuclear antibody, anticardiolipin antibody (because of antiphospholipid antibody syndrome) and procoagulation profile.

Management

This will of course depend on the diagnosis in the particular case. If a TIA is likely, you should plan to discuss vascular risk factor treatments, anti-platelet therapy and the role of carotid endarterectomy.

1. There is a direct relationship between high blood pressure, smoking and cholesterol level and an increased risk of ischaemic stroke as well as coronary artery disease. Therefore, management of risk factors by conservative means or with drugs is essential.

2. Anti-platelet therapy reduces the risk of stroke in patients prone to TIAs. Low-dose aspirin (between 75 and 100 mg per day) is a reasonable regimen to use. Clopidogrel is an adenosine diphosphate (ADP) inhibitor and an expensive alternative to aspirin. Recent studies have suggested a reduction in cerebral events when the combination of aspirin and dipyridamole is used. Aspirin and clopidogrel in combination have not been shown to be more effective than aspirin alone. At least two years of treatment is necessary after a TIA, but many would recommend the lifelong use of anti-platelet agents.

   In those with atrial fibrillation not caused by rheumatic heart disease, aspirin reduces the risk of a recurrent event by one-fifth and warfarin reduces it by one-half. The risk of major haemorrhage with warfarin use is less than 2% per year, especially if the INR is kept below 2.5. Most cardiologists would recommend warfarin to any patient in atrial fibrillation who has had a definite or even a possible embolic event and in patients over the age of 70, or those with hypertension or cardiac failure. In those who have rheumatic heart disease, mechanical prosthetic heart valves or other cardiac sources of emboli, long-term anticoagulation is strongly recommended.

3. Carotid endarterectomy or angioplasty is worth considering in patients with a TIA in the carotid territory within the preceding six months who have documented severe (>70%) stenosis of the origin of the internal carotid artery on the symptomatic side. Surgery in such cases is definitely superior to medical therapy. A decision to operate should be based on the availability of surgical expertise and the complication (stroke) rate of a particular surgical unit.

4. Other treatment will depend on the final diagnosis and can range from anticonvulsants to pacemaker insertion. It is usually unwise to treat these patients without an established diagnosis.

Chapter 13

The infectious disease long case

Humanity has but three great enemies: fever,
famine and war; and of these by far the greatest,
by far the most terrible, is fever.

Harvey Cushing (1869–1939)

Pyrexia of unknown origin

Although not a common long case, pyrexia of unknown origin (PUO) presents both diagnostic and management problems. The term 'pyrexia of unknown origin' is used only for patients with a fever >38.3°C for more than three weeks for whom no diagnosis has been made during a week of intensive study. The common causes of PUO are listed in Table 13.1.

The history

1. Ask about the chronological development of symptoms. Gastrointestinal tract symptoms should be sought (e.g. subphrenic abscess, diverticular abscess, cholangitis, appendiceal abscess, liver abscess, Crohn's disease, metastatic cancer in the abdomen, Whipple's disease). Note any preceding acute infections (e.g. diarrhoeal illness, boils).
   (a) Chest pain may suggest pericarditis, multiple pulmonary emboli or rarely intraluminal dissection of the aorta.
   (b) Joint pain may suggest rheumatoid arthritis, SLE, vasculitis, atrial myxoma or endocarditis.
   (c) Dysuria or rectal pain may indicate prostatic abscess or urinary tract infection.
   (d) Headache and joint or muscle pain may indicate giant cell arteritis.
   (e) Night sweats may indicate lymphoma, tuberculosis, brucellosis, endocarditis or an abscess.
2. Ask about place of residence and overseas travel (e.g. malaria, amoebiasis, fungal infections).
3. Ask about contact with domestic or wild animals or birds (e.g. psittacosis, brucellosis, Q fever, histoplasmosis, leptospirosis, toxoplasmosis).
4. Ask about close contact with persons who have tuberculosis.
5. Enquire about occupation and hobbies—veterinary surgeon, farming (fungal infection, raw milk ingestion, hypersensitivity pneumonitis), intravenous drug use (contaminants e.g. quinine).
6. Enquire about sexual practices (e.g. risk of HIV infection, sexually transmitted disease, pelvic inflammatory disease).

TABLE 13.1 Important causes of pyrexia of unknown origin

1. Neoplasms

(a) Lymphoma, leukaemia

(b) Solid tumours

Primary—renal, lung, atrial myxoma, large bowel, pancreas, liver

Secondary—metastatic disease (including melanoma, sarcoma)

2. Infections

(a) Bacterial—tuberculosis, atypical mycobacteria, abscess (e.g. pelvic, abdominal, dental), brucellosis, endocarditis, pericarditis, osteomyelitis, cholangitis, pyelonephritis, leptospirosis

(b) Viral, rickettsial and chlamydial—hepatitis, HIV, cytomegalovirus, Q fever, psittacosis

(c) Parasitic—malaria, amoebiasis, trichinosis, toxoplasmosis

3. Connective tissue diseases

(a) Rheumatoid arthritis, systemic lupus, rheumatic fever, adult Still's disease

(b) Vasculitis—polyarteritis nodosa, temporal arteritis, Wegener's granulomatosis

4. Miscellaneous

(a) Drug fever e.g. NSAIDs, antibiotics, phenytoin, quinidine

(b) Inflammatory bowel disease, Whipple's disease

(c) Granulomatous disease—granulomatous hepatitis, sarcoidosis (uncommon)

(d) Multiple pulmonary emboli, intraluminal aortic dissection

(e) Thyroiditis

(f) Haematomas—retroperitoneal space (consider especially if on anticoagulants)

(g) Haemolysis

(h) Habitual hyperthermia (usually young women with low-grade fever, but no organic disease)

(i) Thermoregulatory disorders (rare—abnormal temperature-regulating mechanism)

(j) Cyclic neutropenia

(k) Factitious fever

7. Ask about evidence of immunocompromised host (e.g. cytomegalovirus, *Pneumocystis jirovecii*).

8. Find out about medication used—drug fever (antibiotic allergy, e.g. sulfony-lureas, penicillin), arsenicals, iodides, thiouracils, antihistamines, NSAIDs, antihypertensives (methyldopa, hydralazine), antiarrhythmics (procainamide, quinidine).

9. Ask about anticoagulant use (accumulation of old blood in a closed space, e.g. retroperitoneal, perisplenic).

10. Ask about iatrogenic infection (e.g. catheter, arteriovenous fistula, prosthetic heart valve).

11. Ask about factitious fever from injection of contaminated material or tampering with thermometer readings—suspect the former diagnosis if there is an excessively high temperature or the latter in the absence of tachycardia, chills or sweats; this is more common in medical or paramedical personnel.

The examination

1. Look at the temperature chart if available to see whether the fever pattern is characteristic. The temperature tends to fall to normal each day in pyogenic infections, tuberculosis and lymphoma, whereas in malaria the temperature can return to normal for days before rising again.
2. Inspect the patient: note whether he or she appears ill or not, whether there is cachexia (suggesting a chronic disease process) and any skin rash (e.g. erythema multiforme, erythema nodosum, adult Still's disease).
3. Pick up the hands and look for stigmata of infective endocarditis or any vasculitic changes, and for finger clubbing.
4. Inspect the arms for injection sites (intravenous drug abuse).
5. Palpate for epitrochlear and axillary lymphadenopathy (e.g. lymphoma, solid tumour spread, focal infections).
6. Examine the eyes for iritis or conjunctivitis (e.g. connective tissue disease, sarcoidosis) or jaundice (e.g. cholangitis, liver abscess). Look in the fundi for choroidal tubercles (miliary tuberculosis), Roth's spots (infective endocarditis), retinal haemorrhages or infiltrates (e.g. leukaemia). Note any facial rash (e.g. SLE). Feel the temporal arteries (temporal arteritis).
7. Examine the mouth for ulcers and gum disease and the teeth and tonsils for infection. Feel the parotids for parotitis and the sinuses for sinusitis.
8. Palpate the cervical lymph nodes.
9. Examine for thyroid enlargement and tenderness (subacute thyroiditis).
10. Examine the chest. Palpate for bony tenderness over the sternum and shoulders.
11. Examine the respiratory system (e.g. for signs of tuberculosis, abscess, empyema, carcinoma) and the heart for murmurs (e.g. infective endocarditis, atrial myxoma) or prosthetic heart sounds or rubs (e.g. pericarditis).
12. Examine the abdomen. Inspect for skin rash (e.g. the rose-coloured spots of typhoid [an uncommon long case]). Palpate for tenderness (e.g. abscess), hepatomegaly (e.g. granulomatous hepatitis, hepatoma, cirrhosis, metastatic deposits), splenomegaly (e.g. haemopoietic malignancy, infective endocarditis, malaria), renal enlargement (e.g. obstruction, renal cell carcinoma).
13. Feel the testes for enlargement (e.g. seminoma, tuberculosis). Feel for inguinal adenopathy. Always ask for the results of the rectal examination (e.g. prostatic abscess, rectal cancer, Crohn's disease) and pelvic examination (pelvic pus). Look at the penis and scrotum for a discharge or rash.
14. Finally examine the nervous system for signs of meningism (chronic meningitis) or focal neurological signs (e.g. brain abscess, mononeuritis multiplex in polyarteritis nodosa). Check the results of the urine analysis.

Investigations

1. Determine how many blood cultures have been obtained and the results. Ask to review the blood count and smear (e.g. for neutropenia, eosinophilia, atypical lymphocytes), liver function tests, electrolytes and creatinine. Look at the chest X-ray. Rule out urinary tract disease if suspected.
2. Selected serological tests may be helpful depending on the clinical setting (e.g. fungal, HIV, Q fever). An autoimmune screen—ANA, ESR, CRP, an EPG and complement levels—should be assessed if a connective tissue disease is suspected. However, remember that malignancy and infection can also cause an increase in acute phase reactants and a low-titre ANA. Check the purified protein derivative (PPD) for tuberculosis exposure (see Table 13.2).
3. If abdominal disease is suspected or other tests have not provided a clue, obtain a CT scan.

TABLE 13.2 Tuberculin skin testing*
Positive†
A. ≥ 5 mm (high-risk)
1. Abnormal chest X-ray consistent with prior TB
2. Close contact with a documented case
3. Immunosuppressed: HIV, transplant patient or on ≥ 15 mg/day prednisone
B. ≥ 10 mm (intermediate-risk)
1. Health-care workers, nursing home patients
2. Recent immigrants from high-prevalence regions
3. Prisoners, IV drug users
4. Diabetic patients
5. Prednisone (<15 mg/day)
C. ≥15 mm (low-risk)
Everyone else
If positive and no active disease on chest X-ray and by sputum for acid-fast bacteria: treat for latent TB (isoniazid for nine months).
*Contraindicated if history of necrotic skin reaction to previous testing. Prior BCG vaccination does not invalidate the results.
†False negatives occur in anergy or with recent exposure (recheck after 12 weeks) or in the elderly (recheck after three weeks).

4. Biopsy of involved tissue (e.g. bone marrow, liver, lymph node, skin, muscle) may lead to a definitive diagnosis. The clinical setting determines what should be biopsied.

5. Exploratory laparotomy when all other tests are negative and in the absence of any evidence of abdominal disease is usually unproductive.

Treatment

Therapy directed at the underlying disease should be the goal of assessment. Therapeutic trials in the absence of a diagnosis (e.g. antibiotics, antituberculosis therapy, NSAIDs, steroids) may result in resistant bacterial infection or drug toxicity and may make accurate diagnosis difficult. If the patient is thought to have a fever caused by a drug—a *drug fever*—it may be worth stopping the drug or using an alternative one. A possible drug fever makes trialling a change of drug worthwhile.

HIV/AIDS

Patients with HIV infection or the acquired immunodeficiency syndrome (AIDS) have become increasingly available for long-case examinations. Remember that the diagnosis of AIDS can be made when someone infected with HIV has a CD4+ cell count of <200 cells/μL or an HIV-associated disease. These patients present numerous diagnostic and management problems. The candidate will be expected to display a logical approach to the case and, of course, show a sympathetic attitude to the patient with this chronic disease. There needs to be a strong emphasis in the discussion on the psychological and social effects of the illness. Public health implications may also have to be addressed. Candidates should have an approach to pretest counselling for patients being tested for HIV.

The history

1. Ask about the presenting symptoms. As usual for long cases, the candidate must find out what symptoms or complications are currently affecting the patient. These must be assessed in the context of possible longstanding disease affecting many systems of the body.

2. Enquire when the virus was acquired. This is especially important in helping predict the likely level of immunosuppression.

   (a) Find out about symptoms of a possible seroconversion illness in the past (see Table 13.3). Approximately 50% of people have a seroconversion illness. It occurs three to six weeks after infection and often resembles glandular fever. Remember that, without treatment, the development of AIDS takes roughly seven to 10 years from the time of seroconversion. The occurrence of a seroconversion illness does not seem to be associated with a worse prognosis.

   (b) Note from the history any of the conditions likely to occur during the period of mild-to-moderate immunosuppression that precedes the development of AIDS and those related to severe immunosuppression that define the development of AIDS (see Table 13.4).

3. Ask about the mode of acquisition of infection. Co-morbidity differs between subgroups, so specific questions about risk factors are essential. For example, Kaposi's sarcoma is often found in the homosexual male subgroup, whereas viral hepatitis, endocarditis, heroin nephropathy and other disorders related to drug abuse may complicate the disease in the intravenous drug-using group. Many haemophilia A patients acquired HIV from pooled blood products.

4. Ask about sexual contacts. Contact tracing must be mentioned and the possibility of infection of sexual partners without their knowledge addressed. Ask the patient whether family and friends are aware of the diagnosis.

5. Ask about general constitutional symptoms. Symptoms of fever, lethargy and weight loss may indicate the AIDS-related complex or suggest an underlying opportunistic infection or malignancy.

TABLE 13.3 Features of the seroconversion illness

A seroconversion illness occurs in more than 50% of cases. There is usually some combination of the following symptoms:

- fever
- lymphadenopathy
- maculopapular rash
- arthralgia
- myalgia
- pharyngitis
- nausea
- vomiting
- diarrhoea
- headache
- meningism
- weight loss
- oral candidiasis.

TABLE 13.4 HIV-related conditions with severe immunosuppression
Pneumocystis jirovecii pneumonia
Kaposi's sarcoma
Non-Hodgkin's lymphoma
Disseminated *Mycobacterium avium* complex infection
Cytomegalovirus infection
Cerebral toxoplasmosis
Oesophageal candidiasis
AIDS dementia complex
Note: This is a representative rather than an exhaustive list.

6. Enquire about specific symptoms:
    (a) respiratory—cough, dyspnoea, sputum—these may result from *Pneumocystis jirovecii* pneumonia, lymphoid interstitial pneumonitis, tuberculosis, bacterial pneumonia or fungal pneumonia
    (b) gastrointestinal—diarrhoea or weight loss as a result of cryptosporidiosis, microsporidiosis, mycobacterial infection or cytomegalovirus (CMV) colitis; odynophagia as a result of oesophageal candidiasis, herpes simplex or CMV ulceration; vomiting and abdominal pain owing to biliary tract disease; drug side effects (e.g. didanosine-induced pancreatitis)—diarrhoea is usual when patients are treated with protease inhibitors
    (c) neurological—meningism caused by cryptococcal meningitis, focal neurological symptoms or seizures as a result of space-occupying lesions, toxoplasmosis or non-Hodgkin's lymphoma; cognitive decline as a result of HIV dementia or multifocal leucoencephalopathy; peripheral nervous system disease owing to peripheral neuropathy, CMV radiculopathy or myopathy
    (d) renal—nephrotic syndrome from HIV-associated nephropathy; renal failure owing to sepsis or drug side effects
    (e) ocular—deteriorating vision, which usually suggests advanced CMV retinitis
    (f) dermatological—rashes may be caused by drug reactions, viral infection (e.g. herpes zoster virus [HZV] or herpes simplex virus [HSV]) or fungal infection; itch may be caused by scabies or drug reaction; and nodules can be caused by Kaposi's sarcoma or bacillary angiomatosis
    (g) mouth—ulcers (aphthous or viral), gingivitis, periodontal disease, hairy leucoplakia or candidiasis
    (h) cardiac—dyspnoea, chest pain or palpitations owing to myocarditis or pericarditis
    (i) haematological—anaemia (bone marrow suppression or infiltration, treatment with zidovudine); thrombocytopenia and neutropenia are less common.
7. Ask about previous treatment. Find out about antiretroviral drug and antibiotic treatment and about any adverse effects of these. Enquire about specific side effects (see Table 13.5).
8. Ask about previous investigations. The patient may be able to give much helpful information on previous investigations, including viral load results, T cell CD4⁺ counts, MRI scans, CT scans, lumbar punctures, bone marrow biopsies and endoscopy.
9. Enquire about social, drug and alcohol history. The examiners will expect quite detailed knowledge of the patient's social, economic and family circumstances.

TABLE 13.5 Side effects of selected antiretroviral drugs

Drug	Side effects
A. Nucleoside reverse transcriptase inhibitors	
Zidovudine (AZT)	Headache, nausea, myopathy, bone marrow suppression; used in pregnant HIV-positive patients
Didanosine (dI)	Diarrhoea, pancreatitis, peripheral neuropathy
Zalcitabine (ddc)	Mouth and oesophageal ulcers, pancreatitis, peripheral neuropathy
Lamivudine (3TC)	Side effects uncommon
Stavudine (d4T)	Peripheral neuropathy, pancreatitis; do not use in pregnant women with d4T (fatal lactic acidosis)
Abacavir	Hypersensitivity syndrome (3%)—linked to HLAB-5701
B. Non-nucleoside reverse transcriptase inhibitors	
Nevirapine	Rash, hepatitis (can be fatal)
Efavirenz	Dizziness, cognitive disturbance, insomnia, fatigue, rash; teratogenic
Delavirdine	Rash
C. Protease inhibitors	
Indinavir	Nausea, diarrhoea, lipodystrophy, insulin resistance, hepatitis, renal calculi, hair and nail changes
Saquinavir	Diarrhoea, lipodystrophy, insulin resistance, hepatitis
Nelfinavir	Diarrhoea, lipodystrophy, insulin resistance, hepatitis
Amprenavir	Diarrhoea, nausea, perioral paraesthesia, lipodystrophy, insulin resistance
Ritonavir	Nausea, diarrhoea, taste disturbance, perioral paraesthesia, lipodystrophy, insulin resistance
D. Entry/fusion inhibitors	
Enfuvirtide	Increased risk of pneumonia, local reaction at injection site
E. Integrase inhibitors	
Raltegravir	Cholesterol increased, myopathy

The examination

Note especially:

1. temperature
2. nutritional state (wasting is common in advanced disease); there may be fat loss on the face and fat gain over the limbs (retroviral drug effect)
3. skin (e.g. rashes—seborrhoeic dermatitis, molluscum contagiosum—pigmentation and the lesions of Kaposi's sarcoma)
4. mouth (e.g. hairy leucoplakia, Kaposi's sarcoma lesions, periodontal disease, HSV mouth ulcers)
5. eyes—acuity, visual fields and fundoscopy (e.g. CMV retinal lesions)
6. cognition, gait and coordination (e.g. AIDS dementia)
7. chest—cough, sputum, crackles (e.g. opportunistic chest infection)
8. heart—cardiac failure, pericardial disease (e.g. AIDS cardiomyopathy)

9. abdomen—rectal examination, perianal disease (especially warts and HSV)
10. haematological system—lymph nodes and spleen.

Investigations

The patient is likely to have had many tests.

1. The standard screening test for HIV is an ELISA or enzyme immunoassay (EIA) test. It tests against antigens of both HIV1 and HIV2 (very rare in Australia). It has a sensitivity of more than 99%. Its specificity in low-risk populations is only about 90%. False positives can occur related to recent vaccinations, other viral infections and autoimmune diseases. The earliest detectable test is an HIV PCR DNA (within a few days of inoculation).
2. The western blot test is more specific and a negative western blot means a positive EIA test is a false positive.
3. Other tests are used to assess the severity of the illness and immunocompromisation, and to look for associated conditions (e.g. syphilis) and complications. The currently relevant tests will depend on the clinical presentation; however, certain tests are essential for all patients, either as a baseline or for monitoring (see Table 13.6).

TABLE 13.6 Routine initial investigations for HIV patients
All patients
1. CD4+ count
2. Viral load
3. Hepatitis B surface antigen and core antibody
4. Hepatitis C antibody
5. Hepatitis A antibody (IgG)
6. Chest X-ray, which may reveal cardiac or pulmonary complications especially in acutely ill patients (see Figs 13.1–13.3)
7. Cytomegalovirus antibody (IgG)
8. Serological tests for syphilis
9. Toxoplasma antibody
10. Liver function tests, eGFR
Patients with CD4+ count < 200 cells/µL
1. Hepatitis C RNA
2. Cryptococcal antigen
3. Stool examination for cysts, ova and parasites
Patients with CD4+ count < 100 cells/µL
1. Cytomegalovirus PCR
2. Mycobacterial blood cultures
3. Fundoscopy (pupils dilated)
4. ECG

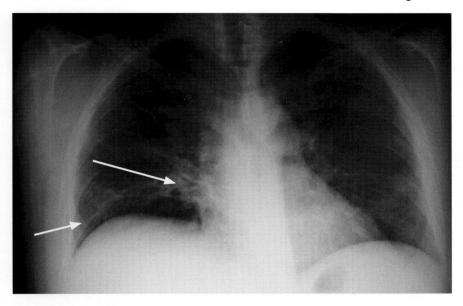

Figure 13.1 Chest X-ray of a patient with HIV and pneumocystis pneumonia. Note the perihilar and basilar reticular airspace opacities (arrows).
Figure reproduced courtesy of The Canberra Hospital.

Figure 13.2 Lateral chest X-ray of a patient with HIV showing left lower lobe consolidation (arrow).
Figure reproduced courtesy of The Canberra Hospital.

Figure 13.3 Chest X-ray of a patient with HIV showing a large pericardial effusion.
Figure reproduced courtesy of The Canberra Hospital.

Baseline
1. Immune function needs to be established at this point with a full blood count, CD4+ level (levels >200 cells/μL are associated with opportunistic infections) and HIV plasma serum viral load.
2. A delayed-type hypersensitivity skin test will help define cellular immune function. The lower the CD4+ (T helper cell) level (see Table 13.7) and the higher the HIV viral load, the more advanced the infection. CD4+ levels may fall progressively to undetectable levels. Aggressive treatment of infections may allow continued survival of patients despite these low CD4+ levels. Antiviral treatment may slow CD4+ depletion or stabilise it for many years. About 5% of infected patients do not develop a reduction in CD4+ counts even after more than 10 years without treatment. These patients are called 'non-progressors'.
3. It should also be established whether the patient has concurrent sexually transmitted disease (syphilis serology, hepatitis B serology) or tuberculosis (tuberculin test), and whether he or she is at risk of activation of latent infection (CMV, toxoplasma serology).
4. Renal and liver function should be checked prior to commencing antiviral drugs.

Monitoring
The key investigations for monitoring progress are the HIV plasma viral load and the CD4+ T cell count. Serial full blood counts and biochemistry will help assess any complications of disease or therapy.

TABLE 13.7 CD4+ level and common clinical features

CD4+ count >500 cells/μL

1. Primary infection
2. Generalised lymphadenopathy
3. Vaginal candidiasis

CD4+ count 200–500 cells/μL

1. Herpes zoster
2. Oral candidiasis
3. Hairy leucoplakia (caused by Epstein-Barr virus)
4. Kaposi's sarcoma (caused by human herpes virus 8)
5. Pulmonary TB
6. Lymphoid interstitial pneumonitis
7. HIV-associated idiopathic thrombocytopenia

CD4+ count < 200 cells/μL

1. *Pneumocystis* pneumonia
2. Microsporidium and cryptosporidium infection
3. Oesophageal candidiasis
4. Peripheral neuropathy
5. Wasting
6. Miliary or extrapulmonary TB
7. Herpes simplex

CD4+ count < 100 cells/μL

1. Cryptococcal meningitis
2. Cerebral toxoplasmosis
3. CNS lymphoma
4. Dementia
5. Non-Hodgkin's lymphoma
6. Multifocal leucoencephalopathy

CD4+ count < 50 cells/μL

1. Disseminated *Mycobacterium avium*
2. Disseminated cytomegalovirus infection—retinitis, gastrointestinal disease

Treatment

1. Candidates will be expected to know the clinical features and general treatment options for common complications of HIV infection, especially opportunistic infection and malignancy. This list would include *P. jiroveci* (*carinii*) pneumonia, Kaposi's sarcoma, cerebral toxoplasmosis, CMV infection, *Mycobacterium avium* complex (MAC) infection, diarrhoeal syndromes and cryptococcal meningitis.
2. Prophylaxis for *P. jirovecci* with cotrimoxazole or pentamidine (if CD4+ count <200 cells/μL) and MAC with azithromycin (if CD4+ count <50 cells/μL) is an important consideration. If the CD4+ count is >200 cells/μL for three months,

prophylaxis can be ceased. Pneumococcal vaccination is routine even when the CD4$^+$ count remains >300 cells/μL.

3. Herpes simplex prophylaxis with acyclovir and *Candida* prophylaxis with fluconazole or ketoconazole are appropriate for prevention after one episode has occurred.

4. Multiple antiretroviral agents are now available for the treatment of HIV (see Table 13.5). Known as HAART (highly active antiretroviral therapy), these drugs have dramatically improved quality of life and life expectancy in HIV disease.

5. Some doubt remains as to the optimal time to commence therapy. It is clear that symptomatic patients, or those with an increasing viral load (>20,000 copies/mL) or a falling CD4$^+$ count (<350 cells/μL) are definite indications, but many clinicians prefer to commence treatment before this. Pregnancy, HIV-associated nephropathy and co-infection with hepatitis B are other indications. Drugs should be used only in combination to prevent emergence of resistance and most regimens contain three or more drugs. Treatment is not curative and must be continued indefinitely.

6. Regimens can be changed if there is evidence of disease progression. HAART reduces the risk of vertical transmission and probably also the risk of seroconversion following occupational exposure (e.g. needlestick injury), if given promptly.

7. Resistance testing is indicated for the treatment of the naive patient, or if treatment is failing and will be changed.

8. In pregnancy, the aim of therapy is to make the patient's viral load undetectable. If the HIV RNA is more than 1000 copies, recommend caesarean section. Treat the mother with zidovudine as an infusion during labour, and treat the infant for six weeks.

9. Patients whose disease is well controlled by antiviral agents are more likely to die of cardiovascular disease than infection. This is partly as a result of their drug treatment (e.g. with protease inhibitors). Aggresive control of cardiovascular risk factors is indicated. Hyperlipidaemia should be treated with pravastatin (which has less interaction with antiviral drugs).

Chapter 14

The short case

> You see, but you do not observe.
> *Sir Arthur Conan Doyle (1859–1930)*

The short case is a test of the candidate's ability to examine a patient smoothly, confidently and accurately. There is rarely the opportunity to go back and repeat the examination. It takes a long time to get used to being watched critically while examining. This is why it is important to practise short cases of every conceivable type so that the physical examination is performed automatically in the correct way. While proceeding, the candidate should be consciously synthesising the results, not trying to remember what to do next.

Written introductions (or *stems*) were introduced for the short cases in 2008. These have a standardised format, including the patient's name and age followed by a brief description of the patient's symptoms, if there are any, and then a request to perform a particular examination. The stem is chosen by the examiners after they have assessed the patient. The written stem is given to the candidate or displayed on the door 1 or 2 minutes before the start of the case and is repeated verbally to the candidate when he or she enters the room. The idea is to give the candidate time to decide what to do. The possible trade-off is that the stems are becoming more subtle.

If the patient has no symptoms, the stem may state this. If the case is an obvious 'spot diagnosis', the stem may give the diagnosis and ask for an appropriate examination to assess the severity, activity or functional effect of the condition on the patient. For example: 'Mrs Jones is a 60-year-old woman who has a long history of rheumatoid arthritis. Please make an assessment of the activity of the disease.'

There has been a trend towards using more oblique stems. For example: 'Mrs Jones is a 60-year-old woman who finds she is continually dropping plates. Please assess her hands and go on from there.' This stem would involve a neurological and joint assessment of the hands. The presentation of the findings should include an explanation for the plate dropping.

If the stem contains specific instructions, these must be followed. For example, if asked to examine a patient's gait, it is vital to get the patient to walk first. This may appear obvious, but many candidates have failed because they have not followed the examiners' instructions. Time is a major factor here—it is limited and you do not want to run out of time before getting to the problem the examiners have raised.

The time allowed for each short case is 15 minutes. This means that time should be available for both examination and discussion. Patients are not included just as quick 'spot diagnosis' cases alone, but if you do 'spot the diagnosis' it will be a golden opportunity to demonstrate systematically the associated signs in full. The examiners will expect a higher standard of examination when the diagnosis is fairly obvious.

With the current marking system, a candidate can fail a short case and still pass the examination. The most common short cases are cardiovascular and neurological problems. Abdominal examinations are probably next in importance. We suggest that candidates aim to examine each short case proficiently within 8 minutes.

It is a good idea, when introduced to the patient, to step over and shake his or her hand firmly. This may endear you to the patient (and exclude dystrophia myotonica). Always position the patient properly (e.g. at 45° for the cardiovascular examination or flat for the abdominal examination) and make sure that the patient is appropriately undressed for the relevant examination.

It is always worthwhile taking a moment to stand back and look at the whole patient. This may prevent you from missing an obvious spot diagnosis, such as myxoedema, a thymectomy scar in a patient with muscle weakness (myasthenia), a psoriatic rash in a patient with arthropathy or a cushingoid appearance in a hypertension examination. Practice really does help improve ability to see clinical associations. A candidate will almost always fail the case if a major sign is missed. The examiners decide what signs they feel are most important and, although they often resolve not to pass a candidate unless these are all found, in practice finding the majority of the agreed signs will result in a pass.

Do not ask the patient any questions, although it is prudent to say 'Let me know if I hurt you' and, when examining the abdomen directly, to ask 'Are you tender anywhere?' This is a test of bedside manner (and may give you a clue!). Always try to make the patient comfortable and avoid totally exposing the patient or exposing parts that are not being examined.

Remember that you are, in fact, demonstrating the signs (particularly in the case of a neurological short case) to the examiners. It is important to perform each manoeuvre accurately and deliberately. Be seen to be smooth and confident, as if you have done the examination a thousand times before. Also try to be confident of each sign before moving on to another area (e.g. on finding an abdominal mass, concentrate on excluding the various possibilities and coming to a firm conclusion) and do not worry too much about the time it takes. Practice will facilitate formation of conclusions accurately and quickly.

Very occasionally the examiners will pull a candidate away in the middle of an examination. This is why it is important to synthesise the data as you go. Do not get flustered by this—it usually means enough of the examination has been completed for you to have discovered the important signs. Examiners no longer require the interpretation of a particular sign in isolation (e.g. the collapsing carotid pulse in aortic regurgitation or the double apex beat in hypertrophic cardiomyopathy).

Usually there is no interruption until the examination is almost finished. We suggest that candidates keep on examining until told to stop and then list all the other things they would like to have done and why (e.g. urine analysis, rectal examination).

Before presenting the findings, listen closely to the examiners' instructions. Candidates will often be asked 'What did you find?', when they are expected to describe the relevant signs first and then comment on possible causes. Sometimes candidates will be asked 'What is your diagnosis?', when they are expected to give a diagnosis or differential diagnosis first and then list the signs supporting the contention.

One useful method of presentation is to first repeat the examiners' introduction, then give the provisional diagnosis and relevant findings. For example: 'I was asked to examine Mr Jones, a 60-year-old man who presented with dyspnoea. On examination of his cardiovascular system, I found ...' When describing the signs it is probably easiest to present them in the order that they were looked for (e.g. for the cardiovascular system—pulse rate, then blood pressure, then jugular venous pressure). It is important to state all the positive signs and the important negative ones. Be definite about each sign mentioned or do not mention the sign at all. There is no place for expressions such as 'slightly asymmetrical', 'minor', 'early clubbing' etc. Never use the phrase 'I think'—it will always be interpreted as uncertainty.

Alternatively, you may talk as you go. This is usually acceptable to the examiners, but we recommend such an approach only in special cases in adult medicine, because the processing of information is more difficult for candidates (see Ch 15).

Confidence is critical to success in the short cases. Do not lose confidence if you make a minor error, just go on—the examiners may not even have noticed.

A short differential diagnosis is usually expected even if the diagnosis is obvious. For example, a patient with fasciculation, plus upper and lower motor neurone signs in the legs and no sensory loss almost certainly has motor neurone disease, but a non-metastatic manifestation of carcinoma must be considered. Always mention common before rare diseases and always consider the patient's age and sex. Never reel off any old list; the differential diagnosis must be tailored to the particular patient. Sometimes patients will have signs of two different problems. This should not be ignored. For example, a patient with proximal muscle weakness as a result of polymyositis may have unrelated Dupuytren's contractures.

After presentation of the signs, a few minutes or more are set aside for discussion. The examiners are not encouraged to take the candidate back for a second look at a sign, but this does happen and presents a genuine second chance. If a candidate has done well in a case and there are a few minutes left for extra questions, the score can only go up, not down. Relevant X-rays or an ECG may be shown to the candidate. Some diagnostic and therapeutic aspects may be discussed in the short case.

The College has moved away from the traditional 'spot' short case (e.g. acromegaly) and now concentrates more on 'realistic' cases (e.g. heart murmurs, abdominal masses). However, all types still crop up—candidates must try to prepare for most possibilities. It is also true that the more straightforward the case, the higher the standard of examination that will be expected, and vice versa. Trick cases are deliberately avoided.

The value of some traditional clinical signs is now being questioned as *evidence-based* approaches to clinical examination help establish the validity and utility of signs. There is much work still to be done in this area, but an understanding of the value of signs is increasingly important. Some useful references that might assist the candidate are listed at the end of the book. A tactful approach may be needed with the examiners to prevent any resentment at the candidate's failing to look for a traditional sign that is a particular favourite of theirs.

Four golden rules for the short cases

1. Do *everything* properly when you examine the patient—*never* take short cuts.
2. *Think* and *synthesise* as you examine the patient—be alert.
3. *Never* make up signs and *never* ignore signs because they don't fit neatly together.
4. Always *be sure of your facts* when presenting—it's better to say that you don't know than to guess.

Chapter 15

Common short cases

> The trouble with doctors is not that they don't
> know enough, but that they don't see enough.
>
> *Corrigan (1802–80)*

In the short cases, candidates may be asked to examine a system or a particular part of the patient. Now that 15 minutes is available for each case, 'spot' diagnoses alone are not likely to be asked for by the examiners. The following pages outline a system for examining major short-case possibilities. Use this information to help develop your own system. Many useful lists are also included in this section.

We have also provided examples of typical X-rays and scans related to particular short-case examinations. At the end of each short-case discussion, the examiners will often ask 'What investigations might be helpful in this case?', and in many cases X-rays, CT scans or MRI scans will be indicated and available for you to look at and comment on.

In all cases, before beginning a specific examination, you should stand back for a moment and carefully observe the patient. It is still important to look for an associated 'spot' diagnosis, such as peripheral neuropathy in a myxoedematous patient or aortic regurgitation in a patient with Marfan's syndrome.

The patient will normally be positioned and undressed ready for you to examine. However, if either positioning or undressing is unsatisfactory, you must insist on having this corrected.

The cardiovascular system

The cardiovascular examination

'This 50-year-old man presents with dyspnoea on exertion and orthopnoea. Please examine his cardiovascular system.'

Method *(see Table 15.1)*

1. Make sure the patient is positioned at 45° and that the patient's chest and neck are fully exposed. For a woman, the requirements of modesty dictate that you cover her breasts with a towel or loose garment.
2. While standing back, inspect for the appearance of Marfan's, Turner's or Down syndrome. Also look for dyspnoea and cyanosis.
3. Pick up the patient's hand. While feeling the radial pulse, ask whether you may take the blood pressure. The examiners will usually supply you with the reading: be sure to remember this value. Inspect the patient's hands for

TABLE 15.1 Cardiovascular system examination

1. GENERAL INSPECTION (lying at 45°)
Marfan's, Turner's, Down syndrome
Rheumatological disorders—ankylosing spondylitis (aortic regurgitation)
Acromegaly etc.
Dyspnoea

2. HANDS
Radial pulses—right and left
Radiofemoral delay (if indicated)
Clubbing
Signs of infective endocarditis—splinter haemorrhages, Osler's nodes etc.
Peripheral cyanosis
Xanthomata

3. BLOOD PRESSURE

4. FACE
Eyes
    Cornea: arcus cornea
    Sclerae: pallor, jaundice
    Pupils: Argyll Robertson (aortic regurgitation)
    Xanthelasma
Malar flush (mitral stenosis, pulmonary stenosis)
Mouth
    Cyanosis
    Palate (high arched—Marfan's)
    Dentition

5. NECK
Jugular venous pressure
    Central venous pressure height
    Wave form (especially large *v* waves)
Carotids
    Pulse character

6. PRAECORDIUM
Inspect
    Scars—whole chest, back
    Deformity
    Apex beat—position, character
    Abnormal pulsations

Palpate
    Apex beat—position, character
    Thrills
    Abnormal impulses
Note: Beware of dextrocardia
Auscultate
    Heart sounds
    Murmurs
    Position patient left lateral position sitting forward (forced expiratory apnoea)
    Note: Palpate for thrills again on positioning.
Dynamic auscultation
    Respiratory phases
    Valsalva manoeuvre
    Exercise (isometric, e.g. handgrip)

7. BACK (sitting forward)
Scars, deformity
Sacral oedema
Pleural effusion (percuss)
Left ventricular failure (auscultate)

8. ABDOMEN (lying flat—1 pillow only)
Palpate liver (pulsatile etc.), spleen, aorta
Percuss for ascites (right heart failure)
Femoral arteries—palpate, auscultate

9. LEGS
Clubbing toes
Cyanosis, cold limbs, trophic changes, ulceration (peripheral vascular disease)
All peripheral pulses
Oedema
Xanthomata
Calf tenderness

10. OTHER
Urine analysis (infective endocarditis)
Fundi (endocarditis)
Temperature chart (endocarditis)

clubbing. Also look for the peripheral stigmata of infective endocarditis—splinter haemorrhages are common (and are also caused by trauma), whereas Osler's nodes and Janeway lesions are rare. Look quickly, but carefully, at each nail bed, otherwise it is easy to miss key signs. Note the presence of an intravenous cannula and, if an infusion is running, look at the bag to see what it is. There will usually be a peripheral or central line in situ if the patient is being treated for infective endocarditis. Note any tendon xanthomata (type II hyperlipidaemia).

HINT BOX
Radiofemoral delay should be assessed very quickly or not at all unless the stem suggests the patient has hypertension.

4. The pulse at the wrist should be timed for rate and rhythm. Pulse character is poorly assessed here. This is also the time to feel for radiofemoral delay (which occurs in coarctation of the aorta) and radial–radial inequality.
5. Next inspect the face. Look at the eyes briefly for jaundice (valve haemolysis) and xanthelasma (type II or III hyperlipidaemia). You may also notice the classic 'mitral facies' (owing to dilation of malar capillaries associated with severe mitral stenosis and caused by pulmonary hypertension and a low cardiac output). Then inspect the mouth using a torch for a high-arched palate (Marfan's syndrome and the possibility of aortic regurgitation and mitral valve prolapse), petechiae and the state of dentition (endocarditis). Look at the tongue or lips for central cyanosis.
6. The neck is very important, so take time to examine here. The jugular venous pressure (JVP) must be assessed for height and character (see Table 15.2 and Fig 15.1). Use the right internal jugular vein to assess this. Look for a change with inspiration (Kussmaul's sign).
7. Now feel each carotid pulse separately (never together!). Assess the pulse character (see Table 15.3).
8. Proceed to the praecordium. Always begin by inspecting for scars, deformity, the site of the apex beat and visible pulsations. Do not forget about pacemaker and cardioverter-defibrillator boxes.

TABLE 15.2 JVP

1. Wave form

    (a) Causes of dominant *a* wave:

        (i)   tricuspid stenosis (also causes a slow *y* descent) (very rare)

        (ii) pulmonary stenosis

        (iii) pulmonary hypertension

    (b) Causes of dominant *v* wave:

        (i)   tricuspid regurgitation (important and common)

    (c) Causes of cannon *a* waves:

        (i)   complete heart block

        (ii) paroxysmal nodal tachycardia with retrograde atrial conduction

        (iii) ventricular tachycardia with retrograde atrial conduction or atrioventricular dissociation

2. Causes of an elevated central venous pressure:

    (a) right ventricular failure

    (b) tricuspid stenosis or regurgitation

    (c) pericardial effusion or constrictive pericarditis

    (d) superior vena caval obstruction

    (e) fluid overload

    (f) hyperdynamic circulation (e.g. fever, anaemia, thyrotoxicosis, arteriovenous fistula, pregnancy, exercise, beri beri, hypoxia, hypercapnia)

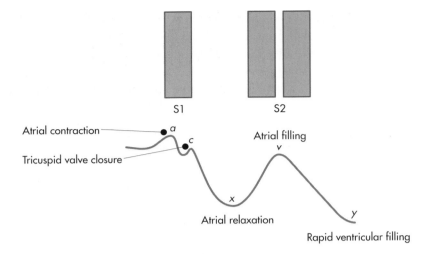

S1   S2

Atrial contraction — a

Tricuspid valve closure

Atrial filling — v

x

Atrial relaxation

y

Rapid ventricular filling

Figure 15.1 The JVP and its relationship to the first (S1) and second (S2) heart sounds.

TABLE 15.3 Arterial pulse character	
Anacrotic	Small volume, slow upstroke, plus *a* wave on the upstroke Cause: aortic stenosis
Plateau	Slow upstroke Cause: aortic stenosis
Bisferiens	Anacrotic plus collapsing Cause: aortic stenosis plus aortic regurgitation
Collapsing	Cause: aortic regurgitation, hyperdynamic circulation, arteriosclerotic aorta (elderly patients particularly), patent ductus arteriosus, peripheral arteriovenous aneurysm
Small volume	Cause: aortic stenosis, pericardial effusion
Alternans	Alternating strong and weak beats Cause: left ventricular failure

HINT BOX
Mitral valvotomy scars (under the left or right breast) can be quite lateral and easily missed (with ghastly repercussions in the test).

9. Palpate for the apex beat position. Be seen to count down the correct number of intercostal spaces. The normal position is the fifth intercostal space, 1 cm medial to the midclavicular line. The character of the apex beat is important. There are a number of types:
   (a) A *pressure-loaded* (hyperdynamic, systolic overloaded) apex beat is a forceful and sustained impulse (e.g. in aortic stenosis, hypertension).
   (b) A *volume-loaded* (hyperkinetic, diastolic overloaded) apex beat is a forceful but unsustained impulse (e.g. in aortic regurgitation, mitral regurgitation).

Don't miss the tapping apex beat of mitral stenosis (a palpable first heart sound) or the dyskinetic apex beat caused by a previous large myocardial infarction. The double or triple apical impulse in hypertrophic cardiomyopathy is very important too. Feel also for an apical thrill and time it.

10. Palpate with the heel of your hand for a left parasternal impulse, which indicates right ventricular hypertrophy or left atrial enlargement. Now feel at the base of the heart for a palpable pulmonary component of the second heart sound (P2) and aortic thrills. Percussion is usually unnecessary.

11. Auscultation begins with listening in the mitral area with both the bell and the diaphragm. Spend most time here. Listen for each component of the cardiac cycle separately. Identify the first and second heart sounds (see Table 15.4) and decide whether they are of normal intensity and whether they are split. Now listen for extra heart or prosthetic heart sounds (see Table 15.4) and murmurs (see Table 15.5). Mechanical valves include bileaflet, ball case and tilting disc. Ball case valves have a sharp opening sound and may rattle. Tilting disc valves have soft opening sounds and sharp closing sounds. All mechanical valves require anticoagulation. Biologic valves may have a systolic murmur; anticoagulation is not required. Do not be satisfied at having identified one abnormality—it is more common to get complex rather than simple lesions in the examination.

12. Repeat the approach at the left sternal edge and then at the base of the heart (aortic and pulmonary areas). Time each part of the cycle with the carotid pulse. Listen below the left clavicle for a patent ductus arteriosus murmur, which may be audible here and nowhere else.

13. It is now time to reposition the patient, first in the left lateral position. Again feel the apex beat for character (particularly tapping). Auscultate carefully for mitral stenosis with the bell. Next sit the patient forward and feel for thrills (with the patient in full expiration) at the left sternal edge and base. Then listen in those areas, particularly for aortic regurgitation.

14. Dynamic auscultation should always be done if there is any doubt about the diagnosis. The Valsalva manoeuvre should be performed whenever there is a pure systolic murmur, otherwise hypertrophic cardiomyopathy is easily missed (p 281).

HINT BOX

The patient who seems familiar with the Valsalva manoeuvre may well have a murmur affected by it.

---

15. The patient is now sitting up. Percuss the back quickly to exclude a pleural effusion (e.g. due to left ventricular failure) and auscultate for inspiratory crackles (left ventricular failure). If there is radiofemoral delay, also listen for a coarctation murmur here. Feel for sacral oedema and note any back deformity (e.g. ankylosing spondylitis [p 275] with aortic regurgitation).

16. Next lay the patient flat and examine the abdomen properly (p 310) for hepatomegaly (e.g. as a result of right ventricular failure) and a pulsatile liver (tricuspid regurgitation). Perform the hepatojugular reflux test. Press over the upper abdomen for 30 seconds or so and watch for a rise in the JVP. This is a reliable sign of heart failure. Feel for splenomegaly (endocarditis) and an aortic aneurysm. Palpate both femoral arteries. Then examine all the peripheral pulses. Look particularly for peripheral oedema, clubbing of the toes, Achilles tendon xanthomata, signs of peripheral vascular disease and the stigmata of infective endocarditis.

TABLE 15.4 Heart sounds

First heart sound (S1)

Loud—mitral stenosis, tricuspid stenosis, tachycardia, hyperdynamic circulation

Soft—mitral regurgitation, calcified mitral valve, left bundle branch block, first-degree heart block

Second heart sound (S2)

Aortic (A2)

Loud—congenital aortic stenosis, systemic hypertension

Soft—calcified aortic valve, aortic regurgitation (when the leaflets cannot coapt)

Pulmonary (P2)

Loud—pulmonary hypertension

Soft—pulmonary stenosis

Increased normal splitting (wider on inspiration)

Right bundle branch block, pulmonary stenosis, ventricular septal defect, mitral regurgitation (earlier A2)

Fixed splitting

Atrial septal defect

Reversed splitting (P2 first)

Left bundle branch block, aortic stenosis (severe), coarctation of aorta, patent ductus arteriosus (large)

Third heart sound (S3)

Mechanism: possibly tautening of the mitral or tricuspid cusps at the end of rapid diastolic filling

Causes

Left ventricular third heart sound (S3) (louder at apex and on expiration) Physiological (under 40 years of age or during pregnancy), left ventricular failure, aortic regurgitation, mitral regurgitation, ventricular septal defect, patent ductus arteriosus

Right ventricular third heart sound (S3) (louder at left sternal edge and on inspiration) Right ventricular failure, constrictive pericarditis

Fourth heart sound (S4)

Mechanism: a high atrial pressure wave is probably reflected back from a poorly compliant ventricle; is always abnormal.

Causes

Left ventricular fourth heart sound Aortic stenosis, acute mitral regurgitation, systemic hypertension, ischaemic heart disease, hypertrophic cardiomyopathy

Right ventricular fourth heart sound Pulmonary hypertension, pulmonary stenosis

17. At the end, ask the examiners for the results of the urine analysis (haematuria in endocarditis) and a temperature chart (fever in endocarditis), and examine the fundi (for Roth's spots in endocarditis and for hypertensive changes).

Note

• It is fairly unlikely that you will have time to complete all aspects of your examination. If you are stopped, mention the list of things you would still like to do that are particularly relevant.

TABLE 15.5 Differential diagnosis of murmurs

Pansystolic	Mitral regurgitation, tricuspid regurgitation, ventricular septal defect, aortopulmonary shunts
Midsystolic	Aortic stenosis, pulmonary stenosis, hypertrophic cardiomyopathy, pulmonary flow murmur of an atrial septal defect
Early systolic	Ventricular septal defect (either very small, or large plus pulmonary hypertension), acute mitral regurgitation, tricuspid regurgitation
Late systolic	Mitral valve prolapse, papillary muscle dysfunction (e.g. hypertrophic cardiomyopathy)
Early diastolic	Aortic regurgitation, pulmonary regurgitation
Mid-diastolic	Mitral stenosis, tricuspid stenosis, atrial myxoma, Austin Flint murmur of aortic regurgitation, Carey Coombs murmur of acute rheumatic fever
Presystolic	Mitral stenosis, tricuspid stenosis, atrial myxoma
Continuous*	1. Patent ductus arteriosus 2. Arteriovenous fistula (coronary artery, pulmonary, systemic) 3. Venous hum (situated over the right supraclavicular fossa and abolished by ipsilateral compression of the internal jugular vein) 4. Rupture of a sinus of Valsalva into the right atrium or ventricle 5. Aortopulmonary connection (e.g. Blalock shunt) 6. 'Mammary soufflé' (in late pregnancy or early postpartum period)

*Aortic stenosis and aortic regurgitation or mitral stenosis and mitral regurgitation may be confused with a continuous murmur.

- If you have auscultated and there is nothing obvious at first, consider the following and exclude them:
  1. mitral stenosis (see Fig 15.2) (position and exercise if necessary)
  2. atrial septal defect (listen carefully for fixed splitting)
  3. mitral valve prolapse (perform a Valsalva manoeuvre)
  4. pulmonary hypertension
  5. constrictive pericarditis.

Notes on valve diseases

After you have made a diagnosis of a valve lesion, the following are the types of facts you should know. An assessment of the lesion's severity is usually required.

Candidates should be able to make some recommendation as to appropriate follow-up. Most patients with valve abnormalities should be reviewed regularly and have repeat echocardiograms. For patients with mild abnormalities about every three to four years is sufficient, but for more severe cases annual review is usually recommended. Patients who are not symptomatic but have severe disease may need six-monthly review, usually with a repeat echocardiogram. Patients should be advised to return for earlier review if symptoms (e.g. dyspnoea, chest pain or exertional dizziness) occur.

Mitral stenosis

Valve area: normal, 4–6 cm^2; severe mitral stenosis, <1 cm^2.

Causes

1. Rheumatic (in women more often than men).
2. Congenital very rarely (e.g. parachute valve, with all chordae inserting into one papillary muscle).

Clinical signs of severity
1. Small pulse pressure.
2. Early opening snap (owing to raised left atrial pressure).
3. Length of the mid-diastolic rumbling murmur (persists as long as there is a gradient).
4. Diastolic thrill at the apex (rare).
5. Presence of pulmonary hypertension, the signs of which are:
   (a) prominent *a* wave in the JVP
   (b) right ventricular impulse
   (c) loud pulmonary component of the second heart sound (P2)
   (d) pulmonary regurgitation
   (e) tricuspid regurgitation.

Results of investigations
1. ECG:
   (a) *P* mitrale in sinus rhythm
   (b) atrial fibrillation (a sign of chronicity)
   (c) right ventricular systolic overload (severe disease)
   (d) right-axis deviation (severe disease).
2. Chest X-ray film (see Fig 15.2):
   (a) mitral valve calcification
   (b) big left atrium:
       (i) double left atrial shadow
       (ii) displaced left main bronchus
       (iii) big left atrial appendage
   (c) signs of pulmonary hypertension:
       (i) large central pulmonary arteries
       (ii) pruned peripheral arterial tree
   (d) signs of cardiac failure.
   Note: If the investigations suggest that left ventricular dilatation is present in the presence of a mitral stenosis murmur, consider these other possibilities:
   • associated mitral regurgitation
   • associated aortic valve disease
   • associated hypertension
   • associated ischaemic heart disease.

Echocardiograph (M mode, 2D Doppler and colour flow mapping)
The posterior mitral leaflet maintains its anterior position in diastole and this is pathognomonic. A delayed mitral closure with decreased ejection fraction slope (an M mode index of mitral valve opening) is not pathognomonic but is very suggestive. There may be heavy echoes from thickened or calcified mitral leaflets. On two-dimensional (2D) scanning the valve can be seen doming in diastole. The mitral valve area can be quite accurately determined by 2D echocardiography and Doppler measurements. The valve area is estimated using the pressure half-time measurement. This analysis of Doppler left ventricular inflow is performed routinely when mitral stenosis is suspected. Colour flow mapping makes finding the inflow jet easier and is very sensitive for the detection of any associated mitral regurgitation.

Indications for surgery
These include progressive dyspnoea, pulmonary oedema or major haemoptysis that has failed to respond to medical therapy. This usually occurs when the valve area falls to about 1 cm^2.

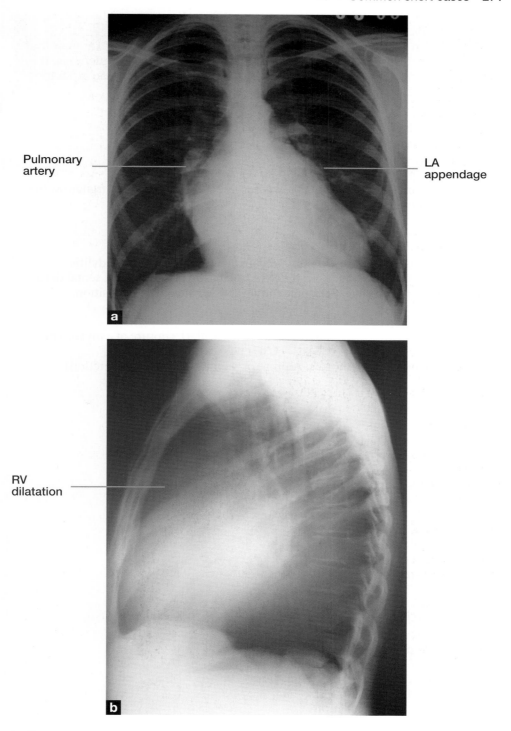

Pulmonary
artery

LA
appendage

RV
dilatation

a

b

Figure 15.2 (a) and (b) Mitral stenosis on PA film. The left atrial appendage is dilated and there are prominent pulmonary arteries. The heart appears enlarged because of right ventricular enlargement, which is more obvious on the lateral film.

Figures reproduced courtesy of The Canberra Hospital.

HINT BOX
A declaration that the apex beat is 'tapping' in quality tells the examiner that you have made the diagnosis of mitral (or very rarely tricuspid) stenosis. It is unwise to allow the word 'tapping' to escape your lips unless you are happy that this is the diagnosis.

Mitral regurgitation

Causes—chronic
1. Degenerative disease.
2. Mitral valve prolapse.
3. Rheumatic (men more often than women)—rarely is mitral regurgitation the only murmur present.
4. Papillary muscle dysfunction:
   (a) left ventricular failure
   (b) ischaemia.
5. Connective tissue disease—rheumatoid arthritis, ankylosing spondylitis.
6. Congenital—endocardial cushion defect (including primum atrial septal defect (ASD) and cleft mitral leaflet), parachute valve, corrected transposition.

Causes—acute
1. Infective endocarditis (perforation of anterior leaflet), rupture of a myxomatous cord.
2. Myocardial infarction (chordae rupture or papillary muscle dysfunction).
3. Surgery.
4. Trauma.

Clinical signs of severity
1. Enlarged left ventricle.
2. Pulmonary hypertension (a late sign).
3. Third heart sound (not always reliable).
4. Early diastolic rumble.
5. Soft first heart sound.
6. Aortic component of second heart sound (A2) is earlier.
7. Small-volume pulse (very severe).
8. Left ventricular failure.

Results of investigations
1. ECG:
   (a) *P* mitrale
   (b) atrial fibrillation
   (c) left ventricular diastolic overload
   (d) right-axis deviation.
2. Chest X-ray film:
   (a) large (sometimes gigantic) left atrium
   (b) increased left ventricular size
   (c) mitral annular calcification
   (d) pulmonary hypertension (much less common).
3. Echocardiography (see Fig 15.3)—this will give information about the possible aetiology, the severity and any associated valve or structural abnormalities:
   (a) thickened leaflets—rheumatic aetiology
   (b) prolapsing leaflet(s)
   (c) left atrial size (a sign of chronicity and severity)

Echocardiography Report

Reason for study: Middle and late systolic murmur ?MVP
Study quality: <u>Good</u> Satisfactory Poor

RV	18	(mm)	(N 10–26)
Sept.	8	(mm)	(N 7–11)
LVEDD	63	(mm)	(N 36–56)
LVESD	28	(mm)	(N 20–40)
LVPW	10	(mm)	(N 7–11)
Aorta	22	(mm)	(N 20–35)
LA	46	(mm)	(N 24–40)
FS	55	%	(N 27–40)
EF	85	%	(N 55–70)

Valves

Mitral	MR, prolapse posterior MV leaflet
Tricus.	Trivial TR
Aortic	Thickened, not stenosed
Pulm.	Appears normal

Doppler–2D
The left ventricle is dilated. LV systolic function is preserved. LA is dilated. Severe prolapse of posterior MV leaflet. Possible flail segment.

Doppler—colour flow mapping
There is a large jet of mitral regurgitation extending into the left atrium.

Conclusions
Severe MR, possible flail mitral valve segment, severe MVP.

Comment
The echocardiography criteria for MVP have been tightened over the last several years. Redundancy of one or both of the MV leaflets is common and probably represents a variation of normal in many cases. Bowing of the leaflet into the left atrium of at least 1 cm must be present before the diagnosis of MVP can be made. In this case, the posterior leaflet appears very abnormal and seems to move into the left atrium in an unrestrained fashion. This suggests its chordal attachment may have been severed. The chords may be involved in the abnormality of the mitral leaflets in patients with prolapse and are at risk of rupture.

The left ventricle is dilated, suggesting that the mitral regurgitation is of haemodynamic significance. Left ventricular ejection remains high in cases of mitral regurgitation until late in the illness. This is because the left ventricular afterload is low. Part of the left ventricular ejection is into the left atrium, which is a low-resistance chamber.

The left atrial enlargement, present here, suggests that some mitral regurgitation has been present for some time. A large left atrium pleases the cardiac surgeons who have trouble getting their hands into the mitral valve through a normal-sized atrium.

Key
EF = ejection fraction; FS = fractional shortening; LA = left atrium; LV = left ventricle; LVEDD = left ventricular end-diastolic dimension; LVESD = left ventricular end-systolic dimension, LVPW = left ventricular posterior wall; MR = mitral regurgitation; MV = mitral valve; MVP = mitral valve prolapse; Pulm. = pulmonary; RV = right ventricle; Sept. = septal thickness; TR = tricuspid regurgitation; Tricus. = tricuspid.

Figure 15.3 Echocardiography report in a patient with mitral regurgitation and mitral valve prolapse.

(d) left ventricular size and function
(e) Doppler detection of the regurgitant jet in the left atrium; colour mapping of jet size and detection of reversal of flow in the pulmonary veins
(f) other abnormalities (e.g. aortic valve disease as a result of rheumatic carditis or an ASD associated with mitral valve prolapse)
(g) calcification of the mitral annulus—common in elderly people.
   Note: the valve leaflets may not appear abnormal.

Indications for surgery
In chronic mitral regurgitation, consider surgery if there are class III or IV symptoms, or if there is left ventricular dysfunction or the left ventricular dimensions have increased progressively. In acute mitral regurgitation, operate if there is haemodynamic collapse (there usually is). Repair of a prolapsing posterior leaflet is now undertaken earlier than valve replacement. The short- and long-term results (1% recurrence per year) are so good that the operation should be recommended for even mild symptoms or once left ventricular dilatation occurs. Mitral valve replacement is usually with a mechanical valve. Tissue valves in the mitral position have a relatively short life (sometimes only five to seven years).

Mitral valve prolapse (systolic click–murmur syndrome)
This is the most common heart lesion in the community (3% of adults) and is more common in women. When it occurs in men it is more likely to progress to cause significant regurgitation.

Dynamic auscultation
The click murmur is affected by the:
1. Valsalva manoeuvre (decreases preload)—murmur longer, click earlier
2. handgrip (increases afterload) or squatting (increases preload)—murmur shorter.

Echocardiography
There is now thought to be a considerable variation in the normal range of the appearance of the mitral leaflets on echocardiography. Some redundancy of one or both leaflets is seen commonly in normal people. Prolapse of a leaflet of 1 cm or more into the left atrium behind the attachment point of the valve is considered abnormal. Antibiotic prophylaxis, however, is not necessary for these patients unless mitral regurgitation is detected on Doppler interrogation.

Associations
1. Marfan's syndrome.
2. ASD (secundum).
3. Anorexia nervosa (disproportion between normal-sized valve ring and small left ventricle).

Complications (more common for men with mitral valve prolapse)
1. Mitral regurgitation.
2. Infective endocarditis.
Arrhythmias, embolism and sudden death are probably not complications of mitral valve prolapse.

Aortic regurgitation
Causes of chronic aortic regurgitation
Valvular
1. Rheumatic (rarely the only murmur in this case).
2. Congenital (e.g. bicuspid valve; ventral septal defect (VSD)—an associated prolapse of the aortic cusp is not uncommon).
3. Seronegative arthropathy, especially ankylosing spondylitis.

Aortic root (murmur may be maximal at the right sternal border)
1. Marfan's syndrome.
2. Aortitis (e.g. seronegative arthropathies, rheumatoid arthritis, tertiary syphilis).
3. Dissecting aneurysm.
4. Old age.

Causes of acute aortic regurgitation
Note: Murmur may be soft because of increased left ventricular end-diastolic pressure.
1. Valvular—infective endocarditis.
2. Aortic root—Marfan's syndrome, hypertension, dissecting aneurysm.

Clinical signs of severity in chronic aortic regurgitation
1. Collapsing pulse.
2. Wide pulse pressure.
3. Length of the *decrescendo* diastolic murmur.
4. Third heart sound (left ventricular).
5. Soft aortic component of the second heart sound (A2).
6. Austin Flint murmur (a diastolic rumble caused by limitation to mitral inflow by the regurgitation jet).
7. Left ventricular failure.

HINT BOX
A loud systolic murmur, rarely with a thrill, may be present in patients with severe aortic regurgitation without any organic aortic stenosis being associated. The peripheral signs of aortic regurgitation are the clue that this is the real lesion in this situation.

Results of investigations
1. ECG—left ventricular hypertrophy (diastolic overload).
2. Chest X-ray film:
   (a) left ventricular dilation
   (b) aortic root dilatation or aneurysm (see Fig 15.4)
   (c) valve calcification.
3. Echocardiography:
   (a) left ventricular dimensions and function
   (b) Doppler estimation of size of regurgitant jet
   (c) vegetations (endocarditis can be a cause of acute aortic regurgitation)
   (d) aortic root dimensions
   (e) valve cusp thickening or prolapse.

Figure 15.4 Massive dilatation of the thoracic aorta (arrow) is seen in this patient with Marfan's syndrome and aortic regurgitation.
Figure reproduced courtesy of The Canberra Hospital.

Indications for surgery
1. Symptoms—dyspnoea on exertion.
2. Worsening left ventricular function, such as low ejection fraction (in aortic regurgitation this is increased until late, severe disease intervenes) measured on a gated blood pool scan.
3. Progressive left ventricular dilatation on serial echocardiograms: left ventricular end-systolic dimension of >5.5 cm.

Aortic stenosis
Valve area: 1.5–2.0 cm². Significant stenosis at <1 cm². In critical aortic stenosis, less than 0.7 cm²/m² or a valve gradient >70 mmHg.

Causes
1. Degenerative senile calcific aortic stenosis (the most common cause in the elderly).
2. Rheumatic (rarely isolated).
3. Calcific bicuspid valve.

Clinical signs of severity
1. Plateau pulse.

HINT BOX
The pulse character has been shown not to be useful in elderly patients; this fact may need to be put tactfully to the examiners.

2. Aortic thrill (very important sign of severe stenosis).
3. Length, harshness and lateness of the peak of the systolic murmur.
4. Fourth heart sound (S4).
5. Paradoxical splitting of the second heart sound (delayed left ventricular ejection and aortic valve closure).
6. Left ventricular failure (a late sign—right ventricular failure is preterminal).

Results of investigations
1. ECG—left ventricular hypertrophy (systolic overload).
2. Chest X-ray film (see Fig 15.5):
   (a) left ventricular hypertrophy
   (b) valve calcification.
3. Echocardiography (see Fig 15.6):
   (a) Doppler estimation of gradient (*note:* Doppler estimation of peak gradient usually overestimates the value compared with cardiac catheterisation)
   (b) valve cusp mobility
   (c) left ventricular hypertrophy
   (d) left ventricular dysfunction.

Indications for surgery
1. Symptoms—exertional angina, exertional dyspnoea, exertional syncope (urgent).
2. Critical obstruction (based on catheterisation data) and severe left ventricular hypertrophy even if asymptomatic.

Choice of valve
Tissue (bovine pericardial or porcine, or occasionally homograft) valves are usually offered to patients over the age of about 65 or to younger patients who wish to avoid warfarin. Their life expectancy before failing is up to 15 years or more.

Tricuspid regurgitation
Look for the following signs:
1. the JVP—large *v* waves: the JVP is elevated if right ventricular failure has occurred
2. palpation—right ventricular heave
3. auscultation—a pansystolic murmur, maximal at the lower end of the sternum and on inspiration, may be present, but the diagnosis can be made on the basis of the peripheral signs alone; multiple systolic clicks are characteristic of Ebstein's anomaly of the tricuspid valve

Figure 15.5 Chest X-ray of a patient with calcific aortic stenosis; valve calcification is visible (arrow).
Figure reproduced courtesy of The Canberra Hospital.

4. abdomen—a pulsatile, large and tender liver is usually present; ascites and oedema with pleural effusions may also occur.

Causes
1. Functional (no disease of the valve leaflets)—right ventricular failure.
2. Rheumatic—only very rarely does tricuspid regurgitation occur alone; usually mitral valve disease is also present.
3. Infective endocarditis (right-sided endocarditis in intravenous drug abusers).
4. Congenital—Ebstein's anomaly.
5. Tricuspid valve prolapse (rare).
6. Right ventricular papillary muscle infarction.
7. Trauma (usually a steering-wheel injury to the sternum).

Echocardiography Report

Reason for study: Systolic ejection murmur ?AS
Study quality: <u>Good</u> Satisfactory Poor

RV	13	(mm)	(N 10–26)
Sept.	13	(mm)	(N 7–11)
LVEDD	53	(mm)	(N 36–56)
LVESD	25	(mm)	(N 20–40)
LVPW	12	(mm)	(N 7–11)
Aorta	22	(mm)	(N 20–35)
LA	38	(mm)	(N 24–40)
FS	53	%	(N 27–40)
EF	83	%	(N 55–70)

Valves

> **Mitral**   Trivial MR
> **Tricus.**   Mild TR
> **Aortic**   Thickened, calcified, reduced cusp movement.
> **Pulm.**   Appears normal

Doppler—2D

There is mild symmetrical LV hypertrophy. The aortic valve is thickened and heavily calcified; it appears trileaflet. The mitral valve appears normal.

Doppler—colour flow mapping

The aortic outflow velocity is 4.6 m/s. The calculated peak aortic gradient is 85 mmHg. The mean gradient is 60 mmHg. Mild aortic regurgitation was detected. Mild MR is present. Mild TR. RV pressure = 24 mmHg.

Conclusions

Severe calcific aortic stenosis and mild LVH.

Comments

This echocardiography report gives considerable information about the patient's murmur. A candidate who had not diagnosed AS would be in some difficulty.

In AS the aortic valve is usually thickened and calcified unless the patient is young and has congenital AS. Stenosed aortic valves are often congenitally bicuspid and so the echocardiographer will often report the number of valve leaflets. Sometimes there is a comment about reduction in valve cusp movement. An almost immobile valve is more likely to be severely stenosed.

LVH is common when AS is significant. This LVH is mild; dimensions of 14 mm or more indicate severe LVH. Left ventricular dilatation and reduced fractional shortening are late signs.

Doppler measurement of the velocity of blood in the ascending aorta in systole allows calculation of the peak pressure difference across the valve (usually almost 0). This gradient tends to be higher than the gradient measured at cardiac catheterisation. The mean gradient is often closer to the catheter gradient.

Some AR is very often detected in the presence of significant AS. It is unlikely this mild AR would be audible and its presence on the report should not lead the candidate to panic.

Key

AR = aortic regurgitation; AS = aortic stenosis; EF = ejection fraction; FS = fractional shortening; LA = left atrium; LV = left ventricular; LVEDD = left ventricular end-diastolic dimension; LVESD = left ventricular end-systolic dimension; LVH = left ventricular hypertrophy; LVPW = left ventricular posterior wall; MR = mitral regurgitation; Pulm. = pulmonary; RV = right ventricle; Sept. = septal thickness; TR = tricuspid regurgitation; Tricus. = tricuspid.

Figure 15.6 Echocardiography report for a patient with aortic stenosis.

Figure 15.7 Chest X-ray of a patient with Ebstein's anomaly, showing a narrow cardiac pedicle.
Figure reproduced courtesy of The Canberra Hospital.

Results of investigations
The chest X-ray film may show right ventricular enlargement or biventricular enlargement if the tricuspid regurgitation is secondary to heart failure. Patients with Ebstein's anomaly may have the characteristic box-shaped heart and narrow cardiac base (see Fig 15.7). Echocardiography enables detection of structural valve abnormality and estimation of the size of the regurgitant jet in the right atrium. Measurement of the velocity of this jet allows estimation of the pressure gradient across the valve. As right atrial pressure is usually 5–10 mmHg, the right ventricular pressure can be estimated in any patient with tricuspid regurgitation by adding 5 to this pressure gradient. Trivial tricuspid regurgitation is a common and normal Doppler echocardiogram finding.

Pulmonary stenosis (in adults)
Look for the following signs:
1. general signs
   (a) peripheral cyanosis because of a low cardiac output

(b) the pulse—normal or reduced because of a low cardiac output
(c) the JVP—giant *a* waves because of right atrial hypertrophy; the JVP may be elevated
(d) palpation—right ventricular heave; thrill over the pulmonary area (common)
(e) auscultation—the murmur may be preceded by an ejection click; a harsh ejection systolic murmur maximal in the pulmonary area and on inspiration is present; S4 may be present (owing to right atrial hypertrophy)
(f) abdomen—presystolic pulsation of the liver may be present
2. signs of severe pulmonary stenosis
(a) an ejection systolic murmur peaking late in systole
(b) absence of an ejection click (also absent when the pulmonary stenosis is infundibular, i.e. below the valve level)
(c) presence of S4
(d) signs of right ventricular failure.

Causes
1. Congenital.
2. Carcinoid syndrome.

Chronic constrictive pericarditis
This diagnosis must not be missed. The patient may appear cachectic. Look for the following signs:
1. pulse and blood pressure—a low blood pressure and pulsus paradoxus are typical
2. JVP—this is raised; Kussmaul's sign is rare; the *x* and *y* descents are prominent
3. apex beat—impalpable
4. heart sounds—these are distant; there may be an early third heart sound and an early pericardial knock (as rapid ventricular filling is abruptly halted)
5. hepatosplenomegaly, ascites and oedema provide important clues
6. underlying aetiology (e.g. radiation, tumour, tuberculosis, connective tissue disease, chronic renal failure, trauma).

Hypertrophic cardiomyopathy
It is always important to consider this diagnosis—it is a popular 'trap'! The classical signs are as follows.
1. Pulse—this is typically sharp, rising and jerky, owing to rapid ejection by a hypertrophied ventricle early in systole, followed then by obstruction; it is not like the pulse of aortic stenosis.
2. The JVP—there is a prominent *a* wave owing to forceful atrial contraction against a non-compliant ventricle.
3. Apex beat—there is typically a double or triple impulse owing to presystolic ventricular expansion following atrial contraction.
4. Auscultation:
(a) late systolic ejection murmur (left sternal edge)
(b) pansystolic murmur (apex) from mitral regurgitation
(c) fourth heart sound.
   Note: there are no diastolic murmurs.
5. Dynamic manoeuvres—the murmur is louder with the Valsalva manoeuvre, standing and isotonic exercise (e.g. jogging—not usually possible under examination conditions). The murmur is softer with squatting, raising the legs and isometric exercise (e.g. forceful handgrip).

Results of investigations
1. ECG:
   (a) left ventricular hypertrophy and lateral ST segment and T wave changes
   (b) deep Q waves
   (c) conduction defects.
2. Chest X-ray film:
   (a) left ventricle enlarged with a hump along the border
   (b) no valve calcification.
3. Echocardiography (see Fig 15.8):
   (a) asymmetrical hypertrophy (ASH) of the ventricular septum
   (b) systolic anterior motion (SAM) of the anterior mitral valve leaflet
   (c) midsystolic closure of the aortic valve
   (d) Doppler detection of mitral regurgitation
   (e) Doppler estimation of the gradient in the left ventricular outflow tract.

Non-cyanotic congenital heart disease
These are difficult examination cases that not infrequently crop up in the test.

Atrial septal defect
There are two types (sinus venosus defects are not often seen in adults): ostium secundum and ostium primum.

ASD: ostium secundum
This is the most common and presents in adult life with:
1. fixed splitting of the second heart sound (*note*: unfortunately, an ASD is still a possible diagnosis when some variation in splitting is detectable during the respiratory cycle)
2. pulmonary systolic ejection murmur (increasing on inspiration)
3. pulmonary hypertension (late).

Results of investigations
1. ECG:
   (a) right-axis deviation
   (b) right bundle branch block pattern
   (c) right ventricular hypertrophy (systolic overload).
2. Chest X-ray film (see Fig 15.9):
   (a) increased pulmonary vasculature
   (b) enlarged right atrium and ventricle
   (c) dilated main pulmonary artery
   (d) small aortic knob.
3. Echocardiography:
   (a) paradoxical septal motion, right ventricular dilation
   (b) echo dropout in atrial septum
   (c) Doppler detection of a shunt at the atrial level
   (d) shunt (bubble) study using agitated saline
   (e) transoesophageal echocardiogram.

Indication for surgery
Almost all ASD need to be surgically closed when the left-to-right shunt is measured to be at least 1.5 to 1 (unless there is reversal of the shunt). A nuclear cardiac shunt study may help estimation of the shunt size.

Echocardiography Report

Reason for study: Systolic murmur, family history of hypertrophic cardiomyopathy
Study quality: <u>Good</u> Satisfactory Poor

RV	13	(mm)	(N 10–26)
Sept.	18	(mm)	(N 7–11)
LVEDD	54	(mm)	(N 36–56)
LVESD	30	(mm)	(N 20–40)
LVPW	10	(mm)	(N 7–11)
Aorta	22	(mm)	(N 20–35)
LA	40	(mm)	(N 24–40)
FS	44	%	(N 27–40)
EF	75	%	(N 55–70)

Valves

Mitral	Mild-to-moderate MR, SAM
Tricus.	Appears normal
Aortic	Appears normal
Pulm.	Appears normal

Doppler—2D
There is asymmetrical septal hypertrophy. LV systolic function appears normal. LA upper limit of normal size.

Doppler—colour flow mapping
There is a gradient in the left ventricular outflow tract of 80 mmHg. Moderate MR jet —½ LA.

Conclusions
Hypertrophic cardiomyopathy with LVOT gradient of 80 mmHg. Systolic anterior motion of anterior mitral valve leaflet. Moderate MR.

Comment
The typical echocardiograph findings in this condition are seen here. The septum is thicker than 11 mm and there is abnormal anterior movement of the anterior mitral valve leaflet in systole—SAM. This movement is, in part, responsible for any LVOT gradient. The LVOT gradient only correlates roughly with symptoms and prognosis in this condition. In some cases of hypertrophic cardiomyopathy there may be no LVOT gradient.

Key
EF = ejection fraction; FS = fractional shortening; LA = left atrium; LV = left ventricle; LVEDD = left ventricular end-diastolic dimension; LVESD = left ventricular end-systolic dimension, LVOT = left ventricular outflow tract; LVPW = left ventricular posterior wall; MR = mitral regurgitation; Pulm. = pulmonary; RV = right ventricle; SAM = systolic anterior motion; Sept. = septal thickness; Tricus. = tricuspid.

Figure 15.8 Echocardiography report for a patient with hypertrophic cardiomyopathy.

ASD: ostium primum
This is an endocardial cushion defect adjacent to the atrioventricular valves. The signs are the same as for ostium secundum, but associated mitral regurgitation, tricuspid regurgitation or VSD is common. The ECG is particularly helpful as there is left-axis deviation and right bundle branch block (and sometimes a prolonged P–R interval). Look also for the presence of Down syndrome and skeletal upper limb defects (Holt-Oram syndrome).

Figure 15.9 Chest X-ray of a patient with an ASD and right atrial and ventricular enlargement. The pulmonary arteries are very prominent (arrow).
Figure reproduced courtesy of The Canberra Hospital.

Ventricular septal defect
The clues to the diagnosis of VSD are a thrill and a harsh pansystolic murmur confined to the left sternal edge. Sometimes mitral regurgitation is also present. Down syndrome is associated.

Results of investigations
The ECG and chest X-ray film may show left ventricular hypertrophy. The chest X-ray film may also show increased pulmonary vasculature and an enlarged right ventricle. The echocardiogram will show the defect and detect the shunt. Estimation of the pressure gradient between the ventricles will allow detection of right ventricular hypertension. As right ventricular pressure rises, the gradient across the defect falls (right ventricular pressure is closer to left ventricular)—a sign that the shunt is causing trouble.

Indication for surgery

Closure is indicated when the left-to-right shunt is moderate to large, with the pulmonary-to-systemic flow being >1.5 to 1.

Patent ductus arteriosus

In patent ductus arteriosus (PDA) there is a vessel from the bifurcation of the pulmonary artery to the aorta. The shunt is usually from the aorta to the pulmonary artery. Reversal of the shunt leads to differential cyanosis and clubbing (toes, *not* fingers). Often a continuous murmur is heard. Confusion with aortic stenosis and regurgitation commonly occurs when candidates examine these patients.

Results of investigations

1. The ECG may show left ventricular hypertrophy (diastolic overload).
2. The chest X-ray film may show:
   (a) increased pulmonary vasculature
   (b) calcification of the duct (trumpet-shaped calcification)
   (c) an enlarged left ventricle.
3. Doppler echocardiography will demonstrate continuous flow in the main pulmonary artery. Left atrial size will be increased.

Indication for surgery

The indication for surgery or use of a closure device (surgery for this condition in adults is difficult and is now largely replaced by the use of percutaneous catheter closure devices) is the diagnosis of PDA with more than a trivial shunt (unless there is pulmonary hypertension).

HINT BOX

The detection of a trivial shunt at echocardiography in a patient with a PDA but without a significant murmur or any symptoms is not an indication for closure.

Coarctation of the aorta

The most common site for this lesion is just distal to the origin of the left subclavian artery. Look for a better developed upper body, radiofemoral delay, hypertension in the arms only, chest collateral vessels, a midsystolic murmur over the praecordium and back, and changes of hypertension in the fundi. Turner's syndrome may be associated in some cases.

Results of investigations

1. The ECG may show left ventricular hypertrophy (systolic overload).
2. The chest X-ray film (see Fig 15.10) may show:
   (a) enlarged left ventricle
   (b) enlarged left subclavian artery
   (c) dilated ascending aorta
   (d) aortic indentation
   (e) aortic prestenotic and poststenotic dilation
   (f) rib notching—second to sixth ribs on the inferior border.
3. Echocardiography may show:
   (a) left ventricular hypertrophy
   (b) coarctation shelf in the descending aorta
   (c) abnormal flow patterns in the same area.

Figure 15.10 Chest X-ray showing coarctation of the aorta. Note the small aortic knuckle (1) and rib notching (2).
Figure reproduced courtesy of The Canberra Hospital.

Cyanotic congenital heart disease

This is a very difficult area. You probably will not be expected to identify the exact lesion. A cardiac cause should be suspected if the patient shows clubbing and cyanosis.

The common causes of the problem in adults are:

1. Eisenmenger's syndrome—pulmonary hypertension plus a large communication between the left and right circulations (e.g. VSD, PDA, ASD)
2. tetralogy of Fallot
3. complex lesions—univentricular heart, Ebstein's anomaly (if there is an associated atrial septal defect with a right-to-left shunt).

You must decide while examining the patient whether pulmonary hypertension is present, as this distinguishes Eisenmenger's syndrome from the tetralogy of Fallot.

Eisenmenger's syndrome

This syndrome may be found in older adults who had right-to-left shunting before the availability of open-heart surgery. The physical signs may include cyanosis, clubbing and polycythaemia. The JVP pattern may have a dominant *a* wave and sometimes a prominent *v* wave. A right ventricular heave and a palpable pulmonary component of the second heart sound (P2) may be found. On auscultation there may be a loud P2 (S2 is split and the second component is loud), a fourth heart sound, a pulmonary ejection click, pulmonary regurgitation and sometimes tricuspid regurgitation (but there may be no murmurs). The signs all add up to pulmonary hypertension in a cyanosed patient.

To work out the level of the shunt, pay close attention to the second heart sound:

1. wide fixed split—ASD
2. single second sound—VSD
3. normal second sound or reversed splitting—PDA (look for differential cyanosis).

HINT BOX
Despite traditional teaching, a loud P2 has little correlation with the presence of pulmonary hypertension, but a palpable P2 correlates well.

Results of investigations
1. The ECG may show:
   (a) right ventricular hypertrophy
   (b) *P* pulmonale.
2. The chest X-ray film (see Fig 15.11) may show:
   (a) right ventricular and right atrial enlargement
   (b) pulmonary artery prominence
   (c) increased hilar vascular markings but attenuated peripheral vessels
   (d) a heart that is *not* boot-shaped.
3. Echocardiography will define the anatomy and enable measurement of pulmonary pressures.

Figure 15.11 Chest X-ray of a patient with Eisenmenger's syndrome due to an untreated VSD: the pulmonary arteries are enormous centrally (arrow) but small in the periphery.
Figure reproduced courtesy of The Canberra Hospital.

Tetralogy of Fallot

There are four features:

1. VSD
2. right ventricular outflow obstruction (which determines severity)
3. overriding aorta
4. right ventricular hypertrophy.

   The physical signs may include cyanosis, clubbing, polycythaemia, a right ventricular heave and a thrill at the left sternal edge, but not cardiomegaly. On auscultation there may be a single second heart sound (A2) and a short pulmonary ejection murmur.

Results of investigations

1. The ECG may show:
   (a) right ventricular hypertrophy
   (b) right-axis deviation.
2. The chest X-ray film (see Fig 15.12) may show:
   (a) a normal-sized heart with a boot shape (i.e. a left concavity where the pulmonary artery is normally situated plus a prominent elevated apex)
   (b) right ventricular enlargement
   (c) decreased vascularity of lung vessels
   (d) right-sided aortic knob, arch and descending aorta (25%).
3. Echocardiography will demonstrate the anatomical abnormalities.

Figure 15.12 Chest X-ray of a child with tetralogy of Fallot.
Figure reproduced courtesy of The Canberra Hospital.

The hypertensive examination

'This 30-year-old man has hypertension. Please examine him.'

Method

1. Stand back and inspect the patient. Look for evidence of Cushing's syndrome, acromegaly, polycythaemia and uraemia (see Table 15.6). If one of these is present, modify your examination appropriately.

TABLE 15.6 Causes of hypertension

Essential (>95%); secondary (<5%)

Renal disease	Renovascular disease (renal artery atherosclerosis, fibromuscular disease, aneurysm, vasculitis) Diffuse renal disease
Endocrine	Conn's syndrome (primary aldosteronism) Cushing's syndrome (especially steroid treatment) 17- and 11-beta-hydroxylase defects Phaeochromocytoma Acromegaly Myxoedema Contraceptive pill
Coarctation of the aorta	
Other	Polycythaemia rubra vera Toxaemia of pregnancy Neurogenic (increased intracranial pressure, lead poisoning, acute intermittent porphyria) Hypercalcaemia Alcohol Sleep apnoea

Note: Alcohol consumption and obesity are associated with essential hypertension.

2. Next, confirm that the blood pressure is elevated. Ask to measure it in both arms, and with the patient both lying and standing. Measurement in the legs in a young patient may be important.
3. Feel the radial pulse and very carefully feel for radiofemoral delay. Palpate for radial–radial asymmetry and inspect both hands for vasculitic changes.
4. Now look at the face. Inspect the conjunctivae for injection (polycythaemia), and then examine the fundi for hypertensive changes (see Table 15.7). Describe what you see when presenting rather than just giving a grade.
5. Examine the rest of the cardiovascular system, looking especially for left ventricular failure and coarctation of the aorta. Usually a fourth heart sound is present in severe hypertension.
6. The abdomen should be examined for renal masses, adrenal masses and an abdominal aneurysm. Auscultate for renal bruits (as a result of fibromuscular dysplasia or atheroma). These may have a diastolic component. Listen first just to the right or left of the midline above the umbilicus. Then sit the patient up and listen in the flanks (a systolic–diastolic bruit in the costovertebral area suggests a renal arteriovenous fistula).
7. At the end, ask for the results of urine analysis (signs of renal disease). Also remember that cerebrovascular accidents, secondary to hypertension, may cause other physical signs.

TABLE 15.7 Fundoscopy changes in hypertension

Grade	Changes
Grade I	Silver wiring
Grade II	Above change plus arteriovenous nipping
Grade III	Above changes plus haemorrhages (characteristically flame-shaped) and exudates: soft exudates, also called cotton wool spots, owing to ischaemia; hard exudates owing to lipid residues from leaky vessels
Grade IV	Above changes plus papilloedema

Marfan's syndrome

'This 37-year-old man has a heart murmur. Please examine him.'

Method

Fortunately, you notice a Marfanoid habitus.
1. While performing your normal cardiovascular examination, look also for the following signs.
   (a) *Hands and arms*. Look for arachnodactyly (spider fingers) and joint hypermobility, as well as long, thin limbs.
   (b) *Face*. You may notice a long and narrow face. Look for lens dislocation or lens replacement. The sclerae may be blue. Look in the mouth for a high-arched palate.
   (c) *Chest*. Note any pectus carinatum or excavatum.
   (d) *Heart*. Auscultate for aortic regurgitation and mitral valve prolapse. Also look for the signs of dissecting aneurysm or coarctation of the aorta.
   (e) *Back*. Look for kyphoscoliosis and hypermobility.
2. At the end, always ask to measure the arm span, which will exceed the height. The upper segment to lower segment ratio will be less than 0.85 (the upper segment is from the crown to the symphysis pubis and the lower segment is from the symphysis pubis to the ground).

Investigations

1. Many of these patients will have had serial echocardiograms in the hope that progressive aortic root dilation will warn of an increased risk of dissection before this occurs.
2. A slit-lamp examination may be required to diagnose lens dislocation.

Oedema

'This 70-year-old man has oedema. Please assess him.'

Method

1. First, stand back and look at the patient. Note whether the oedema is localised or generalised and whether it is gravitational or not.
2. Assess nutrition quickly (as hypoalbuminaemia and also beri beri owing to vitamin B_1 deficiency can cause oedema). Also, any obvious signs of myxoedema (p 321) must never be missed.
3. If necessary, ask the patient to undress as appropriate and then further define the areas affected. Palpate for pitting.
   Proceed, depending on your findings (see Table 15.8).

Pitting lower limb oedema

1. Define the extent of the oedema.
2. Look for signs of DVT (2 cm difference in calf swelling, prominent superficial veins and increased warmth have minor diagnostic value; Homans' sign is unhelpful). Note the presence of varicose veins (a common cause of mild peripheral oedema) and the presence of vein-harvesting scars (for coronary artery surgery).
3. Feel the inguinal nodes. Go to the abdomen and look for abdominal wall oedema, prominent abdominal wall veins (inferior vena caval obstruction), ascites, any abdominal masses and evidence of liver disease. A pulsatile liver (tricuspid regurgitation) or malignant involvement should be particularly looked for.
4. Next examine the JVP. Then examine for signs of right ventricular failure and constrictive pericarditis. Feel all the node groups.

TABLE 15.8 Causes of oedema
1. Cardiac—congestive cardiac failure, constrictive pericarditis
2. Hepatic—cirrhosis
3. Renal—nephrotic syndrome (see Table 11.2)
4. Drugs—calcium channel blockers
5. Malabsorption or starvation
6. Protein-losing enteropathy
7. Beri beri ('wet')
8. Myxoedema
9. Cyclical oedema

5. Finally examine for delayed ankle jerks (to exclude hypothyroidism) and look at the urine analysis. Remember that vasodilating drugs used for hypertension or angina are very common causes of oedema.

Non-pitting lower limb oedema
Consider the various causes, including lymphoedema (from malignant infiltration, congenital disease, filariasis, Milroy's disease) and myxoedema.

Superior vena caval obstruction (see Table 15.9)
1. The patient may appear cushingoid, from either a tumour or treatment with steroids. Note the plethoric cyanosed face with periorbital oedema. There may be exophthalmos and conjunctival injection. Examine the pupils: a mass in the chest may have caused Horner's syndrome. Examine the fundi for venous dilation. Examine the neck, which is enlarged.
2. The JVP is raised, but the vein is not pulsatile.
3. Decide whether the thyroid gland is enlarged. Check Pemberton's sign (p 319).
4. Feel for supraclavicular lymphadenopathy and listen over the trachea for inspiratory stridor.
5. Examine the chest carefully for distended venous collaterals.
6. One or both arms may be oedematous.
7. Look for all the peripheral manifestations of lung carcinoma.

TABLE 15.9 Causes of superior vena caval obstruction
1. Lung carcinoma (90%)
2. Retrosternal tumours—lymphoma, thymoma, dermoid
3. Retrosternal goitre
4. Massive mediastinal lymphadenopathy
5. Aortic aneurysm

The respiratory system

The respiratory examination

'This 69-year-old man presented with breathlessness. Please examine him.'

Method (see Table 15.10)

TABLE 15.10 Respiratory system examination

Sitting up	

1. GENERAL INSPECTION
Sputum mug contents (blood, pus etc.)
Type of cough
Rate and depth of respiration
Accessory muscles of respiration
	Expansion
	Vocal fremitus
	Percuss
	    Supraclavicular region
	    Back
	    Axillae
	    Tidal percussion (diaphragm)
	Auscultate
	    Breath sounds
	    Adventitial sounds
	    Vocal resonance

2. HANDS Clubbing Cyanosis (peripheral) Nicotine staining Wasting, weakness—finger abduction Wrist tenderness (HPO) Pulse (tachycardia; pulsus paradoxus) Flapping tremor (CO_2 narcosis)	

	7. CHEST ANTERIORLY
	Inspect
	Palpate
	    Supraclavicular nodes
	    Vocal fremitus
	    Axillary nodes
	Percuss
	Auscultate
	Pemberton's sign (SVC obstruction)

3. FACE
Eyes—Horner's syndrome (apical
    tumour), jaundice, anaemia
Mouth—central cyanosis
Voice—hoarseness (recurrent laryngeal
    nerve palsy)	

4. TRACHEA	**8. CARDIOVASCULAR SYSTEM (lying at 45°)** JVP (SVC obstruction etc.) Apex beat Pulmonary hypertension Cor pulmonale
5. FORCED EXPIRATORY TIME	

6. CHEST POSTERIORLY
Inspect
    Shape of chest and spine
    Scars
    Radiotherapy marks
    Prominent veins (determine direction
    of flow)
Palpate
    Cervical lymph nodes
	9. OTHER
	Temperature chart (infection)
	Fundi (CO_2 narcosis)
	Evidence of malignancy or pleural
	    effusion: examine breasts, abdomen,
	    rectum, lymph nodes etc.

HPO = hypertrophic pulmonary osteoarthropathy; SVC = superior vena cava.

1. If necessary, ask the patient to undress to the waist and sit over the side of the bed.
2. While standing back to make your usual inspection, ask whether sputum is available for you to look at. A large volume of purulent sputum is an important clue to bronchiectasis. Haemoptysis suggests lung carcinoma or pulmonary infection. Look for evidence of dyspnoea at rest and count the respiratory rate. Note the use of the accessory muscles of respiration and any intercostal indrawing of the lower ribs anteriorly (a sign of emphysema). General cachexia should also be noted.
3. Pick up the patient's hands. Note clubbing (see Table 15.11), peripheral cyanosis, nicotine (actually, tar) staining and anaemia, and look for wasting of the small muscles of the hands and weakness of finger abduction (which may be caused by a lower trunk brachial plexus lesion from apical lung carcinoma involvement). Palpate the wrists for tenderness but only if there is clubbing (hypertrophic pulmonary osteoarthropathy [HPO]) (see Fig 15.18 (b) and

TABLE 15.11 Causes of clubbing

1. Respiratory:
   (a) lung carcinoma (usually *not* small cell carcinoma)
   (b) chronic pulmonary suppuration (e.g. bronchiectasis, lung abscess, empyema)
   (c) idiopathic pulmonary fibrosis, asbestosis
   (d) cystic fibrosis
   (e) pleural fibroma or mesothelioma
   (f) mediastinal disease (e.g. thymoma, lymphoma, carcinoma)
2. Cardiovascular:
   (a) infective endocarditis
   (b) cyanotic congenital heart disease
3. Other:
   (a) inflammatory bowel disease
   (b) cirrhosis
   (c) coeliac disease
   (d) thyrotoxicosis
   (e) brachial arteriovenous aneurysm or arterial graft sepsis (unilateral)
   (f) neurogenic diaphragmatic tumours
   (g) familial (usually before puberty) or idiopathic
   (h) hemiplegic stroke (unilateral)

Note: Clubbing does *not* occur with COPD, sarcoidosis, extrinsic allergic alveolitis, coal worker's pneumoconiosis or silicosis. With this important sign decide whether it is definitely present or absent. Don't call it 'early' if in doubt.

(c)). While holding the patient's hand, palpate the radial pulse for tachycardia or obvious pulsus paradoxus.

4. Go on to the face. Look closely at the eyes for ptosis and constriction of the pupils (Horner's syndrome, p 354). Inspect the tongue for central cyanosis.
5. Palpate the position of the trachea.

HINT BOX
Deviation of the trachea is a most important sign, so spend time on it. If the trachea is displaced, concentrate on the upper lobes for physical signs. Upper lobe fibrosis causes tracheal deviation to the same side.

6. Also note the presence of a tracheal tug, which indicates gross overexpansion of the chest with airflow obstruction. Ask the patient to cough and note whether this is a loose cough, a dry cough or, because of recurrent laryngeal nerve palsy, a bovine cough. Next measure the forced expiratory time (FET). Tell the patient to take a maximal inspiration and blow out as rapidly and completely as possible. Note audible wheeze. Prolongation of expiration beyond 3 seconds is evidence of chronic airflow limitation.
7. The next step is to examine the chest. You may wish to examine this anteriorly first or go around to the back initially. The advantage of the latter is that there are usually more signs there, unless the trachea is obviously displaced.

8. Inspect the back. Look for kyphoscoliosis. Do not miss ankylosing spondylitis (p 345), which causes decreased chest expansion and upper lobe fibrosis. Look for thoracotomy scars and prominent veins. Also note any skin changes from radiotherapy.

HINT BOX

A large thoracotomy scar in a patient who looks cushingoid suggests the possibility of a lung transplant. A unilateral transplant may leave signs on the other side, such as the crackles of ILD (pulmonary fibrosis), while the side with the scar sounds normal.

---

9. Palpate the cervical nodes from behind. Then examine for expansion. First, upper lobe expansion is best seen by looking over the patient's shoulders at clavicular movement during moderate respiration. The affected side will show a delay or decreased movement. Then examine lower lobe expansion by palpation. Note asymmetry and reduction of movement.

10. Ask the patient to bring his elbows together in front of him to move the scapulae out of the way. Examine for vocal fremitus. Then percuss the back of the chest and include both axillae. Do not miss a pleural effusion (see Table 15.12).

11. Auscultate the chest. Note breath sounds (whether bronchial or vesicular) and their intensity (normal or reduced) (see Table 15.13). Listen for adventitial sounds (crackles and wheezes) (see Table 15.14). Finally examine for vocal resonance. If a localised abnormality is found, try to determine the abnormal lobe and segment.

TABLE 15.12 Pleural effusion

Causes

1. Transudate (pleural:serum protein <0.5, and pleural LDH <2/3 upper limit of normal, and pleural:serum LDH <0.6):

   (a) cardiac failure

   (b) nephrotic syndrome

   (c) liver failure

   (d) Meigs' syndrome (ovarian fibroma and pleural effusion)

   (e) hypothyroidism (but classically an exudate)

2. Exudate (pleural:serum protein >0.5 or pleural LDH >2/3 upper limit of normal or pleural:serum LDH >0.6):

   (a) pneumonia

   (b) neoplasm—lung carcinoma, metastatic carcinoma, mesothelioma

   (c) tuberculosis, sarcoidosis

   (d) pulmonary infarction

   (e) subphrenic abscess

   (f) pancreatitis

   (g) connective tissue disease—rheumatoid arthritis, SLE

   (h) drugs—nitrofurantoin (acute), methysergide (chronic), drugs causing lupus, chemotherapeutic agents, bromocriptine

   (i) radiation

TABLE 15.12 Pleural effusion (Continued)

Pleural fluid analysis: differential diagnosis

pH <7.2	Empyema, tuberculosis, neoplasm, rheumatoid arthritis, oesophageal rupture
Glucose <3.33 mmol/L	Infection, carcinoma, mesothelioma, rheumatoid arthritis
Red blood cells >5000/mL	Pulmonary infarction, neoplasm, trauma, asbestosis, tuberculosis, pancreatitis
Amylase >2000 U/L	Pancreatitis, abdominal viscera rupture, oesophageal rupture
Complement decreased	Rheumatoid arthritis, SLE
Chylous	Tumour (usually lymphoma), thoracic duct trauma, tuberculosis, tuberous sclerosis
LDH = lactate dehydrogenase.	

TABLE 15.13 Breath sounds

1. *Vesicular*. Normal, likened to wind rustling in the leaves.
2. *Bronchial*. The expiratory phase is prolonged and has a blowing quality. The breath sounds heard over the trachea and right and left main bronchi are sometimes rather bronchial in quality.

   Causes:

   (a) lobar pneumonia (common) (see Fig 15.14)

   (b) localised fibrosis or collapse

   (c) above a pleural effusion

   (d) large lung cavity.

3. *Reduced*. Use this term rather than 'air entry'.

   Causes:

   (a) emphysema

   (b) large lung mass

   (c) collapse, fibrosis or pneumonia

   (d) effusion

   (e) pneumothorax.

TABLE 15.14 Added sounds

1. Wheezes (rhonchi)

Inspiratory wheezes—characteristic of asthma or upper airway extrathoracic obstruction.

Expiratory wheezes—occur in asthma and COPD.

Fixed inspiratory wheeze (monophonic—does not change with respiration)—an important sign of fixed bronchial obstruction, usually due to a carcinoma.

2. Crackles (crepitations)

Late or pan inspiratory crackles:

* fine—caused by fibrosis—dry crackles
* medium—caused by left ventricular failure
* coarse—caused by bronchiectasis or retained secretions.

Early inspiratory crackles: coarse—caused by COPD.

12. Return to the front of the chest. Inspect again for chest deformity, symmetry of chest wall movement, distended veins, radiotherapy changes and scars. Palpate the supraclavicular nodes carefully. Palpate the apex beat and measure chest expansion. Then test for vocal fremitus and proceed with percussion and auscultation as before. Listen high up in the axillae too. Before leaving the chest, feel the axillary nodes and breasts.

HINT BOX

If COPD seems likely, test for Hoover's sign: place your hands along the costal margins with your thumbs close to the xiphisternum. Normally inspiration causes your thumbs to separate, but the overinflated chest of the COPD patient cannot expand any further and so the diaphragm pulls the ribs and your thumbs closer together.

---

13. Ask the patient to lie down at 45° and then visually measure the JVP.
14. Examine the praecordium for signs of pulmonary hypertension and cor pulmonale. Finally, examine the liver and look for peripheral oedema. Check for Pemberton's sign (p 319).
15. Before leaving the patient, ask whether you may see the temperature chart.

HINT BOX

Try to put the signs together. Common respiratory short cases include:
1. ILD (dry cough, crackles and clubbing)
2. Bronchiectasis (loose cough, full sputum mug, coarse crackles and wheezes, clubbing)
3. COPD (overinflated chest, possible cyanosis, pursed lips breathing, reduced breath sounds and wheezes, Hoover's sign)
4. Pleural effusion (stony dullness, bronchial breathing on top, needle marks from previous aspirations)
5. Thoracoplasty (gross unilateral chest deformity, big scar)
6. Cystic fibrosis (often young patient with signs of bronchiectasis and cachexia)
7. Treated carcinoma (sometimes clubbing, scar, radiotherapy marks, signs of effusion or collapse, lymph nodes)

Chest X-ray films
Hints on how to read a chest X-ray film (see Fig. 15.13)

This is a very valuable investigation and some even consider a chest X-ray as an extension of the physical examination. It is essential to be familiar with the various radiographic appearances. As a physician, you should feel personally responsible for viewing all the patient's radiographs.

1. When first viewing the chest radiograph, check:
   (a) film date, to ensure that it is current
   (b) type of film—posteroanterior (PA) or anteroposterior (AP) film; the latter (which may be labelled 'portable') magnifies heart size, making assessment of cardiac diameter difficult
   (c) correct orientation—the left side is most reliably determined by the position of stomach gas
   (d) film 'centring'—the medial ends of each clavicle should be equidistant from the spines of the vertebrae; rotation affects mediastinal and hilar shadows,

causing undue prominence on the side opposite that to which the patient was turned.

2. Next, systematically examine the PA film, comparing right and left sides carefully for abnormalities of:
   (a) soft tissues (e.g. mastectomy, subcutaneous emphysema) and bony skeleton (e.g. rib fractures, malignant deposits)
   (b) tracheal displacement, paratracheal masses
   (c) heart size, borders and retrocardiac density
   (d) aorta and upper mediastinum (count the ribs, look for mediastinal shift, mediastinal masses—see Figs 15.20 and 15.21)

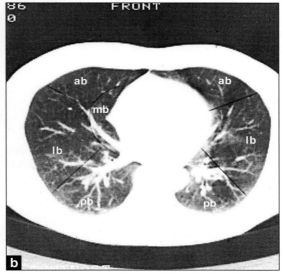

Figure 15.13 The lung segments. (a) PA view (b) CT scan through lung bases.

(Continues)

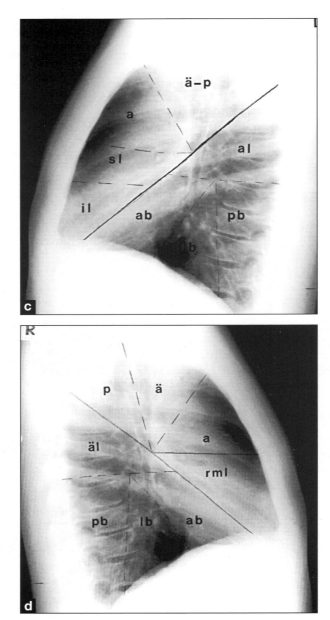

Figure 15.13 **Continued. (c) Left lateral view. (d) Right lateral view**
Right upper lobe: ä = apical segment; a = anterior segment; p = posterior segment. **Left upper lobe:** ä-p = apico-posterior segment; a = anterior segment; sl = superior lingular segment; il = inferior lingular segment. **Right lower lobe:** äl = apical segment; mb = medial basal segment; lb = lateral basal segment; ab = anterior basal segment; pb = posterior basal segment. **Left lower lobe:** äl = apical segment; lb = lateral basal segment; ab = anterior basal segment; pb = posterior basal segment.

(e) diaphragm (right higher than left by 1–3 cm normally), cardiophrenic and costophrenic angles

(f) lung hila (left normally above right by up to 3 cm, usually no larger than an average thumb)

(g) lung fields—upper zone (to lower border of second rib), midzone (from upper zone to lower border of fourth rib) and lower zone (from midzone to diaphragm)

(h) pleura

(i) gastric bubble (normally there should be no opacity >0.5 cm above the air bubble)

(j) the presence of monitoring leads, a permanent or temporary pacemaker, central lines or other 'hardware'.

Learn to do all this rapidly and accurately.

3. Finally, always ask to look at a lateral film. Examine it just as carefully. The lateral film is used to help decide the exact anatomical site of an abnormality.

Candidates must learn the normal position of the fissures (the horizontal fissure, seen sometimes on the PA and lateral film, is a fine horizontal line at the level of the fourth costal cartilage, whereas the oblique fissure is only seen sometimes on the lateral, beginning at the level of the fifth thoracic vertebra and running downwards to the diaphragm at the junction of its anterior and middle thirds).

The lung segments must also be memorised (see Fig 15.13). Remember, abnormalities in the lung fields are described by terms such as 'mottling', 'opacity' or 'shadow'—it is usually unwise to attempt to make a precise diagnosis of the underlying pathology in your initial assessment of the chest X-ray (see Table 15.15).

TABLE 15.15 Differential diagnosis of radiological appearances in chest X-ray film

Homogeneous opacity
Pneumonia—lobar or segmental
Collapse
Effusion (see Fig 15.23)
Localised non-homogeneous opacity
Pneumonia (see Fig 15.14)
Pulmonary infarct
Carcinoma (see Fig 15.18 (a) and (d))
Tuberculosis (see Fig 15.16)
Diffuse opacities
Miliary (<2 mm):
• miliary tuberculosis
• miliary metastases (especially breast, thyroid, melanoma, pancreas)
• sarcoidosis
• pneumocoiosis
• lymphoma, often with prominent hilar lymph nodes (see Fig 15.24(b))
• lymphangitis
• vital pneumonia
• vasculitis (e.g. polyarteritis, Wegener's granulomatosis—see Fig 15.22)
• pulmonary haemorrhage (see Fig 15.19)

(Continues)

TABLE 15.15 Differential diagnosis of radiological appearances in chest X-ray film (Continued)

Diffuse opacities (continued)

Nodular (3–10 mm):

- pneumonia
- pneumoconiosis
- tuberculosis
- metastatic carcinoma (see Fig 15.21)
- sarcoidosis (see Fig 15.24(a))

Reticular (linear opacities)

Fibrosis (see Fig 15.17), bronchiectasis (thickened bronchial walls—see Fig 15.15)

Cavitated lesion

Lung abscess

Carcinoma (usually squamous cell) or Hodgkin's disease

Tuberculosis

Fungi (e.g. coccidioidomycosis)

Calcificied lesions in the lung fields

Tuberculosis

Pneumoconiosis

Post-chickenpox pneumonia

Tularaemia

Miliary calcification

Post-chickenpox pneumonia

Histoplasmosis

Coccidioidomycosis

Eptopic calcification in renal failure, hyperparathyroidism

Coin lesion

Carcinoma (primary or metastatic—look closely for any rib lesion)

Tuberculoma

Hamartoma

Granuloma (e.g. fungus)

Arteriovenous fistula

Rheumatoid nodule

Lung abscess

Hydatid cyst

Some common radiological abnormalities
The following X-rays and scans (Figs 15.14–15.24) show some important changes associated with pulmonary disease.

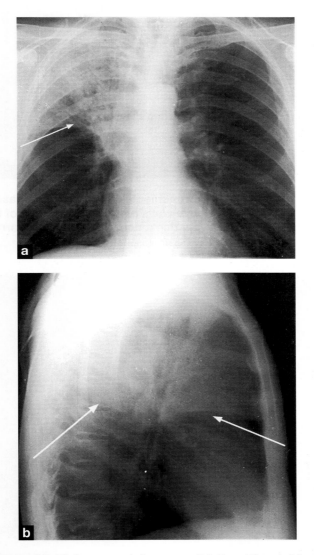

Figure 15.14 (a) and (b) Right upper lobe consolidation. The right upper lobe is opacified and is limited inferiorly by the horizontal fissure (arrows). There must be some collapse as well, as the fissure shows some elevation.
Figures reproduced courtesy of The Canberra Hospital.

Figure 15.15 (a) Right middle lobe bronchiectasis. Note the increased lung markings and the thickened bronchial walls (arrow). (b) CT scan of the chest of a patient with bronchiectasis. Note the thickened bronchial walls (arrow).
Figures reproduced courtesy of The Canberra Hospital.

Figure 15.16 Right upper lobe scarring; old TB infection (arrow).
Figure reproduced courtesy of The Canberra Hospital.

Figure 15.17 Right upper lobe fibrosis. Note the loss of volume and increased lung markings (arrow).
Figure reproduced courtesy of The Canberra Hospital.

Figure 15.18 (a) Recurrent carcinoma of the lung following right upper lobectomy. Note mass and rib destruction.
Figure reproduced courtesy of The Canberra Hospital.

(Continues)

Figure 15.18 Continued. (b) Hypertophic pulmonary osteoarthropathy (HPOA) of the ulna in the same patient as in (a) (arrow). (c) HPOA of the tibia in the same patient as in (a) (arrows).

Figures reproduced courtesy of The Canberra Hospital.

Figure 15.18 Continued. (d) CT scan of the chest showing a right upper lobe tumour—Pancoast tumour. (e) Chest X-ray of the same patient as in (d) showing right upper lobe tumour (arrow).

Figures reproduced courtesy of The Canberra Hospital.

Figure 15.19 CT chest showing pulmonary haemorrhage in a patient with Goodpasture's syndrome.
Figure reproduced courtesy of The Canberra Hospital.

Figure 15.20 Retrosternal mass goitre (arrow).
Figure reproduced courtesy of The Canberra Hospital.

Figure 15.21 Retrosternal mass thoracic aortic aneurysm (1) and pulmonary metastases (2).
Figure reproduced courtesy of The Canberra Hospital.

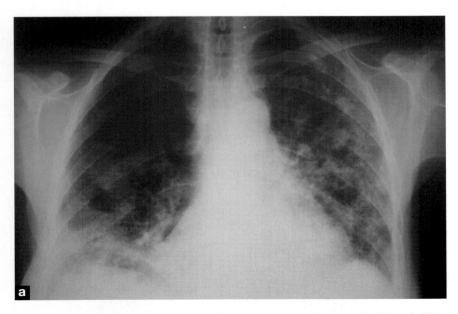

Figure 15.22 (a) Chest X-ray showing Wegener's granulomatosis. Note infiltrates and destructive changes.
Figure reproduced courtesy of The Canberra Hospital.

(Continues)

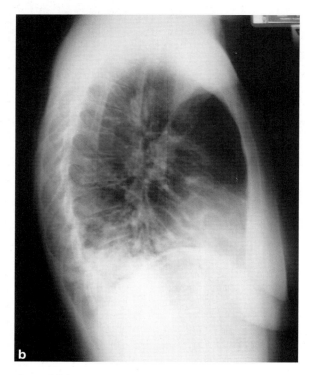

Figure 15.22 Continued (b) Lateral view. Note infiltrates and destructive changes.
Figure reproduced courtesy of The Canberra Hospital.

Figure 15.23 Large left pleural effusion (arrow). Note previous left mastectomy.
Figure reproduced courtesy of The Canberra Hospital.

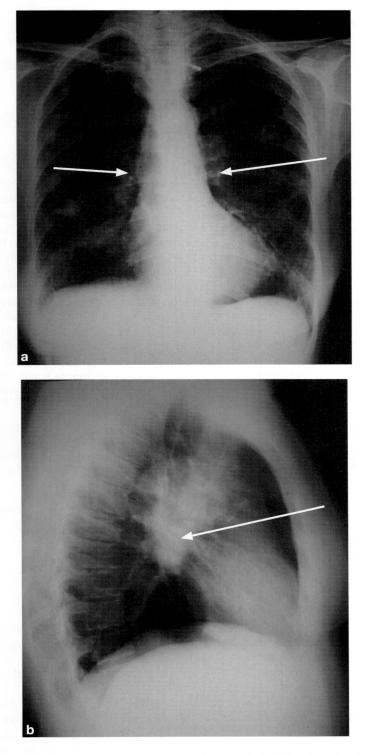

Figure 15.24 (a) Sarcoidosis basal infiltrate (arrows). (b) Hilar lymphadenopathy (arrow).
Figures reproduced courtesy of The Canberra Hospital.

The gastrointestinal system

The abdominal examination

'This 60-year-old man has had episodes of abdominal discomfort. Please examine his abdomen.'

Method (see Table 15.16)

1. Position the patient correctly, with one pillow for the head and complete exposure of the abdomen.
2. Briefly look at the patient's general appearance and inspect particularly for signs of chronic liver disease and renal disease.
3. Inspect the abdomen from the side, squatting to the patient's level. Large masses may be visible. Ask the patient to take slow, deep breaths. Stand up and look for scars, distension, prominent veins, striae, bruising and pigmentation.
4. Palpate lightly in each quadrant for masses (see Tables 15.17–15.22). Ask first whether any particular area is tender (to avoid causing pain and also to obtain a clue to the site of possible pathology). Next palpate more deeply in each quadrant and then feel specifically for hepatomegaly and splenomegaly. A palpable liver may be a result of enlargement or ptosis. If there is hepatomegaly (see Table 15.17), confirm with percussion and estimate the span (normal span is approximately 12.5 cm). The same procedure is followed for splenomegaly (use a two-handed technique) (see Table 15.21). Percussion is useful to exclude splenomegaly (over the lowest intercostal space in the left anterior axillary line: if dull in full inspiration, suspect splenomegaly and palpate again). Always roll the patient on to the right side and palpate again if no spleen is palpable.
5. Carefully feel for the kidneys bimanually. Remember that any left-sided mass may arise from a number of sites.

HINT BOX

If you have found hepatosplenomegaly, always consider the possibility of associated polycystic kidneys (a common trap for young players in the test).

---

6. The usual distinguishing features of a spleen compared with a kidney are as follows:
   (a) The spleen has no palpable upper border.
   (b) The spleen has a notch.
   (c) The spleen moves inferomedially on respiration.
   (d) There is usually no resonance over a splenic mass.
   (e) The spleen is not bimanually palpable (i.e. not ballottable).
   (f) A friction rub may occasionally be heard over the spleen.
7. Percuss for ascites as a routine. If the abdomen is resonant out to the flanks on percussion, do not roll the patient over. Otherwise, look for shifting dullness. The technique is usually performed by percussing away from your side of the bed until you reach a dull note, then rolling the patient towards you and waiting at least a short time before percussing again for resonance.
8. Always auscultate briefly over the liver, spleen and renal areas. Listen for bruits, rubs and a venous hum. Note the presence of bowel sounds. An arterial systolic bruit over the liver is usually caused by either hepatocellular carcinoma or acute alcoholic hepatitis. A friction rub over the liver may be caused by tumour, recent liver biopsy, infarction or gonococcal perihepatitis (rather unusual); splenic rubs indicate infarction. A venous hum occurs uncommonly in portal hypertension.

TABLE 15.16 Gastrointestinal system examination

Lying flat (1 pillow)

1. GENERAL INSPECTION
Jaundice (liver disease etc.)
Pigmentation (e.g. haemochromatosis)
Xanthomata (e.g. primary biliary cirrhosis, chronic biliary tract obstruction)
Mental state (encephalopathy)

2. HANDS
Nails—clubbing
    —leuconychia (white nails)
Palmar erythema
Dupuytren's contractures (alcohol)
Arthropathy
Hepatic flap

3. ARMS
Spider naevi
Bruising
Wasting
Scratch marks (chronic cholestasis)

4. FACE
Eyes—sclera: jaundice, anaemia, iritis
    —cornea: Kayser-Fleischer rings (Wilson's disease)
Parotids (alcohol)
Mouth—breath: fetor hepaticus
    —lips: stomatitis, leucoplakia, ulceration, localised pigmentation (Peutz-Jeghers syndrome), telangiectasia (hereditary haemorrhagic telangiectasia)
    —gums: gingivitis, bleeding, hypertrophy, pigmentation, *Candida*
    —tongue: atrophic glossitis, leucoplakia, ulceration

5. CERVICAL/AXILLARY LYMPH NODES

6. CHEST
Gynaecomastia
Spider naevi

7. ABDOMEN
Inspect
    Scars
    Distension
    Prominent veins—determine direction of flow (caput medusae; inferior vena caval obstruction)
    Striae
    Bruising
    Localised masses
    Visible peristalsis
Palpate
    Superficial palpation—tenderness, rigidity, outline of any mass
    Deep palpation—organomegaly (liver, gallbladder, spleen, kidney), abnormal masses

Roll on to right side (spleen)
Percuss
    Viscera outline
    Ascites—shifting dullness
Auscultate
    Bowel sounds
    Bruits, hums
    Rubs

8. GROIN
Genitalia
Lymph nodes
Hernial orifices (standing up and coughing)

9. LEGS
Bruising
Oedema
Neurological signs (alcohol)

10. OTHER
Rectal examination—inspect (fistulae, tags, blood on glove etc.), palpate (masses)
Urine analysis (bile etc.)
Blood pressure (renal disease)
Cardiovascular system (cardiomyopathy)
Neurological system (Wernicke's encephalopathy etc.)
Temperature chart (infection)

HINT BOX
If you are asked to examine the gastrointestinal system rather than the abdomen, begin by examining the hands and go on to the arms, face, chest, abdomen and legs as described (see Table 15.16).

TABLE 15.17 Differential diagnosis in liver palpation

Hepatomegaly

1. Massive
   (a) metastases
   (b) alcoholic liver disease with fatty infiltration
   (c) myeloproliferative disease
   (d) right heart failure
   (e) hepatocellular carcinoma

2. Moderate
   (a) the above causes
   (b) haemochromatosis
   (c) haematological disease—chronic myeloid leukaemia, lymphoma
   (d) fatty liver—obesity, diabetes mellitus, toxins

3. Mild
   (a) the above causes
   (b) hepatitis (viral, drugs)
   (c) cirrhosis
   (d) biliary obstruction
   (e) granulomatous disorders
   (f) hydatid disease
   (g) amyloidosis and other infiltrative diseases
   (h) HIV infection
   (i) ischaemia

Firm and irregular liver

1. Cirrhosis
2. Metastatic disease
3. Hydatid disease, granuloma, amyloid, cysts, lipoidoses

Tender liver

1. Hepatitis
2. Rapid liver enlargement—right heart failure, Budd-Chiari syndrome
3. Hepatocellular carcinoma

Pulsatile liver

1. Tricuspid regurgitation
2. Hepatocellular carcinoma
3. Vascular abnormalities

TABLE 15.18 Causes of renal masses

Bilateral

1. Polycystic kidneys (see Table 15.19)

2. Hydronephrosis or pyonephrosis (bilateral)

3. Hypernephroma (bilateral renal cell carcinoma)

4. Acute renal vein thrombosis (bilateral)

5. Amyloid, lymphoma and other infiltrative diseases

6. Acromegaly

Unilateral

1. Renal cell carcinoma

2. Hydronephrosis or pyonephrosis

3. Polycystic kidney (asymmetrical enlargement)

4. Acute renal vein thrombosis

5. Normal right kidney or a solitary kidney (uncommon)

Note: In very thin patients, bilateral renal enlargement owing to early diabetic nephropathy or nephrotic syndrome is occasionally detectable.

TABLE 15.19 Adult polycystic kidneys

If you find polycystic kidneys, remember these very important points:

1. Take the blood pressure (75% have hypertension).

2. Examine the urine for haematuria (owing to haemorrhage into a cyst) and proteinuria (usually less than 2 g/day when measured).

3. Look for evidence of anaemia (as a result of chronic renal failure) or polycythaemia (owing to high erythropoietin levels). *Note:* The haemoglobin level is higher than expected for the degree of renal failure.

4. Note the presence of hepatic cysts (present in 30% of cases of polycystic renal disease) and splenic cysts (rare). These may cause confusion when examining the abdomen.

Note: Subarachnoid haemorrhage occurs in 3% of patients as a result of intracranial aneurysm. As this is an autosomal dominant condition, all family members of patients with polycystic kidney disease should be assessed for kidney disease. Cerebral aneurysms can be screened for in patients with kidney disease by MRI, in the absence of a previous history of subarachnoid haemorrhage.

TABLE 15.20 Some other causes of abdominal masses

Right iliac fossa

Appendiceal abscess

Carcinoma of the caecum

Crohn's disease

Pelvic kidney

Ovarian tumour or cyst

Carcinoid tumour

Amoebiasis

(Continues)

TABLE 15.20 Some other causes of abdominal masses (Continued)

Right iliac fossa (continued)
Psoas abscess
Ileocaecal tuberculosis

Left iliac fossa
Faeces (*note:* can be indented)
Carcinoma of sigmoid or descending colon
Diverticular disease
Ovarian tumour or cyst
Psoas abscess

Upper abdomen
Retroperitoneal lymphadenopathy (e.g. lymphoma, teratoma)
Abdominal aortic aneurysm (pulsatile)
Carcinoma of stomach
Pancreatic pseudocyst or tumour
Pyloric stenosis
Carcinoma of transverse colon

TABLE 15.21 Causes of splenomegaly

1. Massive
(a) chronic myeloid leukaemia
(b) myelofibrosis
(c) primary lymphoma of spleen, hairy cell leukaemia, malaria, kala-azar (all rare)

2. Moderate
(a) the above causes
(b) portal hypertension
(c) lymphoma
(d) leukaemia (chronic or acute)
(e) thalassaemia
(f) storage diseases (e.g. Gaucher's disease)

3. Small
(a) the above causes
(b) other myeloproliferative disorders—polycythaemia rubra vera, essential thrombocythaemia
(c) haemolytic anaemia
(d) megaloblastic anaemia (rarely)
(e) infection—viral (infectious mononucleosis [glandular fever], hepatitis), bacterial (infective endocarditis)
(f) connective tissue disease or vasculitis—rheumatoid arthritis, systemic lupus erythematosus, polyarteritis nodosa
(g) infiltration—amyloidosis, sarcoidosis
Note: Secondary carcinomatosis is a rare cause of splenomegaly.

TABLE 15.22 Causes of hepatosplenomegaly

1. Chronic liver disease with portal hypertension
2. Haematological disease—myeloproliferative disease, lymphoma, leukaemia, pernicious anaemia, sickle cell anaemia
3. Infection—acute viral hepatitis, glandular fever, cytomegalovirus
4. Infiltration—amyloidosis, sarcoidosis
5. Connective tissue disease—systemic lupus erythematosus
6. Acromegaly
7. Thyrotoxicosis

9. Examine the groin next. Palpate for inguinal lymphadenopathy. Always ask if you may palpate the testes.
10. If you now suspect liver disease, you must go on and look for the peripheral stigmata of chronic liver disease. In this instance, it is probably better to proceed from the abdomen to the chest wall. Look for gynaecomastia, spider naevi, hair loss (in men) and breast atrophy (in women). Examine the breasts if you suspect intra-abdominal malignant disease.
    (a) Now sit the patient at 45° and measure the JVP so as not to miss constrictive pericarditis as a cause of cirrhosis. Palpate anteriorly for supraclavicular nodes, then sit the patient forwards and feel posteriorly for the other cervical nodes. Look at the back for sacral oedema and spider naevi. If ascites is present, examine the chest for pleural effusions.
    (b) Look at the face next. Note any scleral abnormality (jaundice, anaemia or iritis) and look at the corneas for Kayser-Fleischer rings. Xanthelasma are common in patients with advanced primary biliary cirrhosis. Feel for parotid enlargement, which may be present soon after an acute alcoholic binge. Inspect the mouth with a torch and spatula for angular stomatitis, ulceration and atrophic glossitis. Smell the breath for fetor hepaticus.
    (c) Look at the arms for bruising and spider naevi. Next examine the hands. Ask the patient to extend his arms and hands and look for evidence of hepatic flap. Look also at the nails for clubbing and white nails (leuconychia), and note any palmar erythema and Dupuytren's contractures (the latter are associated with alcohol or trauma). The arthropathy of haemochromatosis may also be present (a degenerative arthritis that particularly involves the second and third metacarpophalangeal joints).
    (d) Next examine the legs for oedema and bruising. Look for the nervous system signs of alcoholism—namely, peripheral neuropathy, proximal myopathy, cerebellar syndrome, Wernicke's encephalopathy (bilateral VI nerve palsies) and Korsakoff's psychosis.
    (e) Candidates are almost always stopped well before this stage. Do not forget to ask to perform a rectal examination and urine analysis. Also ask to look at the temperature chart. Ask whether you may further examine for hernias by asking the patient to stand and cough.
11. If, on the other hand, you have found signs consistent with a haematological problem, proceed as described in that section.
12. If you find a pulsatile liver, examine the cardiovascular system and particularly note any other signs of tricuspid regurgitation.
13. If an enlarged kidney is present (see Table 15.19), ask to check the blood pressure and the urine.

14. If malignant disease is suspected, examine all the node groups, the lungs and the breasts after a thorough abdominal examination. Non-haematological malignant disease that causes hepatomegaly rarely leads to splenomegaly unless the portal vein is directly involved.

HINT BOX

Haemochromatosis, an autosomal recessive disorder, is an important cause of liver disease and is common in the examination. Consider this diagnosis if any of the following signs are present:

- pigmentation (bronze)
- arthropathy (typically degenerative arthritis of the MCP joints of the index and middle fingers, but any other joint may be involved; pseudogout may occur)
- testicular atrophy (owing to iron deposition in the pituitary gland)
- dilated cardiomyopathy
- glycosuria (as a result of diabetes mellitus).

The haematological system

The haemopoietic examination

'This 75-year-old man has had problems with tiredness. Please examine his haemopoietic system.'

Method (see Table 15.23)

1. If necessary, position the patient as for a gastrointestinal examination. Make sure he is fully undressed. Look for bruising, pigmentation, cyanosis, jaundice, scratch marks (owing to myeloproliferative disease or lymphoma) and leg ulceration (see below). Also note the presence of frontal bossing and the racial origin of the patient (thalassaemia is more common in people of Asian or Greek background).
2. Pick up the patient's hands. Look at the nails for koilonychia (spoon-shaped nails, which are rarely seen today and which indicate iron deficiency) and the changes of vasculitis. Pale palmar creases indicate anaemia (usually the haemoglobin level is <90 g/L). Evidence of arthropathy may be important—for example, rheumatoid arthritis and Felty's syndrome, recurrent haemarthroses in bleeding disorders or secondary gout in myeloproliferative disorders.
3. Examine the epitrochlear nodes. Do this by placing your palm under the patient's elbow—your thumb will be placed over the appropriate area (proximal and slightly anterior to the medial epicondyle). A palpable node is usually pathological and may indicate non-Hodgkin's lymphoma. Note any arm bruising. Remember petechiae are pinhead haemorrhages, whereas ecchymoses are larger bruises. Palpable purpura suggests vasculitis, dysglobulinaemia or bacteraemia.
4. Go to the axillae and palpate the axillary nodes. Do this by raising the patient's arm and placing your fingers as high as possible in the axilla. Then position the patient's forearm comfortably over your own forearm. Use your left hand for the patient's right axilla, and vice versa. There are four main areas: central, lateral (above and lateral), pectoral (most medial) and subscapular (most inferior).
5. Look at the patient's face. Inspecting the eyes, note jaundice, pallor or haemorrhage of the sclera, or the injected sclera of polycythaemia.

TABLE 15.23 Haematological system examination

Lying flat (1 pillow)

1. **GENERAL INSPECTION**
   Bruising (thrombocytopenia, scurvy etc.)
   —petechiae (pinhead bleeding)
   —ecchymoses (large bruises)
   Pigmentation (lymphoma)
   Rashes and infiltrative lesions (lymphoma)
   Ulceration (neutropenia)
   Cyanosis (polycythaemia)
   Plethora (polycythaemia)
   Jaundice (haemolysis)
   Scratch marks (myeloproliferative disease)
   Racial origin

2. **HANDS**
   Nails—koilonychia
   Palmar crease pallor (anaemia)
   Arthropathy (haemophilia; secondary gout; drug treatment etc.)
   Pulse

3. **ARMS**
   Epitrochlear nodes (non-Hodgkin's lymphoma, chronic lymphocytic leukaemia, intravenous drug use, sarcoid)
   Axillary nodes

4. **FACE**
   Sclera—jaundice, pallor, conjunctival suffusion (polycythaemia)
   Mouth—gum hypertrophy (acute leukaemia), ulceration, infection, haemorrhage (marrow aplasia etc.); atrophic glossitis, angular stomatitis (iron, vitamin deficiencies)
   Tonsils—enlarged (lymphoma)

5. **CERVICAL NODES (sitting up)**
   Palpate from behind

6. **BONY TENDERNESS**
   Sternum
   Clavicles
   Shoulders
   Spine

7. **ABDOMEN (lying flat) and GENITALIA**
   Detailed examination

8. **INGUINAL NODES**

9. **LEGS**
   Vasculitis (Henoch-Schönlein purpura—buttocks, thighs)
   Bruising
   Pigmentation
   Ulceration
   Neurological signs (subacute combined degeneration, peripheral neuropathy)

10. **OTHER**
    Fundi (hyperviscosity, haemorrhages, infection etc.)
    Temperature chart (infection)
    Urine analysis (haematuria, bile etc.)
    Rectal examination (blood loss)

HINT BOX

Anaemia is most accurately detected by pulling down one of the patient's lower eyelids and comparing the colour of the anterior part of the conjunctiva with the pearly white of the palpebral conjunctiva more posteriorly. The anterior conjunctiva should be distinctly more red in colour unless significant anaemia (<100 g/L) is present.

6. Examine the mouth. Note gum hypertrophy (differential diagnosis includes acute myeloid leukaemia—especially monocytic—and scurvy), ulceration, infection (e.g. *Candida*), haemorrhage, atrophic glossitis (secondary to iron, vitamin B_{12} or folate deficiency) and angular stomatitis. Look for tonsillar and adenoid enlargement (Waldeyer's ring).

7. Now sit the patient up. Examine the cervical nodes from behind. There are seven groups: submental, submandibular, jugular chain, posterior triangle, postauricular, preauricular and occipital. Then feel the supraclavicular area from the front. Tap the spine with your fist for bony tenderness (which can be caused by an enlarging marrow—e.g. in myeloma, carcinoma). Also gently press the sternum, clavicles and shoulders for bony tenderness.

8. Lay the patient flat again. Examine the abdomen, particularly for splenomegaly (see Table 15.21) and hepatomegaly (see Tables 15.17 and 15.22).

9. Spring the hips for pelvic tenderness.

10. Palpate the inguinal nodes. There are two groups—along the inguinal ligament and along the femoral vessels. Do not forget to feel the testes and ask to do a rectal examination (e.g. for melaena).

11. Examine the legs. Note particularly leg ulcers, which may occur with hereditary spherocytosis, sickle cell syndromes, thalassaemia, macroglobulinaemia and Felty's syndrome. Ask to examine the legs from a neurological aspect for evidence of vitamin B_{12} deficiency. Remember, hypothyroidism and lead poisoning can cause anaemia and peripheral neuropathy. Do not miss Henoch-Schönlein purpura over the buttocks and legs.

12. Finally, ask to examine the fundi (engorged retinal vessels, papilloedema, haemorrhages etc.) and look at the temperature chart.
      Causes of generalised lymphadenopathy are presented in Table 15.24.

TABLE 15.24 Causes of generalised lymphadenopathy

1. Lymphoma (rubbery and firm)

2. Leukaemia (chronic lymphocytic leukaemia, acute lymphoblastic leukaemia particularly)

3. Malignant disease (metastases or reactive changes usually causing asymmetrical, very firm nodes)

4. Infections—viral (e.g. cytomegalovirus, HIV, infectious mononucleosis [glandular fever]), bacterial (e.g. tuberculosis, brucellosis), protozoal (e.g. toxoplasmosis)

5. Connective tissue diseases—rheumatoid arthritis, SLE

6. Infiltrations—sarcoidosis

7. Drugs—phenytoin (pseudolymphoma)

The endocrine system

The thyroid gland

'This 40-year-old woman has noticed some discomfort in her neck. Please examine her.'

Method (see Table 15.25)

The most likely problem is thyroid disease, but in the neck examination you should also consider the possibilities of superior vena caval obstruction, cervical lymphadenopathy, carotid aneurysm or bruit, JVP abnormalities and tracheal deviation.

1. Glance first at the face for signs of thyrotoxicosis or myxoedema (see below).

2. With the patient sitting up and the neck fully exposed, inspect for scars, swelling and prominent veins. Look at the front and the sides. Ask the patient to swallow a sip of water and look for thyroid enlargement. The thyroid moves up with swallowing.

3. Palpate gently from behind, with the neck flexed, feeling for any thyroid mass (see Table 15.26). Note the shape, consistency and distribution of the thyroid enlargement. If a nodule is palpable, determine whether this is single or part of a multinodular goitre. Ask the patient whether the gland is tender (a clue to subacute thyroiditis) and note any hoarseness of the voice (which may be caused by recurrent laryngeal nerve palsy). Decide whether you can palpate the lower border of the gland (to exclude retrosternal extension) and whether there is a thrill. Feel for cervical lymphadenopathy from behind. Palpate

TABLE 15.25 Neck examination

Sitting up

1. GENERAL INSPECTION

Face—thyrotoxicosis, myxoedema, other diagnostic facies (see Table 15.35)

2. NECK

Inspect
  Scars
  Swelling
  Prominent veins
  Swallowing (a glass of water)
Palpate (from behind with neck flexed)
  Thyroid enlargement—note size, shape, consistency, borders, mobility
  Thyroid tenderness
  Thyroid thrill
  Cervical nodes
Palpate (from in front)
  Thyroid (as above)
  Carotid arteries
  Supraclavicular nodes
  Trachea position
  Sternomastoid function
Percuss
  Upper manubrium
Auscultate
  Thyroid bruit
  Carotid bruit
Pemberton's sign

3. OTHER

Signs of thyrotoxicosis/myxoedema elsewhere

Thyroidectomy scar—test for hypoparathyroidism (Chvostek's and Trousseau's signs)

Jugular venous pressure—superior vena cava obstruction

Causes of localised cervical gland enlargement—chest, abdomen, head and neck examination

TABLE 15.26 Causes of a diffuse goitre

1. Idiopathic (majority)

2. Puberty, pregnancy and postpartum

3. Graves' disease

4. Thyroiditis—Hashimoto's thyroiditis, subacute thyroiditis (tender), chronic fibrosing (Riedel's) thyroiditis (rare)

5. Simple goitre (iodine deficiency)

6. Goitrogens—iodine excess, drugs (e.g. lithium, phenylbutazone)

7. Inborn errors of thyroid hormone synthesis—Pendred's syndrome, an autosomal recessive condition associated with nerve deafness

---

each carotid artery (absence possibly indicating malignant infiltration). Test the sternomastoid function, as malignant disease may infiltrate this muscle. Finally, palpate the gland from in front and note the tracheal position.

4. Percuss over the upper part of the manubrium from one side to the other right across the bone and note any change from resonant to dull (a sign of retrosternal extension).

5. Auscultate over the thyroid gland for bruits (a sign of active thyrotoxicosis) and also over the carotid arteries.

6. Remember Pemberton's sign. Ask the patient to lift her arms over her head. Look for suffusion of the face, elevation of the JVP and inspiratory stridor. Any retrosternal mass may cause these changes.

7. If there is evidence of a goitre and obvious eye disease (indicating the presence of *thyrotoxicosis*; see Table 15.27), proceed to the face. Examine the eyes for exophthalmos by noting the presence of sclera below the cornea when the patient is looking straight ahead. Note lid retraction by looking for the presence of sclera above the cornea. Then test for lid lag by asking the patient to follow your finger descending at a moderate rate. Now examine the conjunctiva for chemosis.

TABLE 15.27 Causes of thyrotoxicosis
Primary
1. Graves' disease
2. Toxic adenoma or multinodular goitre
3. Hashimoto's thyroiditis (early in its course), subacute thyroiditis (transient) and painful (if granulomatous) or painless (if lymphatic)
4. Iodine-induced (after previous iodine deficiency)—termed the Jod-Basedow phenomenon
5. Excess thyroid hormone replacement
6. Postpartum thyroiditis (non-tender)
7. Drugs—amiodarone (via Jod-Basedow), lithium (rare)
Secondary
1. Pituitary or ectopic thyroid-stimulating hormone hypersecretion (very rare)
2. Hydatidiform mole or choriocarcinoma (human chorionic gonadotrophin secretion—rare)
3. Struma ovarii (rare)
4. Factitious
Note: The three components of Graves' disease—viz. eye signs, hyperthyroidism with goitre and pretibial myxoedema—run independent courses.

8. Test eye movements for ophthalmoplegia. The inferior oblique muscle power is lost first, then convergence is affected, followed by the other muscles in thyrotoxicosis. Examine the fundi because optic atrophy can occur late. Then look from behind, over the patient's forehead, when she is looking forward, for proptosis.

9. Examine the patient's outstretched hands for tremor. It is worthwhile placing a sheet of paper over the dorsal aspects of the fingers. Look at the nails for onycholysis (Plummer's nails)—distal separation of the nail from its bed—and thyroid acropachy (this looks like clubbing and is clubbing, but is not called clubbing!). Note any palmar erythema. Feel for warmth and sweating. Feel the radial pulse for sinus tachycardia, atrial fibrillation or a collapsing pulse.

10. Test for proximal myopathy in the arms and tap the arm reflexes for briskness.

11. If there is time, proceed to the legs and look for skin manifestations: pretibial myxoedema—bilateral firm, elevated dermal nodules and plaques that can be pink, brown or skin-coloured and that are caused by mucopolysaccharide accumulation—and vitiligo. Test for proximal myopathy and hyperreflexia in the legs.

12. Ask to examine the chest for evidence of gynaecomastia (in men) and the heart for an ejection systolic murmur and signs of congestive cardiac failure.

13. Although it is rarely of importance, there may also be mild splenomegaly and hepatomegaly on abdominal examination, as well as generalised lymphadenopathy.

14. If a thyroidectomy scar is present, ask to look for the signs of hypocalcaemia (i.e. Chvostek's and Trousseau's signs). Chvostek's sign may be present in normal patients. It is tested by tapping over the facial nerve 3–5 cm below and in front of the ear. The facial muscle twitches briefly in the presence of hypocalcaemia. Trousseau's sign is tested by pumping up a sphygmomanometer cuff above systolic blood pressure and looking for *main d'accoucheur* (a strongly adducted thumb with fingers extended except at the MCP joints) that occurs within 2 minutes.

15. If you suspect *hypothyroidism* (when goitre is unusual) (see Table 15.28), proceed as follows:

(a) Examine the hands. Note peripheral cyanosis, swelling and dry, cold skin. Look at the palmar creases for anaemia (see Table 15.29). Feel the pulse for bradycardia and a small volume. Test for carpal tunnel syndrome. Ask the patient to flex both wrists for 30 seconds—paraesthesiae will often be precipitated in the affected hand if the carpal tunnel syndrome is present (Phalen's wrist flexion test).

(b) Test for delayed relaxation of the biceps jerk. Examine for proximal myopathy, which is rare.

(c) Proceed to the face. Note here any general swelling and periorbital oedema. Look for loss of the outer one-third of the eyebrows and periorbital xanthelasma. Note whether the skin is dry, fine and smooth. There may be signs of carotenaemia, alopecia or vitiligo. Look at the tongue, which may be swollen, then ask the patient to tell you her name and address and note any hoarseness or slowness of speech. Test for nerve deafness, which may be bilateral.

(d) Go to the legs next. Examine them neurologically, starting with the ankle jerks, noting particularly any evidence of slow relaxation, which is best seen with the patient kneeling on a chair. Then examine for peripheral neuropathy and look for other uncommon neurological abnormalities (see Table 15.30).

(e) Finally ask to examine the chest for pleural and pericardial effusions. There may be dry, rough 'sandpaper-like' skin over the chest.

TABLE 15.28 Causes of hypothyroidism
Primary
Without a goitre (decreased or absent thyroid tissue)
Idiopathic atrophy
Treatment (e.g. iodine-131, surgery)
Agenesis or a lingual thyroid
Unresponsiveness to thyroid-stimulating hormone
With a goitre (decreased synthesis)
Chronic thyroiditis (e.g. late Hashimoto's disease, Riedel's thyroiditis)
Drugs (e.g. lithium, amiodarone)
Endemic iodine deficiency
Iodine-induced hypothyroidism
Inborn errors (enzyme deficiency)
Secondary
Pituitary lesions
Tertiary
Hypothalamic lesions
Transient
Thyroid hormone treatment withdrawn
Subacute thyroiditis
Postpartum thyroiditis

TABLE 15.29 Causes of anaemia in patients with hypothyroidism

1. Chronic disease (direct or erythropoietin-mediated depressive effect on bone marrow)
2. Folate deficiency secondary to bacterial overgrowth
3. Pernicious anaemia associated with myxoedema
4. Iron deficiency in women owing to menorrhagia
5. Haemolysis secondary to hypercholesterolaemia-induced spur-cell anaemia

TABLE 15.30 Neurological associations of hypothyroidism

Common

1. Entrapment (e.g. carpal tunnel, tarsal tunnel)
2. Delayed relaxation phase of ankle jerks
3. Nerve deafness

Uncommon

1. Peripheral neuropathy
2. Proximal myopathy (with normal creatine kinase levels)
3. Hypokalaemic periodic paralysis
4. Eaton-Lambert syndrome or deterioration or unmasking of myasthenia gravis
5. Cerebellar syndrome
6. Psychosis
7. Coma
8. Cerebrovascular disease
9. High cerebrospinal fluid protein
10. Muscle cramps

Panhypopituitarism

'This 35-year-old man has lost his libido. Please assess him.'

Method

You cleverly note that this man looks 'panhypopituitary' (see Table 15.31). Proceed as follows.

1. Ask him to stand and make sure he is fully undressed. Note the pale skin and lack of hair.
2. The patient may have short stature (failure of growth hormone secretion before growth is complete) and no secondary sexual characteristics (gonadotrophin failure before puberty).
3. Look at the face more closely. Multiple fine skin wrinkles around the eyes and mouth are characteristic of growth hormone deficiency. Look closely for a hypophysectomy scar on the forehead near the inner canthus of the eye. Examine the eyes for signs of a pituitary tumour (visual fields, especially for bitemporal hemianopia, fundi for optic atrophy) and assess cranial nerves III, IV and VI, as well as the first division of V (affected by tumour extension into the cavernous sinus). Feel the facial hair over the beard area.
4. Go to the chest and look for decreased body hair, pale skin and gynaecomastia. Lay the patient down and look for loss of pubic hair and testicular atrophy (testes are small and soft—the normal size is 15–25 mL in volume).

5. Test the ankle jerks (for slow relaxation in hypothyroidism—there is no myxoedematous appearance) and ask to check the blood pressure lying and standing (hypotension with adrenocorticotrophic hormone [ACTH] deficiency).

TABLE 15.31 Causes of panhypopituitarism

1. Chromophobe adenoma (most common cause in males)
2. Other space-occupying lesion (craniopharyngioma, metastatic carcinoma, granuloma)
3. Iatrogenic (surgery, radiation)
4. Sheehan's syndrome (postpartum necrosis)
5. Head injury
6. Idiopathic

Note: Loss of function (in order)
60% pituitary loss: growth hormone, FSH and LH
80% pituitary loss: TSH
100% pituitary loss: ACTH

ACTH = adrenocorticotrophic hormone; FSH = follicle-stimulating hormone; LH = luteinising hormone; TSH = thyroid-stimulating hormone.

Cushing's syndrome

'This 56-year-old man has noted weight gain. Please examine him.'

Method (see Table 15.32)

TABLE 15.32 Cushing's syndrome examination

Standing

1. GENERAL INSPECTION
Central obesity and thin limbs
Skin bruising, atrophy
Pigmentation (ACTH tumour— rare—or bilateral adrenalectomy)
Poor wound healing

2. ARMS
Purple striae (proximally)
Proximal myopathy

Sitting

3. FACE
Plethora, hirsutism, acne, telangiectasia
Moon shape
Eyes—visual fields (pituitary tumour), fundi (atrophy, papilloedema, signs of hypertension or diabetes)
Mouth—thrush
Neck—supraclavicular fat pads, acanthosis nigricans

4. BACK
Buffalo hump (interscapular fat pad)

Kyphoscoliosis (osteoporosis)
Tenderness of vertebrae (osteoporotic fractures)

5. LEGS
Squat (proximal myopathy)
Striae (thighs)
Bruising, oedema

6. MENTAL STATE
Depression
Psychosis
Irritability

Lying flat

7. ABDOMEN
Purple striae
Adrenal masses, adrenalectomy scars
Liver (tumour deposits)

8. OTHER
Urine analysis (glycosuria, evidence of renal stone disease)
Blood pressure (hypertension)
Signs of ectopic tumour (e.g. lung small cell carcinoma or carcinoid)—rare

This type of introduction may mean Cushing's syndrome in the clinical examination. Make sure that the patient is undressed to his underpants and ask him to stand.

1. Look at the patient from the front, sides and behind. Note central obesity with peripheral sparing and look at the skin for bruising, atrophy and pigmentation of extensor areas. Hyperpigmentation suggests an ectopic ACTH-secreting tumour, or it may indicate an ACTH-secreting pituitary adenoma in a patient who has had a bilateral adrenalectomy (Nelson's syndrome).

2. Test for proximal myopathy of the arms and also of the legs (initially by getting the patient to squat). Examine the back for a buffalo hump and feel it. Look for kyphoscoliosis and tap the spine for bony tenderness as a result of osteoporotic vertebral crush fractures.

3. Ask the patient to sit on the side of the bed. Look at the face for plethora, hirsutism, acne, telangiectasia and a moon shape.

4. Test the eyes for visual field defects (which are uncommon) and look in the fundi for papilloedema (caused by benign intracranial hypertension or a pituitary tumour) and optic atrophy, as well as hypertensive or diabetic changes (see Tables 15.7 and 15.41). Then look at the neck for supraclavicular fat pads and acanthosis nigricans.

5. Ask the patient to lie down. Examine the abdomen for adrenalectomy scars, pigmentation, striae and adrenal masses. Look at the genitalia. Virilisation in women or gynaecomastia in men suggests that adrenal carcinoma is more likely. Next look at the legs for oedema, bruising and poor wound healing.

6. Do not forget to ask for the results of urine analysis (glucose) and take the blood pressure (hypertension). Diagnostic tests are summarised in Table 15.33.

TABLE 15.33 Diagnosis of Cushing's syndrome*

Screening tests

1. Cortisol levels morning and evening (serum or salivary): loss of diurnal rhythm (evening cortisol level should be less than half the morning value) of little diagnostic value.

2. 24-hour urine collection for urinary free cortisol determination (an indirect assessment of cortisol production). Should be threefold increased (above normal).

3. Overnight dexamethasone suppression test (1 mg dexamethasone at midnight causes suppression of cortisol in normal subjects at 9.00 am). No suppression is found in Cushing's syndrome, but this may also occur with alcoholism, induction of hepatic enzymes (e.g. phenytoin) or depression, in patients taking the contraceptive pill and in some obese patients.

4. Blood count (secondary polycythaemia, neutrophil leucocytosis, eosinopenia).

5. Electrolyte levels (hypokalaemic alkalosis, particularly with ectopic ACTH-producing tumours).

6. Blood sugar level (hyperglycaemia).

Definitive tests

1. 2 mg dexamethasone suppression test (0.5 mg six-hourly for 48 hours). No suppression of plasma cortisol or urinary free cortisol occurs in Cushing's syndrome, but usually suppression does occur in normal subjects, obese patients and depressed patients.

2. 8 mg dexamethasone suppression test (2 mg six-hourly for 48 hours). Suppression occurs in Cushing's disease, but no suppression is usually found in adrenal adenoma or carcinoma or in the presence of ectopic ACTH production. False-positive results can occur in patients taking anticonvulsants (which accelerate dexamethasone metabolism).

TABLE 15.33 Diagnosis of Cushing's syndrome* (Continued)

3. ACTH level—high in ectopic ACTH production, low with adrenal adenoma or carcinoma, high or normal in Cushing's disease. Ectopic secretion of CRH by tumours is a very rare cause of Cushing's syndrome.

4. Petrosal sinus ACTH sampling—a central-to-peripheral venous cortisol ratio of >2:1 is diagnostic of Cushing's disease; lateralisation of ACTH production helps the neurosurgeon plan trans-sphenoidal exploration of the sella.

* Cushing's disease is specifically pituitary ACTH overproduction.

To diagnose Cushing's syndrome, at least two definitive tests should be abnormal.

Note: If Cushing's disease is present, pituitary assessment is necessary. If adrenal disease is suspected, CT scanning is useful to assess the anatomy. Remember, ectopic ACTH production by a tumour (e.g. small cell carcinoma of lung, carcinoid of lung or thymus, pancreatic islet cell carcinoma, ovarian carcinoma) does not usually cause Cushingoid clinical features but may present with hyperpigmentation, hypokalaemic alkalosis and hypertension.

Acromegaly

'This 64-year-old man has noted some change in his facial appearance. Please examine him.'

Method (see Table 15.34)

TABLE 15.34 Acromegaly examination

1. GENERAL INSPECTION Diagnostic facies	Visual fields Cranial nerves III, IV, VI, V Fundi
2. HANDS Shape Sweat Phalen's test (carpal tunnel)	**8. NECK** Thyroid gland (diffuse or nodular goitre)
3. ULNAR NERVE Thickened	**9. HEART** Cardiac failure
4. PROXIMAL MYOPATHY	**10. ABDOMEN** Organomegaly
5. AXILLAE Skin tags Acanthosis nigricans Greasy skin	**11. LOWER LIMBS** Hips ⎫ Knees ⎭ osteoarthritis, pseudogout Entrapment neuropathy Heel pad thickening
6. FACE Frontal bossing Hirsutism Macroglossia Prognathism Hoarseness	**12. OTHER** Urine analysis (glycosuria) Rectal examination—colonic polyps (correlate with skin tags) Blood pressure (hypertension) Sleep apnoea
7. EYES	

TABLE 15.35 Common diagnostic facies	
1. Acromegalic	7. Myotonic
2. Thyrotoxic	8. Parkinsonian
3. Myxoedematous	9. Thalassaemic
4. Cushingoid	10. Marfanoid
5. Pagetic	11. Mitral
6. Myopathic	

The order and direction of the examination obviously depend on the stem.

> **HINT BOX**
> The change to a written stem has led to variations on this introduction.
> At one end of the spectrum the examiners may give the diagnosis: 'This
> 64-year-old man has acromegaly. Please examine him to assess the
> extent and activity of the condition.' At the other end of the spectrum the
> introduction may be more oblique: 'This 64-year-old man has had premature
> and severe arthritis. Please examine his knees.'

1. Consider the possible diagnostic facies (see Table 15.35). If the patient looks acromegalic, proceed as follows.
2. Have the patient stand or sit on the side of the bed. Look at the hands. Look for coarse features and spade-like shape, as well as increased sweating and warmth. Osteoarthritis-like changes are frequent in the hands, shoulders, hips and knees. Perform Phalen's wrist flexion test for the carpal tunnel syndrome (median nerve entrapment). Feel the ulnar nerve for thickening at the elbow.
3. Go to the arms and test for proximal myopathy. Also look in the axillae for skin tags (molluscum fibrosum), greasy skin and acanthosis nigricans (brown-to-black velvety elevation of the epidermis owing to multiple confluent papillomas).
4. Go on to the face. Look for frontal bossing as a result of a large supraorbital ridge (which may also occur in rickets, Paget's disease, hydrocephalus or achondroplasia). Note whether there is a large tongue (sometimes too big to fit into the mouth neatly). Enlargement of the lower jaw (called prognathism) and splaying of the teeth may be present. Notice any acne or hirsutism in women (see Table 15.44) and test the voice, which may be deep, husky and resonant.
5. The eyes must be carefully examined. Visual fields should be checked—look particularly for bitemporal hemianopia, but many field defects are possible (see Fig 15.46). Examine the fundi for optic atrophy, papilloedema and angioid streaks (red, brown or grey streaks 3–5 times the diameter of the retinal veins appearing to emanate from the optic disc and owing to degeneration of Bruch's membrane with resultant fibrosis). There may also be diabetic or hypertensive changes.

> **Causes of angioid streaks (PASH)**
> Paget's disease, pseudoxanthoma elasticum, poisoning (lead)
> Acromegaly
> Sickle cell anaemia
> Hyperphosphataemia (familial)

6. Examine the thyroid gland for diffuse enlargement or a multinodular goitre.
7. Examine the cardiovascular system for signs of congestive cardiac failure, the abdomen for organomegaly—of liver, spleen and kidney—and for signs of hypogonadism (secondary to an enlarging pituitary adenoma).
8. Examine the lower limbs for osteoarthritis and pseudogout. Large osteophyte formation and ligamentous laxity are common features. Also look for foot drop (entrapment of common peroneal nerve) and heel pad thickening.
9. If there is time, look for evidence of hypothyroidism and adrenocortical insufficiency (from an enlarging pituitary adenoma).
10. Do not forget to ask for the results of a urine analysis to exclude glycosuria secondary to glucose intolerance and take the blood pressure (hypertension is an association). Decide whether the acromegaly is active (see Table 15.36). Ask whether any photographs taken of the patient over the years are available for inspection (typically, manifestations begin in middle age). See Table 15.37 for the diagnostic evaluation.

TABLE 15.36 Evidence of activity in acromegaly
1. Skin tag number
2. Excessive sweating
3. Presence of glycosuria
4. Increasing visual field loss or development of cranial nerve palsies of III, IV, VI and V
5. Enlarging goitre
6. Hypertension
7. Symptoms of headache, or increasing ring size, shoe size or dentures

TABLE 15.37 Diagnosis of acromegaly
Biochemical
1. Insulin-like growth factor (IGF-1) (somatomedin C) level in plasma (elevated in active acromegaly)
2. Glucose tolerance test (no suppression or a paradoxical rise in growth hormone level)
Anatomical (99% pituitary adenoma)
1. Skull X-ray film (enlarged sella, double floor)—not routine
2. MRI scan (if normal, exclude extra-pituitary acromegaly)

Addison's disease

'This 65-year-old woman has weakness, anorexia and weight loss. Please assess her.'

Method

Fortunately, you suspect Addison's disease.
1. Ensure the patient is appropriately undressed and look for pigmentation (particularly in the palmar creases, elbows, gums and buccal mucosa, genital areas and scars) and vitiligo, owing to an autoimmune disease association. Ear lobe calcification occurs rarely.

2. Take the blood pressure and test for a postural drop. Ask for the results of a urine analysis, as diabetes is associated with Addison's disease. Remember that the rest of the autoimmune cluster may also be associated (see Table 15.38) and consider the possible causes (see Table 15.39). Diagnostic tests are summarised in Table 15.40.

TABLE 15.38 Autoimmune-associated disease

Addison's disease

Hypoparathyroidism

Mucocutaneous candidiasis

Diabetes mellitus (type 1)

Hashimoto's thyroiditis

Graves' disease

Primary ovarian failure

Pernicious anaemia

Vitiligo

Alopecia

Hypophysitis

Myasthenia gravis

TABLE 15.39 Causes of Addison's disease (chronic adrenal insufficiency)*

1. Iatrogenic

2. Primary

Autoimmune adrenal disease (>80% of all cases)

Polyglandular syndromes:

Type I: Addison's disease, hypoparathyroidism, mucocutaneous candidiasis, primary hypogonadism

Type II: Addison's disease, type 1 diabetes mellitus, Hashimoto's thyroiditis or Graves' disease, primary hypogonadism

Tuberculosis, histoplasmosis

Infiltration (e.g. amyloidosis, sarcoidosis)

Metastatic malignant disease

Demyelinating disease—adrenoleucodystrophy (asymmetrical cortical signs and Addison's disease), adrenomyeloneuropathy (spastic paraparesis and Addison's disease)

Drugs—heparin (bilateral adrenal haemorrhage), aminoglutethimide, ketoconazole, HIV infection

3. Secondary

Pituitary or hypothalamic disease (usually *no* mineralocorticoid deficiency)

*Acute adrenal insufficiency may follow any stress in a patient with chronic hypoadrenalism or abrupt cessation of prolonged high-dose steroid therapy.

TABLE 15.40 Diagnosis of Addison's disease

Screening tests

1. Electrolyte levels (hyponatraemia, hyperkalaemia, hyperchloraemic acidosis, hypercalcaemia)

2. Hypoglycaemia

3. Blood count (lymphocytosis, eosinophilia)

4. Chest X-ray film (tuberculosis, small heart)

5. Plain abdominal X-ray film (adrenal calcification)

Definitive tests

1. Short Synacthen test (0.25 mg synthetic ACTH given intramuscularly)

2. Long Synacthen test (8-hour intravenous infusion or depot administration) if subnormal response

3. Plasma ACTH level

Diabetes mellitus

'This 70-year-old woman has diabetes. Please examine her [or her legs or eyes].'

Method (see Table 15.41)

TABLE 15.41 Diabetes mellitus examination

Lying

1. GENERAL INSPECTION
Weight—obesity
Hydration
Endocrine facies
Pigmentation—haemochromatosis etc.

2. LEGS
Inspect
  Skin—necrobiosis, hair loss, infection, pigmented scars, atrophy, ulceration, injection sites
  Muscle wasting
  Joint destruction—Charcot's joints
Palpate
  Temperature of feet (cold, blue owing to small or large vessel disease)
Peripheral pulses
  Femoral (auscultate)
  Popliteal
  Posterior tibial
  Dorsalis pedis
Oedema
Neurological assessment
  Femoral nerve mononeuritis
  Peripheral neuropathy

3. ARMS
Inspect
  Injection sites
  Skin lesions
Pulse

4. EYES
Fundi—cataracts, rubeosis, retinal disease, III nerve palsy etc.

5. MOUTH AND EARS
Infection

6. NECK
Carotid arteries—palpate, auscultate

7. CHEST
Signs of infection

8. ABDOMEN
Liver—fat infiltration; rarely haemochromatosis
Fat hypertrophy—insulin injection sites

9. OTHER
Urine analysis—glycosuria, ketones, proteinuria
Blood pressure and pulse—lying and standing

1. General inspection may reveal a characteristic facial appearance (e.g. Cushing's syndrome or acromegaly) or pigmentation (e.g. haemochromatosis), which will modify the examination approach. Otherwise, expose the patient's legs. This is the only case in which there is an advantage in starting at the legs.

2. Look for necrobiosis lipoidica over the shins (a central yellow scarred area with a surrounding red margin, if active, owing to atrophy of subcutaneous collagen—it is rare), pigmented scars, skin atrophy, small rounded plaques with raised borders lying in a linear fashion over the shins (diabetic dermopathy), ulceration and infection. Look at the thigh for injection sites, fat atrophy (owing to the use of impure insulin) or fat hypertrophy (owing to repeated injections into the same site, which leads to scarring and hypertrophy) and quadriceps wasting, from femoral nerve mononeuritis—called (inaccurately) diabetic amyotrophy.

3. Inspect the feet and toes very carefully. Look for loss of hair, skin atrophy and blue, cool feet (small vessel vascular disease), ulcers and foot deformity. Feel all the peripheral pulses and note capillary return. Feel for pitting oedema. Auscultate over the femoral artery for bruits.

4. Test proximal muscle power and test the reflexes. Assess for peripheral neuropathy, including dorsal column loss—called diabetic pseudotabes (p 378). Charcot's joints (see Fig 15.25) (owing to proprioceptive loss) may be present. (*Note*: Neuropathic joint disease: sensory loss [e.g. from diabetes, tabes dorsalis, amyloidosis, leprosy, meningomyelocele] allows repeated joint trauma, producing bony overgrowth, synovial effusion and joint distortion and instability.)

5. Go to the upper limbs. Look at the nails for *Candida* infection. Feel the upper arm injection sites. Ask for the blood pressure and take the pulse lying and standing to detect autonomic neuropathy (see Table 15.42).

6. Now examine the eyes for visual acuity. Remember, episodes of poor control cause lens abnormalities acutely. Look for Argyll Robertson pupils (which are rare). Remember, a diabetic third nerve palsy is usually pupil sparing—infarction

Figure 15.25 Gross destructive changes in the ankle joints in a patient with diabetic neuropathy—Charcot's joints.
Figure reproduced courtesy of The Canberra Hospital.

TABLE 15.42 Autonomic neuropathy

Clinical features

Postural hypotension (a blood pressure fall of >30/20 mmHg on standing upright from a supine position)

Loss of sinus arrhythmia

Valsalva manoeuvre causes no slowing of the pulse

Loss of sweating

Erectile dysfunction

Nocturnal diarrhoea

Urine retention, incontinence

TABLE 15.43 Features of diabetic retinopathy

Non-proliferative

Haemorrhages:

1. Dot-haemorrhage into the inner retinal areas
2. Blot-haemorrhage into more superficial nerve fibre layers

Hard exudates have straight edges—leakage of protein and lipids from damaged capillaries

Soft exudates (cotton wool spots) have a fluffy appearance owing to microinfarcts

Microaneurysms

Dilated veins

Proliferative

New vessels

Vitreous haemorrhage

Scar formation

Retinal detachment (opalescent sheet that balloons forward into the vitreous)

Laser scars (small brown or yellow spots)

affects the inner more than the outer fibres, whereas compressive lesions affect the outer fibres first and so involve the pupil early.

7. Look in the fundi (see Table 15.43). While performing fundoscopy, also note the presence of cataracts and any new blood vessel formation over the iris (rubeosis).
8. Always test the III, IV and VI cranial nerves and remember that other cranial nerves may be affected. Periorbital and perinasal swelling with gangrene can occur with rhinocerebral mucormycosis, an opportunistic fungal infection.
9. Look in the mouth for *Candida* and other infections.
10. Look in the ears for infection (e.g. malignant otitis externa caused by *Pseudomonas aeruginosa*).
11. Feel and auscultate the carotid arteries.
12. Examine for hepatomegaly as a result of fatty infiltration and then ask for the results of urine analysis with respect to glucose and protein.
13. There may be signs of chronic renal failure (kidney disease) with advanced diabetes.
14. Ask whether you may weigh the patient.

Hirsutism

A diagnostic approach is summarised in Table 15.44.

TABLE 15.44 Hirsutism
Clinical approach
General appearance—acromegaly, cushingoid
Skin changes of porphyria cutanea tarda
Hair distribution
Face
Midline (front and back)
Genital
Signs of virilisation
Receding hairline and increased oiliness of skin
Breast atrophy
Muscle bulk
Clitoromegaly
Abdomen
Adrenal masses (rarely palpable)
Polycystic ovaries or ovarian tumour (rarely palpable)
Blood pressure
Raised in C–11-hydroxylase deficiency (potassium low)
Causes of hirsutism
1. Constitutional (normal endocrinology)
2. Polycystic ovarian syndrome
3. Adrenal—Cushing's syndrome, congenital adrenal hyperplasia (21- and 11-hydroxylase deficiency), virilising adrenal tumour
4. Ovary (e.g. stromal ovarian cancer)
5. Drugs (e.g. phenytoin, diazoxide, streptomycin, minoxidil, androgen, glucocorticoids)
6. Other (e.g. acromegaly, porphyria cutanea tarda)

The rheumatological system

In this section only the common joints that are encountered in the examination are discussed.

HINT BOX

These rheumatological examinations are ripe for new more subtle stems related to assessment of function. The examiners may assume the diagnosis is obvious.

The hands

'This 67-year-old woman has arthritis. Please examine her hands.'

Method (see Table 15.45)

TABLE 15.45 Hand examination	
Sitting up (hands on a pillow)	**3. FEEL AND MOVE PASSIVELY**
1. GENERAL INSPECTION	Wrists
Cushingoid	Synovitis
Weight	Effusions
Iritis, scleritis etc.	Range of movement
Obvious other joint disease	Crepitus
2. LOOK	Ulnar styloid tenderness
Dorsal aspect	Metacarpophalangeal joints
Wrists	Synovitis
Skin—scars, redness, atrophy, rash	Effusions
Swelling—distribution	Range of movement
Deformity	Crepitus
Muscle wasting	Subluxation
Metacarpophalangeal joints	Proximal and distal interphalangeal joints
Skin	As above
Swelling—distribution	Palmar tendon crepitus
Deformity—ulnar deviation, volar subluxation etc.	Carpal tunnel syndrome tests
Proximal and distal interphalangeal joints	**4. HAND FUNCTION**
Skin	Grip strength
Swelling—distribution	Key grip
Deformity–swan necking, bouton-nière, Z, sausage-shaped etc.	Opposition strength
Nails	Practical ability
Psoriatic changes—pitting, ridging, onycholysis, hyperkeratosis, discolouration	**5. OTHER**
Palmar aspect	Elbows—subcutaneous nodules, psoriatic rash
Skin—scars, palmar erythema, palm creases (anaemia), discolouration	Other joints
Muscle wasting	Signs of systemic disease

When you are asked to examine the hands consider the possibilities of arthropathy, acromegaly, a peripheral nerve lesion, a myopathy or a neuropathy. If there is obvious joint disease, examine as follows.

1. First make the patient comfortable, expose as much of the hands and forearms as possible and place the patient's hands on a pillow, palms down. You may talk as you go. We believe this is the best way to proceed with a joint examination. However, also practise examining this sort of case by presenting at the end of the examination. Be gentle while examining—do not hurt the patient.
2. If the patient has arthropathy with an obvious rheumatoid distribution, start by stating that the patient has a symmetrical deforming polyarthropathy involving the wrists and hands. Then describe the forearms and wrists—look at the skin for erythema, ecchymoses or skin atrophy (this may indicate steroid use), scars and rashes (e.g. psoriasis: look over the elbows, in the scalp and around the umbilicus). Look for rheumatoid nodules.
3. Then look for swelling and its distribution, wrist deformity and muscle wasting involving the forearms and interosseous muscles.
4. Go on to the metacarpophalangeal (MCP) joints. Mention, if present, any skin abnormalities, swelling and deformity, particularly ulnar deviation and volar subluxation.

5. Next describe the proximal and distal interphalangeal (PIP and DIP) joints. Symmetrical wrist, MCP and proximal joint swellings suggest rheumatoid arthritis. Swelling in the PIP joints and DIP joints is suggestive of osteoarthritis. Again mention any skin changes that may be present, swelling over each joint if present and deformity, particularly 'swan necking' and boutonnière deformity of the fingers, and 'Z' deformity of the thumb. Sausage-shaped phalanges and telescoping of the fingers with predominant interphalangeal joint disease usually means psoriatic arthropathy or Reiter's disease. Small joint ankylosis is common. Look for telangiectasiae.

6. Next look at the nails and describe any psoriatic nail changes (present in the great majority of patients with psoriatic arthritis)—namely pitting, onycholysis, hyperkeratosis, ridging and discolouration. Note the signs of vasculitis (splinter haemorrhages or black to brown 1–2 mm skin infarcts, usually in a periungual location) and mention this to the examiners.

7. Now ask the patient to open and close the hands. This will reveal tendon ruptures and fixed flexion deformities.

8. Turn the wrists over and look at the palms for scars, palmar erythema and muscle wasting.

9. Now go on and palpate each joint, starting with the wrists. Feel for synovitis (boggy swelling) and effusions. Describe the range of passive movement of the joint. Also note any joint crepitus. Palpate the ulnar styloid for tenderness. When examining the MCP joints, also feel for subluxation. Test for palmar tendon crepitus (tenosynovitis).

10. Having examined each joint, assess the function of the hand. This is very important. Test grip strength, key grip and opposition strength (thumb and little finger), and ask the patient to perform a practical procedure, such as undoing a button.

11. A formal neurological examination of the hand is not required in assessing arthropathy. However, a ganglion or tenosynovitis may cause the carpal tunnel syndrome. Ask the patient to flex both wrists together for 30 seconds— paraesthesiae will often be precipitated in the affected hand if the carpal tunnel syndrome is present (Phalen's wrist flexion test). Tap over the carpal tunnel while the wrist is held in extension for Tinel's sign (paraesthesiae in the distribution of the median nerve). These tests have similar but limited specificity and sensitivity. After you have finished with the hands, feel at the elbows for rheumatoid nodules and look carefully for any psoriatic rash there also.

12. If function has been mentioned, check sensation in the median and ulna nerve distributions.

    You should now have an idea of the pattern and severity of the deformity, as well as the extent of the loss of function and the activity of the disease.

    Always consider the differential diagnosis of a deforming polyarthropathy:
    *   rheumatoid arthritis (see Figs 15.26 and 15.27)
    *   seronegative arthropathies—particularly psoriatic arthritis (see Figs 15.28 and 15.29)
    *   polyarticular gout or pseudogout (see Fig 15.30)
    *   primary generalised osteoarthritis (where DIP and PIP joint involvement is common) (see Fig 15.31).

    Look carefully while doing your hand examination for any of these possibilities.

    At the end, ask whether you may examine all the other joints that are likely to be involved and the other systems likely to be affected.

Figure 15.26 X-rays of the hands of a patient with early rheumatoid arthritis. Note the erosions of the metacarpal heads, reduced cartilage in the joint spaces and erosion of the ulnar styloid (arrow).
Figure reproduced courtesy of The Canberra Hospital.

Figure 15.27 X-ray of the hands showing advanced destructive changes in a patient with rheumatoid arthritis. Note ulnar deviation, Z deformity of the thumb, destruction of the PIP and MCP joints, and bone erosion.
Figure reproduced courtesy of The Canberra Hospital.

Figure 15.28 X-rays of the hands of a patient with polyarthritis secondary to connective tissue disease (CREST syndrome). There are destructive changes in all the joints (the DIP joints are not spared), and bony erosions are prominent.
Figure reproduced courtesy of The Canberra Hospital.

Figure 15.29 X-ray of the hands of a patient with psoriatic arthritis. Note bone erosion, loss of joint space and 'pencil in cup deformity' of the PIP joints.
Figure reproduced courtesy of The Canberra Hospital.

Figure 15.30 X-ray of the hands of a patient with severe gouty arthritis. Note the large soft-tissue masses and severe joint destruction.
Figure reproduced courtesy of The Canberra Hospital.

Figure 15.31 X-ray of the hands of a patient with severe osteoarthtitis. Note Heberden's nodes and DIP joint involvement.
Figure reproduced courtesy of The Canberra Hospital.

The knees
'This 70-year-old man has had painful knees. Please examine him.'

Method
1. Expose both knees and thighs fully and have the patient lie on his back.
2. Look for quadriceps wasting and then over the knees for any skin abnormalities (scars or rashes), swelling and deformity. Synovial swelling is seen medial to the patella and in the suprapatellar area. Fixed flexion deformity must be assessed. This is looked for by inspecting the knee from the side (a space beneath the knee is seen).
3. Feel the quadriceps for wasting.
4. Ask about tenderness and palpate for warmth and synovitis over the knee joint.
5. Examine for effusions—the patella tap (ballottement) is used to confirm a large effusion. The fluid from the suprapatellar bursa is pushed by the hand into the joint space by squeezing the lower part of the quadriceps and then pushing the patella downwards with the fingers. The patella will be ballottable if fluid is present under it. In patients with a smaller effusion, pressing over the lateral knee compartment may produce a noticeable medial bulge as a result of fluid displacement.
6. Test flexion and extension passively and note the range of movement and the presence or absence of crepitus.
7. Examine for fixed flexion deformity by gently extending the knee.
8. Test the ligaments next. The lateral and medial collateral ligaments are tested by having the knee slightly flexed, holding the leg with the right hand and arm, steadying the thigh with the left hand and moving the leg laterally and medially. Movements of more than 5–10° are abnormal. The cruciate ligaments are tested by steadying the foot with your elbow and moving the leg anteriorly and posteriorly with the other hand. Again, laxity of more than 5–10° is abnormal.
9. Use McMurray's test for meniscal integrity. Hold the lower leg and foot, flex and extend the knee while internally and externally rotating the tibia. Pain or clicking is very suggestive of a meniscal tear.
10. Ask the patient to stand up and examine for a Baker's cyst, which is felt in the popliteal fossa and is more obvious when the knee is extended.
11. Proceed then to examine other joints that may be involved or test function by asking the patient to walk.

HINT BOX
The knees and other hinge joints are commonly affected in patients with arthritis secondary to haemophilia. The pattern of joint involvement and juxta-articular bony sclerosis on X-ray film help to distinguish this from rheumatoid arthritis involving the knees (see Figs 15.32 and 15.33).

The feet
'This 50-year-old woman has painful feet. Please examine her [her feet].'

Method
1. Start by inspecting the ankles. Look at the skin of the feet and toes (for scars, ulcers and rashes), and look for swelling, deformity and muscle wasting. Examine the midfoot and forefoot similarly. Deformities affecting the forefoot include hallux valgus and clawing and crowding of the toes (in rheumatoid arthritis). If pes cavus is present, consider a hereditary motor and sensory neuropathy.

15.32 X-ray of the knee joint of a patient with arthritis secondary to haemophilia. Note loss of joint space. The juxta-articular aspects of the tibia and femur appear sclerotic, but the bones are generally osteoporotic.
Figure reproduced courtesy of The Canberra Hospital.

Figure 15.33 X-ray of the knee of a patient with rheumatoid arthritis. Here there is more severe joint space loss.
Figure reproduced courtesy of The Canberra Hospital.

2. Note any psoriatic nail changes. Look at the transverse and longitudinal arches. Look for callus over the metatarsal heads, which occurs in subluxation. Note any obvious painless deformities or Charcot's joints.
3. Palpate, starting with the ankle, feeling for synovitis and effusion. Passive movement of the talar joints (dorsiflexion and plantarflexion) and subtalar joints (inversion and eversion) must be assessed. The best way to examine the subtalar and midtarsal joints is to fix the os calcaneus and ankle joint with the left hand while inverting and everting the midfoot with the right. Tenderness on movement is more important than range of movement. The midfoot (midtarsal joint) allows rotation of the forefoot on a fixed hindfoot. Squeeze the metatarsophalangeal joints for tenderness.
4. Examining the individual toes is useful in seronegative spondyloarthropathies (a sausage-like swelling of the toe is characteristic in psoriatic arthritis).
5. Feel the Achilles tendon for nodules and palpate the inferior aspect of the heel for tenderness (plantar fasciitis).
6. Consider a neurological examination—test pinprick sensation and proprioception. Go on to examine other joints as appropriate.

   X-rays of the feet are the most likely investigations that will be available (see Figs 15.34–15.38). Patients with rheumatoid arthritis can have involvement of the cervical spine, hips and shoulders, and X-rays of these may also be available (see Figs 15.39–15.41).

Figure 15.34 (a) X-ray of the feet of a patient with early rheumatoid arthritis. Note the joint erosions and deformity of some of the MTP and PIP joints.
Figure reproduced courtesy of The Canberra Hospital.

Figure 15.34 Continued (b) X-ray of the ankles of a patient with rheumatoid arthritis. There is generalised loss of joint spaces, and early destructive changes are present.
Figure reproduced courtesy of The Canberra Hospital.

Figure 15.35 X-ray of the feet of a patient with early psoriatic arthritis. Note the large erosions and absence of osteoporosis. There is already some joint deformity, and a spiculated bony growth is visible.
Figure reproduced courtesy of The Canberra Hospital.

Figure 15.36 X-ray of the feet of a patient with severe psoriatic arthritis: *arthritis mutilans.*
Figure reproduced courtesy of The Canberra Hospital.

Figure 15.37 X-ray of the feet of a patient with severe gouty arthritis. Note the relative preservation of the joint spaces with erosions and overhanging edges. The area of the junction of the forefoot and midfoot has numerous erosions, which is a common finding.
Figure reproduced courtesy of The Canberra Hospital.

Figure 15.38 X-ray of the feet of a patient with diabetic arthropathy. Note the gross joint destruction—Charcot's joints.

Figure reproduced courtesy of The Canberra Hospital.

Figure 15.39 Cervical spine X-ray of a patient with rheumatoid arthritis. Note the erosions and loss of joint space. Special views are needed to exclude erosion of the odontoid process.

Figure reproduced courtesy of The Canberra Hospital.

Figure 15.40 (a) X-ray of the pelvis of a patient with rheumatoid arthritis. Note the severe destructive changes on both sides—very different from (b). (b) Osteoarthritis of the left hip. Note the asymmetrical loss of joint space.
Figures reproduced courtesy of The Canberra Hospital.

Figure 15.41 **X-ray of the chest of a patient with rheumatoid arthritis involving the shoulder. Note the erosions of the humeral heads with subluxation and erosions of the distal clavicles.**
Figure reproduced courtesy of The Canberra Hospital.

The back

'This 47-year-old man has had back pain for many years. Please examine him.'
   Or
'This 47-year-old man has ankylosing spondylitis. Please examine him and assess the severity of his disease.'

Method

1. The initial inspection confirms that this is a case of ankylosing spondylitis (see Table 15.46). Ask the patient to undress to his underpants and stand up. Look for deformity, inspecting from both the back and the side, particularly for loss of kyphosis and lumbar lordosis. Palpate each vertebral body for tenderness and palpate for muscle spasm.

TABLE 15.46 The seronegative spondyloarthropathies	
	HLA-B27
1. Ankylosing spondylitis	95%
2. Psoriatic spondylitis	50%
3. Reactive arthritis, including Reiter's syndrome	80%
4. Enteropathic arthritis	75%

2. Test movement next. Measure the finger–floor distance (inability to touch the toes suggests early lumbar disease).
3. Next look at extension, lateral flexion and rotation of the back. Get him to run each hand down the corresponding thigh to test lateral flexion.

4. Ask whether you may perform a modified Schober's test. This involves identifying the level of the posterior iliac spine on the vertebral body (approximately at L5). Place a mark 5 cm below this point and another 10 cm above this point. Ask the patient to touch his toes. There should normally be an increase of 5 cm or more in the distance between the marks. In ankylosing spondylitis there will be little separation of the marks, since all the movement is taking place at the hips.

> **HINT BOX**
> Small adhesive paper or plastic strips are popular as markers: do not mark the patient with a pen.

5. Next test the occiput-to-wall distance. Ask the patient to place his heels and back against the wall and ask him to touch the wall with the back of his head without raising his chin above the carrying level; inability to touch the wall suggests cervical involvement and the distance from occiput to wall is measured.

> **HINT BOX**
> It is a good idea to know why this test is performed: it is to assess progression of the disease at clinic visits.

6. Before asking the patient to lie down, test for active sacroiliac disease by springing the anterior superior iliac spines. Pain felt in the region of the sacroiliac joints suggests activity. A simple (and unreliable) test for sacroiliac disease is to push with the heel of the hand on the sacrum and note the presence of tenderness in either sacroiliac joint on springing. (*Note:* Usually there is bilateral disease in ankylosing spondylitis.)
7. Ask the patient to lie on his stomach. Examine the heels for Achilles tendinitis and plantar fasciitis, which are characteristic of the spondyloarthropathies. Evaluate the other large joints, particularly the knees, hips and shoulders.
8. Examine the chest for decreased lung expansion (chest expansion of less than 3 cm at the nipple line suggests early costovertebral involvement) and for signs of apical fibrosis. Examine the heart for aortic regurgitation, mitral valve prolapse and evidence of conduction defects, and the eyes for uveitis.
9. Examine the gastrointestinal system for evidence of inflammatory bowel disease and for signs of amyloid deposition (e.g. hepatosplenomegaly, abnormal urine analysis results). Remember also to check for signs of psoriasis and Reiter's syndrome, which may cause spondylitis and unilateral sacroiliitis. Rarely, patients with ankylosing spondylitis have a cauda equina compression. X-ray changes are described in Table 15.47 and illustrated in Figures 15.42–15.44.

> **The cauda equina syndrome**
> Back, buttock and leg pain
> Saddle sensory loss
> Lower limb weakness
> Loss of sphincter control

TABLE 15.47 X-ray changes in ankylosing spondylitis

Sacroiliac joints

1. Cortical outline lost (early)
2. Juxta-articular osteosclerosis
3. Erosions
4. Joint ankylosis

Lumbar spine

1. Loss of lumbar lordosis
2. Squaring of vertebrae
3. Syndesmophytes (thoracolumbar region)
4. Bamboo spine (bony bridging of vertebrae) and osteoporosis
5. Apophyseal joint fusion

Figure 15.42 X-ray of the pelvis of a patient with Reiter's syndrome. Note the loss of joint space in the two sacroiliac joints and lumbar spine ankylosis.
Figure reproduced courtesy of The Canberra Hospital.

Figure 15.43 Lateral chest X-ray of a patient with ankylosing spondylitis. Note the loss of joint space and squaring of the vertebrae.
Figure reproduced courtesy of The Canberra Hospital.

Figure 15.44 X-ray of the pelvis of a patient with ankylosing spondylitis. Note the lateral bridging syndesmophytes (arrow).
Figure reproduced courtesy of The Canberra Hospital.

The nervous system

Cranial nerves

There will usually be some direction from the stem, sometimes to the upper or lower cranial nerves. The introduction may vary, from a problem with vision, speech or swallowing to a history of neck surgery or trauma.

Method

1. Inspect the head and neck briefly first. Have the patient sit over the edge of the bed facing you and look for any craniotomy scars (often well disguised by hair), neurofibromata, Cushing's syndrome, acromegaly, Paget's disease, facial asymmetry and obvious ptosis, proptosis, skew deviation of the eyes or pupil inequality.
2. Look for the characteristic facies of myasthenia gravis or myotonic dystrophy.

First nerve

1. Ask the examiners whether they want you to test smell. They will rarely allow you to proceed as it is time-consuming and not usually fruitful in examinations. If you are required to test smell, a series of sample bottles will be provided by the examiners containing vanilla, coffee and other non-pungent substances. Remember to test each nostril separately (see p 355 for the causes of anosmia).

Second nerve

2. Test visual acuity (with the patient's spectacles on, as refractive errors are not cranial nerve abnormalities) using a visual acuity chart. Test each eye separately, covering the other eye with a small card.
3. Examine the visual fields by confrontation using a red-tipped hatpin, making sure your head is level with the patient's head. A red hatpin enables you to detect earlier peripheral field loss. Test each eye separately. If the patient has such poor acuity that a hatpin is difficult to use, map the fields with your fingers. When you are testing the patient's right eye, he or she should look straight into your left eye. The patient's head should be at arm's length and he or she should cover the eye not being tested with a hand. Bring the hatpin from the four main directions diagonally towards the centre of the field of vision.
4. Next map out the blind spot by asking about disappearance of the hatpin lateral to the centre of the field of vision of each eye. A gross enlargement may be detectable by comparison with your own blind spot.
5. Look into the fundi (p 353).

Third, fourth and sixth nerves

6. Look at the pupils. Note the shape, relative sizes and any associated ptosis. Use your pocket torch and shine the light from the side to gauge the reaction to light on both sides. Do not bore the examiners by shining the light repeatedly into each eye—practise assessing the direct and consensual responses rapidly.
7. Look for the Marcus Gunn phenomenon (afferent pupillary defect) by moving the torch in an arc from pupil to pupil. The affected pupil will paradoxically dilate after a short time when the torch is moved from a normal eye to one with optic atrophy or very decreased visual acuity from other causes.
8. Test accommodation by asking the patient to look into the distance and then at your red hatpin placed about 15 cm from his or her nose.
9. Assess eye movements with both eyes first. Ask the patient to look voluntarily and quickly from left to right and then to follow the red hatpin in each

direction—right and left lateral gaze, plus up and down in the lateral position. Look for failure of movement and nystagmus.

HINT BOX
Sometimes reduced eye movement will be detected only when the patient looks quickly from one side to the other.

---

10. Ask about diplopia (double vision) when the eyes are in each position. With complex lesions then assess each eye separately. Move the patient's head if the patient is unable to follow movements. Beware of strabismus.

Fifth nerve
11. Ask permission first to test the corneal reflexes. Make sure you touch the cornea (not the conjunctiva) gently with a piece of cotton wool. Come in from the side and do this only once on each side. If the nerve pathways are intact, the patient will blink both eyes. Ask whether he or she can actually feel the touch (V is the sensory component).

HINT BOX
Corneal reflex: when there is an ipsilateral seventh nerve palsy, only the contralateral eye will blink—sensation is preserved (nerve VII is the motor component). Also, with an ipsilateral seventh nerve palsy, the eye on the side of the lesion may roll superiorly with the corneal stimulus ('Bell's phenomenon').

---

12. Test facial sensation in the three divisions: ophthalmic, maxillary and mandibular. Use a pin first to assess pain. Map out any area of sensory loss from dull to sharp and check for any loss on the posterior part of the head (C2) and neck (C3). Light touch must be tested also, as there may be some sensory dissociation.

HINT BOX
A medullary or upper cervical lesion of the fifth nerve causes loss of pain and temperature sensation with preservation of light touch. A pontine lesion may cause loss of light touch with preservation of pain and temperature sensation.

---

13. Examine the motor division by asking the patient to clench his or her teeth (feeling the masseter muscles) and open the mouth; the pterygoid muscles will not allow you to force it closed if the nerve is intact. A unilateral lesion causes the jaw to deviate towards the weak (affected) side.
14. Always test the jaw jerk (with the mouth just open, the finger over the jaw is tapped with a tendon hammer). An increased jaw jerk occurs in pseudobulbar palsy.

Seventh nerve
15. Look for facial asymmetry and then test the muscles of facial expression. Ask the patient to look up and wrinkle the forehead. Look for loss of wrinkling and

feel the muscle strength by pushing down on each side. This is preserved in an upper motor neurone lesion because of bilateral cortical representation of these muscles.

16. Next ask the patient to tightly shut the eyes—compare how deeply the eyelashes are buried on the two sides and then try to open each eye. Ask the patient to grin and compare the nasolabial grooves.

17. If a lower motor neurone lesion is detected, quickly check for ear and palatal vesicles of herpes zoster of the geniculate ganglion—the Ramsay Hunt syndrome. Examining for taste on the anterior two-thirds of the tongue is not usually required.

Eighth nerve

18. Whisper a number softly about 0.5 m away from each ear and ask the patient to repeat the number. Perform Rinne's and Weber's tests with a 256-hertz tuning fork. If indicated, ask for an auriscope (wax is the most common cause of conductive deafness).

Ninth and tenth nerves

19. Look at the palate and note any uvular displacement. Ask the patient to say 'aaah' and look for asymmetrical movement of the soft palate. With a unilateral tenth nerve lesion the uvula is drawn towards the unaffected (normal) side.

20. Testing the gag reflex is traditional, but adds little to the examination. If the palate moves normally and the patient can feel the spatula, the same information is obtained (the ninth nerve is the sensory component and the tenth nerve the motor component): touch the back of the pharynx on each side. Remember to ask the patient whether he or she feels the spatula each time. You may not attain top marks if the patient vomits all over the examiners. If the spatula is used correctly, the patient will gag only if the reflex is hyperactive.

21. Ask the patient to speak (to assess hoarseness) and to cough (listen for a bovine cough, which may occur with a recurrent laryngeal nerve lesion). *Note:* You will not usually be required to test taste on the posterior third of the tongue (i.e. ninth nerve).

Eleventh nerve

22. Ask the patient to shrug the shoulders and then feel the trapezius bulk and push the shoulders down. Then instruct the patient to turn his or her head against resistance (your hand) and also feel the muscle bulk of the sternomastoids.

Twelfth nerve

23. While examining the mouth, inspect the tongue for wasting and fasciculation (best seen with the tongue not protruded, and which may be unilateral or bilateral).

HINT BOX

Take time to inspect the tongue. Fasciculations and wasting are easily missed but are very important in the diagnosis of a lower motor neurone twelfth nerve palsy.

---

24. Ask the patient to protrude the tongue. With a unilateral lesion it deviates towards the weaker (affected) side.

25. The way to finish your assessment depends entirely on your findings. For

example, if you discover evidence of a particular syndrome (such as the lateral medullary syndrome), you should proceed to confirm your impressions by examining more peripherally, if allowed (especially for sensory long tract and cerebellar signs, see below).

HINT BOX

If you have discovered multiple lower cranial nerve palsies, you would want to assess, among other features, the nasopharynx for signs of tumour and the neck for scars and radiotherapy changes.

---

26. Auscultating for carotid or cranial bruits (over the mastoids, temples and orbits), as well as taking the blood pressure and testing the urine for sugar, are often relevant.

    Relevant investigations are likely to be CT or MRI scans. These are not always easy for physicians to report. Candidates would hope to have a good idea where in the brain or the spinal cord the abnormality is likely to be present. Only scans with quite obvious abnormalities are likely to be used for the exam (see Fig 15.45).

Figure 15.45 MRI scan of a right-handed woman with right hemiplegia and aphasia. There is a large left middle cerebral artery stroke with haemorrhagic transformation (arrow).

Figure reproduced courtesy of The Canberra Hospital.

Eyes

'Please examine this man's eyes.'

Method *(see Table 15.48)*

TABLE 15.48 Eye examination	
Sitting up	Fields
1. GENERAL INSPECTION Diagnostic facies (see Table 15.35)	Red hatpin confrontation—each eye Central vision Fundi

2. CORNEA
Corneal arcus
Band keratopathy
Kayser-Fleischer rings
	Cornea
	  Lens
	  Humour
	  Colour of disc and state of cup
	  Retina—vessels, exudates,

3. SCLERA
Jaundice
Pallor
Injection
	haemorrhages, pigmentation etc.
	Pupils
	  Shape, size, symmetry
	  Light reflex—direct and consensual

4. PTOSIS	Marcus Gunn phenomenon
5. EXOPHTHALMOS	Accommodation Eye movements

6. EYELIDS
Xanthelasma
	III, IV, VI nerves—movement, diplopia,
	  nystagmus
	  Gaze palsies (e.g. supranuclear

7. LID LAG	lesions)
8. ORBITS Palpate—tenderness—brow (for loss of sweating in Horner's syndrome) Listen for a bruit	Fatiguability (myasthenia) Corneal reflex (V)
	10. OTHER

9. NEUROLOGICAL EXAMINATION
Acuity
    Eye chart—each eye separately
	Depends on findings—other cranial
	  nerves, long tract signs, urine analysis
	  (diabetes)

1. Always inspect the eyes first, with the patient sitting over the end of the bed facing you at eye level if possible. Note any corneal abnormalities, such as band keratopathy (in hypercalcaemic states) or Kayser-Fleischer rings (Wilson's disease). Look at the sclerae for colour (e.g. jaundice, blue in osteogenesis imperfecta), pallor, injection and telangiectasia. Inspect carefully for subtle ptosis or strabismus. Look for exophthalmos from behind and above the patient, as well as in front.

2. Proceed then as for the cranial nerve eye examination, testing acuity, fields and pupils, and then performing fundoscopy.

3. Begin fundoscopy by examining the cornea and lens, and then the retina. Note any corneal, lens or humor abnormalities. Look for retinal changes of diabetes mellitus (see Table 15.43) and hypertension (see Table 15.7). Also carefully inspect for optic atrophy, papilloedema, angioid streaks (see p 326), retinal detachment, central vein or artery thrombosis and retinitis pigmentosa.

4. Test eye movements. Also look for fatiguability of eye muscles by asking the patient to look up at your hatpin for half a minute (myasthenia gravis). Test for lid lag if you suspect hyperthyroidism.

5. Test the corneal reflex.

6. Palpate the orbits for tenderness and auscultate the eyes with the bell of the

stethoscope (the eye being tested is shut, the other is open and the patient is asked to stop breathing).

7. Do not forget that the patient may have a glass eye. Suspect this if visual acuity is zero in one eye and no pupillary reaction is apparent. Lengthy attempts to examine the fundus of a glass eye are embarrassing (and not uncommon).

One-and-a-half syndrome

This is rare but important to recognise. These patients have a horizontal gaze palsy when looking to one side (the 'one') plus impaired adduction on looking to the other side (the 'and-a-half'). Other features often include turning out (exotropia) of the eye opposite the side of the lesion (paralytic pontine exotropia). The one-and-a-half syndrome can be caused by a stroke (infarct), plaque of multiple sclerosis or tumour in the dorsal pons.

Horner's syndrome

If you find a partial ptosis and a constricted pupil (which reacts normally to light), Horner's syndrome is likely (see Table 15.49). Proceed as follows.

TABLE 15.49 Causes of Horner's syndrome
1. Carcinoma of the lung apex (usually squamous cell carcinoma)
2. Neck—thyroid malignancy, trauma
3. Carotid arterial lesion—carotid aneurysm or dissection, pericarotid tumour, cluster headache
4. Brain stem lesions—vascular disease (especially the lateral medullary syndrome), syringobulbia, tumour
5. Retro-orbital lesions
6. Syringomyelia (rare)

1. Test for a difference in sweating over each brow with the back of your finger (even though your brow is usually more sweaty than the patient's); this occurs only when the lesion is proximal to the carotid bifurcation. Absence of sweating differences does not exclude the diagnosis of Horner's syndrome.
2. Next, examine the appropriate cranial nerves to exclude the lateral medullary syndrome:
   (a) nystagmus (to the side of the lesion)
   (b) ipsilateral fifth (pain and temperature), ninth and tenth cranial nerve lesions
   (c) ipsilateral cerebellar signs
   (d) contralateral pain and temperature loss over the trunk and limbs.
3. Ask the patient to speak and note any hoarseness (which may be caused by recurrent laryngeal nerve palsy from a chest lesion or a cranial nerve lesion).
4. Look at the hands for clubbing. Test finger abduction to screen for a lower trunk brachial plexus (C8, T1) lesion.
5. If there are signs of hoarseness or a lower trunk brachial plexus lesion, proceed to a respiratory examination, concentrating on the apices for signs of lung carcinoma.
6. Examine the neck for lymphadenopathy, thyroid carcinoma and a carotid aneurysm or bruit (e.g. fibromuscular dysplasia causing dissection).
7. As syringomyelia may rarely cause this syndrome, finish off the assessment by examining for dissociated sensory loss. Remember, this lesion may cause a *bilateral* Horner's syndrome (a trap for the unwary).

Notes on the cranial nerves
First (olfactory) nerve (p 349)
Causes of anosmia
Bilateral
1. Upper respiratory tract infection (most common)
2. Meningioma of the olfactory groove (late)
3. Ethmoid tumours
4. Head trauma (including cribriform plate fracture)
5. Meningitis
6. Hydrocephalus
7. Congenital—Kallmann's syndrome (hypogonadotrophic hypogonadism)

Unilateral
1. Meningioma of the olfactory groove (early)
2. Head trauma

Second (optic) nerve (p 349)
Light reflex
Constriction of the pupil in response to light is relayed via the optic nerve and tract, the superior quadrigeminal brachium, the Edinger-Westphal nucleus and its efferent parasympathetic fibres, which terminate in the ciliary ganglion. There is no cortical involvement.

Accommodation reflex
Constriction of the pupil with accommodation originates in the cortex (in association with convergence) and is relayed via parasympathetic fibres in the third nerve.

Causes of absent light reflex but intact accommodation reflex
1. Midbrain lesion (e.g. Argyll Robertson pupil)
2. Ciliary ganglion lesion (e.g. Adie's pupil)
3. Parinaud's syndrome
4. Bilateral anterior visual pathway lesions (i.e. bilateral afferent pupil deficits)

Causes of absent convergence but intact light reflex
1. Cortical lesion (e.g. cortical blindness)
2. Midbrain lesions (rare)

Pupil abnormalities
Causes of constriction
1. Horner's syndrome
2. Argyll Robertson pupil
3. Pontine lesion (often bilateral, but reactive to light)
4. Narcotics
5. Pilocarpine drops
6. Old age

Causes of dilation
1. Mydriatics, atropine poisoning or cocaine
2. Third nerve lesion
3. Adie's pupil
4. Iridectomy, lens implant, iritis
5. Post-trauma, deep coma, cerebral death
6. Congenital

Visual field defects (see Fig 15.46)

1. **Tunnel vision:** concentric diminution (e.g. glaucoma, papilloedema)	
2. **Enlarged blind spot:** optic nerve head enlargement	
3. **Central scotomata:** optic nerve head to chiasmal lesion (e.g. demyelination, toxic, vascular, nutritional)	
4. **Unilateral field loss:** optic nerve lesion (e.g. vascular, tumour)	
5. **Bitemporal hemianopia:** optic chiasma lesion (e.g. pituitary tumour, sella meningioma)	
6. **Homonymous hemianopia:** optic tract to occipital cortex, lesion at any point (e.g. vascular, tumour) Note: Incomplete lesion results in macular (central) vision sparing	
7. **Upper quadrant homonymous hemianopia:** temporal lobe lesion (e.g. vascular, tumour)	
8. **Lower quadrant homonymous hemianopia:** parietal lobe lesion	

Figure 15.46 Visual field defects associated with lesions of the visual system.

Adie's syndrome
Cause
Lesion in the efferent parasympathetic pathway.

Signs
1. Dilated pupil
2. Decreased or absent reaction to light (direct and consensual)
3. Slow or incomplete reaction to accommodation with slow dilation afterwards
4. Decreased tendon reflexes
5. Patients are commonly young women
6. Denervation supersensitivity to a weak (e.g. 0.125%) pilocarpine solution

Argyll Robertson pupil
Cause
Lesion of the iridodilator fibres in the midbrain, as in:
1. syphilis
2. diabetes mellitus
3. alcoholic midbrain degeneration (rarely)
4. other midbrain lesions.

Signs
1. Small, irregular, unequal pupil
2. No reaction to light
3. Prompt reaction to accommodation
4. If tabes associated, decreased reflexes
5. Some mydriatics (e.g. atropine, cocaine) dilate slowly; direct sympathetic agonists dilate promptly

Papilloedema versus papillitis

Papilloedema	Papillitis
Optic disc swollen without venous pulsation	Optic disc swollen*
Acuity normal (early)	Acuity poor
Colour vision normal	Colour vision affected (particularly red desaturation)
Large blind spot	Large central scotoma
Peripheral constriction of visual fields	Pain on eye movement
Usually bilateral	Onset usually sudden and unilateral
*In retrobulbar neuritis and old papillitis the optic disc becomes pale.	

Causes of papilloedema
1. Space-occupying lesion (causing raised intracranial pressure) or a retro-orbital mass
2. Hydrocephalus (associated with large ventricles):
   (a) obstructive (block in the third ventricle, aqueduct or outlet to fourth ventricle—e.g. tumour)
   (b) communicating:
       (i) increased formation—choroid plexus papilloma
       (ii) decreased absorption—tumour causing venous compression, subarachnoid space obstruction from meningitis
3. Benign intracranial hypertension (pseudotumour cerebri, associated with small ventricles):
   (a) idiopathic
   (b) contraceptive pill
   (c) Addison's disease
   (d) drugs—nitrofurantoin, tetracycline, vitamin A, steroids
   (e) lateral sinus thrombosis
   (f) head trauma
4. Hypertension (grade IV)
5. Central retinal vein thrombosis
6. Cerebral venous sinus thrombosis
7. High cerebrospinal fluid protein level—Guillain-Barré syndrome

Causes of optic atrophy
1. Chronic papilloedema or optic neuritis
2. Optic nerve pressure or division
3. Glaucoma
4. Ischaemia
5. Familial—retinitis pigmentosa, Leber's disease, Friedreich's ataxia

Causes of optic neuropathy
1. Multiple sclerosis (see Fig 15.47)
2. Toxic—ethambutol, chloroquine, nicotine, alcohol
3. Metabolic—vitamin B_{12} deficiency
4. Ischaemia—diabetes mellitus, temporal arteritis, atheroma
5. Familial—Leber's disease
6. Infective—infectious mononucleosis (glandular fever)

Figure 15.47 MRI of the brain of a patient with multiple sclerosis showing numerous plaques (white patches).
Figure reproduced courtesy of The Canberra Hospital.

Causes of cataract
1. Old age (senile cataract)
2. Endocrine—diabetes mellitus, steroids
3. Hereditary or congenital—dystrophia myotonica, Refsum's disease
4. Ocular disease—glaucoma
5. Irradiation
6. Trauma

Causes of ptosis
1. With normal pupils:
   (a) senile ptosis (common)
   (b) myotonic dystrophy
   (c) fascioscapulohumeral dystrophy
   (d) ocular myopathy
   (e) thyrotoxic myopathy
   (f) myasthenia gravis
   (g) botulism, snake bite
   (h) congenital
   (i) fatigue
2. With constricted pupils:
   (a) Horner's syndrome
   (b) tabes dorsalis
3. With dilated pupils: third nerve lesion

Third (oculomotor) nerve (p 349)

Clinical features of a third nerve palsy
1. Complete ptosis (partial ptosis may occur with an incomplete lesion)
2. Divergent strabismus (eye 'down and out')
3. Dilated pupil unreactive to direct or consensual light and unreactive to accommodation

---

HINT BOX

Always exclude a fourth (trochlear) nerve lesion when a third nerve lesion is present. Do this by tilting the patient's head to the same side as the lesion. The affected eye will intort if the fourth nerve is intact. Or ask the patient to look down and across to the opposite side from the lesion and look for intortion. Remember SIN:

Superior (oblique muscle), supplied by the IV nerve, INtorts the eye

---

Aetiology
Central
1. Vascular (e.g. brain stem infarction)
2. Tumour
3. Demyelination (rare)
4. Trauma
5. Idiopathic

Peripheral
1. Compressive lesions:
   (a) aneurysm (usually on the posterior communicating artery)
   (b) tumour causing raised intracranial pressure (dilated pupil occurs early)
   (c) nasopharyngeal carcinoma
   (d) orbital lesions—Tolosa-Hunt syndrome (superior orbital fissure syndrome—painful lesion of the third, fourth, sixth and the first division of the fifth cranial nerves)
   (e) basal meningitis
2. Infarction—diabetes mellitus, arteritis (pupil is usually spared)
3. Trauma
4. Cavernous sinus lesions

Sixth (abducens) nerve (p 349)

Clinical features of a sixth nerve palsy
1. Failure of lateral movement
2. Affected eye is deviated inwards in severe lesions
3. Diplopia—maximal on looking to the affected side; the images are horizontal and parallel to each other; the outermost image is from the affected eye and disappears on covering this eye (this image is also usually more blurred)

Aetiology
Bilateral
1. Trauma (head injury)
2. Wernicke's encephalopathy
3. Raised intracranial pressure
4. Mononeuritis multiplex

Unilateral
1. Central:
   (a) vascular
   (b) tumour
   (c) Wernicke's encephalopathy
   (d) multiple sclerosis (rare)
2. Peripheral:
   (a) diabetes, other vascular lesions
   (b) trauma
   (c) idiopathic
   (d) raised intracranial pressure

Eye movements

1. With the eye abducted: the elevator is the superior rectus (third nerve). The depressor is the inferior rectus (third nerve).
2. With the eye adducted: the elevator is the inferior oblique (third nerve). The depressor is the superior oblique (fourth nerve).

Causes of nystagmus

Jerky

1. Horizontal:
   (a) vestibular lesion (*Note:* Chronic lesions cause nystagmus to the side of the lesion—fast component.)
   (b) cerebellar lesion (*Note:* Unilateral disease causes nystagmus to the side of the lesion.)
   (c) internuclear ophthalmoplegia (*Note:* Nystagmus is in the abducting eye, with failure of adduction on the affected side. This is a result of a medial longitudinal fasciculus lesion. The most commont cause in young adults with bilateral involvement is multiple sclerosis; in the elderly, consider brain stem infarction. When the medial longitudinal fasciculus and the abducens nucleus on the same side are affected, the only horizontal movement the patient can make is abduction of the contralateral eye—*one-and-a-half syndrome.*)
2. Vertical:
   (a) brain stem lesion
      (i) upbeat nystagmus suggests a lesion in the floor of the fourth ventricle
      (ii) downbeat nystagmus suggests a foramen magnum lesion
   (b) toxic—phenytoin, alcohol (may also cause horizontal nystagmus)

Pendular

1. Retinal (decreased macular vision)—albinism
2. Congenital

Supranuclear palsy ·

Loss of vertical upward gaze and sometimes downward gaze. Clinical features (distinguishing from third, fourth and sixth nerve palsy):
1. both eyes affected
2. pupils often unequal
3. no diplopia
4. reflex eye movements (e.g. on flexing and extending the neck) intact.

Steele-Richardson-Olszewski syndrome (progressive supranuclear palsy)
1. Loss of vertical downward gaze first, later vertical upward gaze and finally horizontal gaze.
2. Associated with pseudobulbar palsy, long tract signs, extrapyramidal signs, dementia and neck rigidity.

Parinaud's syndrome
Loss of vertical upward gaze often associated with convergence–retraction nystagmus on attempted convergence and pseudo Argyll Robertson pupils.

Causes of Parinaud's syndrome
1. Central:
   (a) pinealoma
   (b) multiple sclerosis
   (c) vascular lesions
2. Peripheral:
   (a) trauma
   (b) diabetes mellitus
   (c) other vascular lesions
   (d) idiopathic
   (e) raised intracranial pressure

Fifth (trigeminal) nerve palsy (p 350) (see Fig 15.48)

Figure 15.48 Divisions of the trigeminal nerve and dermatomes of the head and neck.

Aetiology
Central (pons, medulla and upper cervical cord)
1. Vascular
2. Tumour
3. Syringobulbia
4. Multiple sclerosis

Peripheral (posterior fossa)
1. Aneurysm
2. Tumour (skull base, e.g. acoustic neuroma)
3. Chronic meningitis

Trigeminal ganglion (petrous temporal bone)
1. Meningioma
2. Fracture of the middle fossa

Cavernous sinus (associated third, fourth and sixth nerve palsies)
1. Aneurysm
2. Thrombosis
3. Tumour

Other
1. Sjögren's syndrome
2. SLE
3. Toxins
4. Idiopathic

HINT BOX
1. If there is loss of all sensation in all three divisions of the fifth nerve—consider a lesion at the ganglion or sensory root.
2. If there is total sensory loss in one division—consider a postganglionic lesion.
3. If there is loss of pain but preservation of touch—consider a brain stem or upper cervical cord lesion.
4. If there is loss of touch but pain sensation is preserved—consider a pontine nucleus lesion.

Seventh (facial) nerve palsy (p 350)
Aetiology
Upper motor neurone lesion (supranuclear)
1. Vascular
2. Tumour

Lower motor neurone lesion
1. Pontine (often associated with nerves V, VI):
   (a) vascular
   (b) tumour
   (c) syringobulbia
   (d) multiple sclerosis
2. Posterior fossa:
   (a) acoustic neuroma
   (b) meningioma

3. Petrous temporal bone:
   (a) Bell's palsy
   (b) Ramsay Hunt syndrome
   (c) otitis media
   (d) fracture
4. Parotid:
   (a) tumour
   (b) sarcoid

Causes of bilateral lower motor neurone facial weakness
1. Guillain-Barré syndrome
2. Bilateral parotid disease (e.g. sarcoidosis)
3. Mononeuritis multiplex (rare)

> **HINT BOX**
> Myopathy and neuromuscular junction defects can cause bilateral facial weakness.

Eighth (acoustic) nerve (p 351)
To differentiate nerve deafness from conductive deafness, use the following tests.

Rinne's test
A 256-hertz vibrating tuning fork is first placed on the mastoid process, behind the ear and, when the sound is no longer heard, it is placed in line with the external meatus.

> **HINT BOX**
> The tines of the fork should be in line with the external auditory canal, so that the sound waves that leave the fork from two axes do not cancel each other out.

Results
1. Normal—the note is audible at the external meatus.
2. Nerve deafness—the note is audible at the external meatus because air and bone conduction are reduced equally, so that air conduction is better (as is normal); positive result.
3. Conduction (middle ear) deafness—no note is audible at the external meatus; negative result.

Weber's test
A 256-hertz tuning fork is placed on the centre of the forehead.

Results
1. Normal—the sound is heard in the centre of the forehead.
2. Nerve deafness—the sound is transmitted to the normal ear.
3. Conduction deafness—the sound is heard louder in the abnormal ear.
Note: Although these tests are of traditional importance, they are not very accurate and are now rarely used by neurologists. However, candidates must be able to perform them.

Causes of deafness
1. Nerve (sensorineural) deafness:
   (a) degeneration (e.g. presbycusis)
   (b) trauma (e.g. high noise exposure, fracture of the petrous temporal bone)
   (c) toxic (e.g. aspirin, alcohol, streptomycin)
   (d) infection (e.g. congenital rubella syndrome, congenital syphilis)
   (e) tumour (e.g. acoustic neuroma)
   (f) brain stem lesions
   (g) vascular disease of the internal auditory artery
2. Conductive deafness:
   (a) wax
   (b) otitis media
   (c) otosclerosis
   (d) Paget's disease of bone

Ninth (glossopharyngeal) and tenth (vagus) nerve palsy (p 351)
Aetiology
Central
1. Vascular (e.g. lateral medullary infarction owing to vertebral or posterior inferior cerebellar artery disease)
2. Tumour
3. Syringobulbia
4. Motor neurone disease (vagus nerve only)

Peripheral—posterior fossa
1. Aneurysm
2. Tumour
3. Chronic meningitis
4. Guillain-Barré syndrome (vagus nerve only)

Twelfth (hypoglossal) nerve palsy (p 351)
Aetiology
Upper motor neurone lesion
1. Vascular
2. Motor neurone disease
3. Tumour
4. Multiple sclerosis

HINT BOX
The syndrome of bilateral upper motor neurone lesions of the ninth, tenth and twelfth nerves is called *pseudobulbar palsy*.

HINT BOX
It is difficult to detect unilateral twelfth lesions, as the tongue muscles (except the genioglossus) are bilaterally innervated.

Lower motor neurone lesion—unilateral
1. Central:
   (a) vascular—thrombosis of the vertebral artery
   (b) motor neurone disease
   (c) syringobulbia
2. Peripheral (posterior fossa):
   (a) aneurysm
   (b) tumour
   (c) chronic meningitis
   (d) trauma
   (e) Arnold-Chiari malformation
   (f) fracture or tumour of the base of the skull

HINT BOX

The Arnold-Chiari malformation is a protrusion of the cerebellar tonsils through the foramen magnum. The more severe types (II–IV) cause basilar compression with lower cranial nerve palsies, cerebellar limb signs (owing to tonsillar compression) and upper motor neurone signs in the legs.

Lower motor neurone lesion—bilateral
1. Motor neurone disease
2. Arnold-Chiari malformation
3. Guillain-Barré syndrome
4. Polio

Causes of multiple cranial nerve palsies

Think of *cancer* first.
1. Nasopharyngeal *carcinoma*
2. Chronic meningitis (e.g. *carcinoma*, tuberculosis, sarcoidosis)
3. Guillain-Barré syndrome (spares nerves I, II and VIII), including the Miller-Fisher variant
4. Brain stem lesions—these are usually as a result of vascular disease causing crossed sensory or motor paralysis (i.e. cranial nerve signs on one side and contralateral long tract signs); patients with brain stem *gliomas* may have similar signs and may live for many years
5. Arnold-Chiari malformation
6. Trauma
7. Lesion of the base of the skull (e.g. Paget's disease, large *meningioma*, *metastasis*)
8. Rarely, mononeuritis multiplex (e.g. diabetes mellitus)

Higher centres

'Please examine this 78-year-old man's higher centres.'

Method *(see Table 15.50)*

In this assessment especially, you must be guided by your findings. The introduction is important. For example, if you are told the patient also presents with right-sided weakness, you should concentrate on looking for dominant parietal lobe signs.
1. Shake the patient's hand, noting any obvious focal weakness and introduce yourself. Explain that you will be asking him some questions.
2. First, ask whether he is right- or left-handed. Then ask questions about orientation (person, place and time). Ask his name, the present location and the date.

TABLE 15.50 Higher centres' examination

Lying or sitting	Both
1. GENERAL INSPECTION Diagnostic facies (see Table 15.35) Obvious cranial nerve or limb lesions Ask patient about handedness, level of education Shake hands	Sensory inattention Visual inattention Cortical sensory loss (loss of graphaesthesia, two-point discrimination, joint position sense and stereognosis) Constructional apraxia
2. ORIENTATION Time Place Person	**5. MEMORY (temporal lobe)** Short term (e.g. names of flowers) Long term
3. SPEECH Name objects (nominal dysphasia)	**6. FRONTAL LOBE** Reflexes—grasp—pout—palmar mental Proverb interpretation Smell Fundi Gait

4. PARIETAL LOBES
Dominant (AALF or Gerstmann's syndrome)
    Acalculia—(mental arithmetic)
    Agraphia (write)
    Left–right disorientation
    Finger agnosia (name fingers)
Non-dominant
    Dressing apraxia
	7. OTHER
	Visual fields
	Bruits
	Blood pressure etc.

3. This also allows you to test for speech abnormality. Assess any nominal dysphasia by asking the patient to name some objects, such as your watch or a pen (see Table 15.51). Ask the patient to repeat a phrase or sentence, for example: 'The barrister's closing argument convinced him.' This allows you to assess the fluency of speech, as well as comprehension and repetition. Next ask the patient to perform one- and two-step commands, such as 'point to the ceiling, but first take off your spectacles'. This assesses the patient's comprehension.

4. Next, assess the parietal lobes. Begin with the dominant parietal lobe, as Gerstmann's syndrome is common in examinations.

HINT BOX

Dominant parietal lobe evaluation: using the mnemonic AALF, examine for:
  Acalculia (test mental arithmetic)
  Agraphia (test for an inability to write)
  Left–right disorientation (e.g. by asking the patient to put his right palm on his left ear, then vice versa)
  Finger agnosia (inability to name individual fingers), which is caused by a left angular gyrus lesion in right-handed and about half of left-handed patients

---

5. Test general parietal functions (involving either lobe). Examine for sensory and visual inattention. Also test for agraphaesthesia (inability to appreciate numbers drawn on the palm) and astereognosis (inability to name objects placed in the hand). Assess constructional apraxia by asking the patient to draw a clock face and fill in the numbers.

TABLE 15.51 Examination of dysphasia
Fluent speech (usually receptive, conductive or nominal dysphasia)
1. Naming of objects—patients with nominal, conductive or receptive aphasia name objects poorly.
2. Repetition—conductive and receptive aphasics cannot repeat.
3. Comprehension—only receptive aphasic patients cannot follow commands (verbal or written).
4. Reading—conductive and receptive aphasic patients have difficulty reading.
5. Writing—conductive aphasic patients have impaired writing (dysgraphia), whereas receptive aphasic patients have abnormal content. Dysgraphia may also occur with dominant frontal lobe lesions.
Non-fluent speech (usually expressive aphasia)*
1. Naming of objects—poor (but may be better than spontaneous speech).
2. Repetition—may be possible with great effort. Phrase repetition (e.g. 'no ifs ands or buts') is poor.
3. Comprehension—near normal (written and verbal commands are followed).
4. Writing—dysgraphia may be present.
5. Look for hemiparesis—arm more affected than leg.
*As the patient is aware of his deficit, he is often frustrated and depressed.

6. The major specific non-dominant parietal dysfunction is dressing apraxia. This can be tested by turning the patient's pyjama top inside out and asking him to put it on correctly.

7. Assess memory, both short and long term. This is a medial temporal lobe function. Ask the patient to remember the name of three flowers (e.g. **R**ose, **O**rchid and **T**ulip—mnemonic **ROT** for those candidates with a poor memory) and repeat them immediately. Then assess long-term memory, such as by asking when World War II finished. Ask the names of the flowers again at the end of your higher centres' examination.

8. Test frontal lobe problems, first by assessing the primitive reflexes (see Figs 15.49 and 15.50) normally not present in adults. The grasp reflex, pout reflex and palmar–mental reflex are usually all that need be tested. Then ask for interpretation of a common proverb, such as 'A rolling stone gathers no moss'. Test for anosmia (cranial nerve I) and gait apraxia (a frontal gait abnormality is marked by gross unsteadiness in walking—the feet typically behave as if glued to the floor, resulting in a hesitant shuffling gait with freezing).

9. If there is evidence of a frontal lobe lesion, look at the fundi to exclude the rare Foster Kennedy syndrome (optic atrophy on the side of the lesion and papilloedema in the opposite fundus).

10. Any abnormality of the parietal, temporal or occipital lobes may cause a characteristic visual field loss. This should be tested, if appropriate, at the conclusion of your examination. Other important signs to look for are carotid bruits, hypertension and relevant focal neurological signs.

11. MRI and CT scans may show cerebral atrophy consistent with dementia or sometimes a space-occupying lesion.

Figure 15.49 CT of the brain of a patient with early dementia, showing generalised cerebral atrophy. There is obviously more CSF present than normal (arrows).
Figure reproduced courtesy of The Canberra Hospital.

Figure 15.50 A frontal glioma found on MRI scan in a patient with frontal lobe signs (arrow).
Figure reproduced courtesy of The Canberra Hospital.

Speech

'Please assess this man's speech.'

Method

Immediately ask the patient to state his name, age and present location. Then ask him to say 'British Constitution'. By now you should have decided whether the problem is dysphasia, dysarthria or dysphonia.

Dysphasia

1. If the speech is fluent but conveys information imperfectly, often with paraphasic errors (e.g. 'treen' for train—substitution of a word of similar sound), the main possibilities are nominal and receptive aphasia. Test for these by asking the patient to name objects, to repeat a statement after you and then follow commands. Then ask him to read and write if the above are abnormal (see Table 15.51).
2. If the speech is slow and non-fluent (hesitant), exactly the same procedure is followed, but an expressive aphasia is likely. At the end ask to assess for a hemiparesis (see Table 15.51).
3. Remember, large lesions may cause global aphasia, with inability to comprehend or speak, plus hemiparesis (see Table 15.52).

Dysarthria

1. This is a disorder of articulation with no disorder of the content of speech. Consider cerebellar disease and lower cranial nerve lesions particularly. Cerebellar speech is slurred or 'scanning' (i.e. irregular and staccato). Pseudobulbar palsy causes slow, hesitant, hollow-sounding speech with a harsh, strained voice, while bulbar palsy causes nasal speech with imprecise articulation.
2. Ask the patient to say 'British Constitution', 'West Register Street', 'Me Me Me' and 'Lah Lah Lah'.
3. If the speech is cerebellar, go on to this system (p 388).
4. If palsy of a lower cranial nerve is likely, examine the lower cranial nerves carefully.
5. Do not forget to elicit the jaw jerk. Look in the mouth too for ulceration or other local lesions.
6. Less common causes of dysarthria include extrapyramidal disease and myopathies (p 385).

TABLE 15.52 The sites of lesions in aphasia
Receptive aphasia
Wernicke's area—posterior part of first temporal gyrus in the dominant lobe
Expressive aphasia
Broca's area—posterior part of the third frontal gyrus
Conductive aphasia
Arcuate fasciculus (temporal lobe)
Nominal aphasia
Angular gyrus (temporal lobe)—small localised lesion
Other causes: encephalopathies (metabolic, toxic), pressure effects from a distant space-occupying lesion
Recovery phase from any dysphasia

Dysphonia
This is huskiness of the voice from a laryngeal disorder, recurrent laryngeal nerve palsy or focal dystonia. Assess the quality of the cough too.

Upper limbs
'This man has noticed weakness in his arms. Please examine him.'

Method (see Table 15.53)

TABLE 15.53 Upper limb neurological examination	

1. GENERAL INSPECTION
Diagnostic facies (see Table 15.35)
Scars
Skin (e.g. neurofibromata, café-au-lait)
Abnormal movements
 	
2. SHAKE HANDS
 	
3. MOTOR SYSTEM
Inspect arms, shoulder girdle—extend
   both arms
   Wasting
   Fasciculation
   Tremor
   Drift
Palpate
   Muscle bulk
   Muscle tenderness
Tone
   Wrist
   Elbow
Power
   Shoulder
   Elbow
   Wrist
   Fingers
   Ulnar, median nerve function
	Reflexes
	   Biceps
	   Triceps
	   Supinator
	   Finger
	Coordination
	   Finger–nose test—intention tremor,
	   past pointing
	   Dysdiadochokinesis
	   Rebound
	
	4. SENSORY SYSTEM
	Pain (pinprick)
	Vibration (128-Hz tuning fork)
	Proprioception—DIP joint (each hand)
	Light touch (cotton wool)
	
	5. OTHER
	Thickened nerves (wrist, elbow)
	Axillae
	Neck
	Lower limbs
	Cranial nerves
	Urine analysis etc.

1. Look at the whole patient briefly. Note particularly evidence of a myopathic face, Parkinsonian features or stroke.
2. Shake the patient's hand firmly and introduce yourself. If he cannot let go, you have made the diagnosis: myotonia (usually caused by dystrophia myotonica). Ask him to sit over the side of the bed facing you.

Motor system
Examine the motor system systematically every time.
1. Inspect first for wasting (both proximally and distally) and fasciculations. Do not forget to include the shoulder girdle in your inspection (p 373).
2. Ask the patient to hold both his hands out with the arms extended and close his eyes. Look for drifting of one or both arms. There are only three causes for this drift:
   (a) upper motor neurone weakness (usually downwards owing to muscle weakness)
   (b) cerebellar lesion (usually upwards owing to hypotonia)

(c) posterior column loss (any direction owing to joint position sense loss).
3. Also note any tremor and pseudoathetosis as a result of proprioceptive loss.
4. Feel the muscle bulk next, both proximally and distally, and note any muscle tenderness. In the presence of wasting and weakness, fasciculation indicates lower motor neurone degeneration.
5. Test tone at the wrists and elbows by moving the joints at varying velocities.
6. Assess power next.
   (a) Shoulder:
   - abduction (C5, C6): tell the patient to abduct his arms with the elbows flexed and not to let you push them down
   - adduction (C6–C8): tell him to adduct his arms with the elbows flexed and not to let you separate them.
   (b) Elbow:
   - flexion (C5, C6): tell him to bend his elbow and pull so as not to let you straighten it
   - extension (C7, C8): tell him to bend his elbow and push so as not to let you bend it.
   (c) Wrist:
   - flexion (C6, C7): tell him to bend his wrist and not to let you straighten it
   - extension (C7, C8): tell him to straighten his wrist and not to let you bend it.
   (d) Fingers:
   - extension (C7, C8): tell him to straighten his fingers and not to let you push them down
   - flexion (C7, C8): tell him to squeeze two of your fingers
   - abduction (C8, T1): tell him to spread out his fingers and not to let you push them together.
   Grade the power (p 376).
7. Test for an ulnar lesion (loss of finger abduction and adduction) and a median nerve lesion (loss of thumb abduction) (p 380).
8. Examine the reflexes:
   (a) biceps (C5, C6)—biceps muscle
   (b) triceps (C7, C8)—triceps muscle
   (c) supinator (C5, C6)—brachioradialis muscle (elbow flexion)
   (d) inverted supinator jerk—when tapping the lower end of the radius, elbow extension and finger flexion are the only response; associated with an absent biceps and exaggerated triceps jerk, this indicates an intraspinal lesion compressing the spinal cord and nerve roots at C5, C6
   (e) finger (C8)—normally, slight flexion of all fingers occurs.
9. Assess coordination with finger–nose testing and look for dysdiadochokinesis and rebound (p 388).
   Motor weakness can be caused by an upper motor neurone lesion, lower motor neurone lesion, neuromuscular junction disorder or myopathy. If there is evidence of a lower motor neurone lesion, consider anterior horn cell, nerve root and brachial plexus lesions, peripheral nerve lesions or a motor peripheral neuropathy.

Sensory system
Examine the sensory system after motor testing because this can be time-consuming.
1. First test the spinothalamic pathway (pain and temperature). Use a new blunt neurology pin. One candidate accidentally pricked his own finger during the examination with a sharp pin. By the time he stopped bleeding his short case time was up. (In case you believe this might be a good ploy, the candidate failed.)

2. Demonstrate to the patient the sharpness of the pin on the anterior chest wall or forehead. Then ask him to close his eyes and tell you if the sensation is sharp or dull. Start proximally and test each dermatome. As you are assessing, try to fit any sensory loss into dermatomal (cord or nerve root lesion) (see Fig 15.51), peripheral nerve, peripheral neuropathy (glove) or hemisensory (cortical or cord) distribution. Also remember that 'cape' sensory loss (neck, shoulders and arms) suggests syringomyelia, whereas 'shield' sensory loss (front of the chest) may occur with syphilis. It is not usually necessary to test temperature perception in the examination.

3. Next test the posterior column pathway (vibration and proprioception). Use a 128-hertz tuning fork to assess vibration sense. Place this when vibrating on the ulnar head at the wrist when the patient has his eyes closed and ask whether he can feel it. If so, ask him to tell you when the vibration ceases and then stop the vibration. If the patient has deficient sensation, test at the elbow, then the shoulder. Test both arms.

4. Examine proprioception first with the DIP joint of the index finger. When the patient has his eyes open, grasp his distal phalanx from the sides and move it up and down to demonstrate, then ask him to close his eyes and repeat the manoeuvres. Normally, movement through even a few degrees is detectable and he can tell whether it is up or down. If there is an abnormality, proceed to test the wrist and elbows similarly.

> **HINT BOX**
> Proprioceptive loss may be subtle. A normal person can detect movement and usually direction changes of 1 or 2°. Begin with small joint movements.

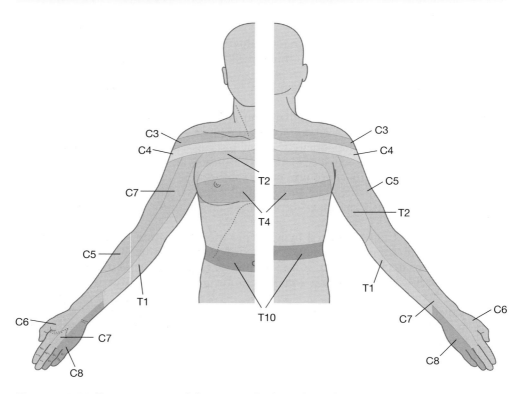

Figure 15.51 **Dermatomes of the upper limb and trunk.**

5. Test light touch with cotton wool. Touch the skin lightly in each dermatome.
6. Feel for thickened nerves—ulnar at the elbow, median at the wrist and radial at the wrist—and feel the axillae if there is evidence of a plexus lesion. Do not forget to mention any scars that may be present. Finally, examine the neck movements, if relevant, and look for surgical scars in the front and back of the neck and in the axillae.
7. To confirm a diagnosis, it may be necessary to examine further afield. Ask the examiners whether you can do this. For example, if there is evidence of motor neurone disease, assess the lower limbs, as well as the tongue. If there is evidence of a C5, C6 root lesion, assess the lower limbs for an upper motor neurone lesion and the neck for cervical spondylosis.

Shoulder girdle examination

'This 48-year-old woman has had difficulty lifting objects above her head. Please examine her shoulder girdle.'

HINT BOX

This introduction is often used for facio-scapulo-humeral (FSH) muscular dystrophy. A careful inspection of the face will reveal wasting of the masseter and temporalis muscles, among others.

Method

This is likely to be a muscular dystrophy or a root lesion. Proceed by inspecting each muscle, palpating its bulk and testing function as follows.
1. From the back:
   (a) trapezius (XI, C3, C4)—ask the patient to elevate her shoulders against resistance and look for winging of the upper scapula
   (b) serratus anterior (C5–C7)—ask her to push her hands against the wall and look for winging of the lower scapula
   (c) rhomboids (C4, C5)—ask her to pull both shoulder blades together with her hands on her hips
   (d) supraspinatus (C5, C6)—ask her to abduct her arms against resistance and begin with her arms less than 15° from her sides
   (e) infraspinatus (C5, C6)—ask her to rotate her upper arms externally against resistance with her arms at her side
   (f) teres major (C5–C7)—ask her to rotate her upper arms internally against resistance
   (g) latissimus dorsi (C7, C8)—ask her to cough and palpate on both sides.
2. From the front:
   (a) pectoralis major, clavicular head (C5–C8)—ask the patient to lift her upper arms above the horizontal and push them forward
   (b) pectoralis major, sternocostal part (C6–T1) and pectoralis minor (C7)—ask her to adduct her upper arms against resistance
   (c) deltoid (C5, C6) (and circumflex nerve)—ask her to abduct her arms against resistance, but begin with her arms more than 15° from her sides.
3. Go on to look for sensory changes, which will be absent if this is a muscular dystrophy.

HINT BOX

If FSH is suspected (facial muscle wasting and winging of the scapulae), look for foot drop and then test for facial weakness (inability to close the eyes tightly, whistle or puff out the cheeks).

Lower limbs

'This 60-year-old man has had difficulty walking. Please examine his lower limbs.'

Method (see Table 15.54)

TABLE 15.54 Lower limb neurological examination

Lying	Knee
	Ankle
1. GENERAL INSPECTION	Plantar
Diagnostic facies (see Table 15.35)	Coordination
Scars, skin	Heel–shin test
Urinary catheter	Toe–finger test
	Foot tapping test
2. GAIT	
	4. SENSORY SYSTEM
3. MOTOR SYSTEM	Pain
Inspect	Vibration
Wasting	Proprioception
Fasciculation	Light touch
Tremor	
Palpate	**5. SADDLE REGION SENSATION**
Muscle bulk	**6. ANAL REFLEX**
Muscle tenderness	
Tone	**7. BACK**
Knee—and test for clonus	Deformity
Ankle—and test for clonus	Scars
Power	Tenderness
Hip	Bruits
Knee	**8. OTHER**
Ankle	Upper limbs
Foot	Cranial nerve
Reflexes	Urine analysis etc.

---

1. Test the gait first. Ask the examiners whether this is possible—sometimes the patient may be unable to walk. If the patient can walk, ask him to walk across the room, turn around and walk back. If he looks to be in difficulty, ask the bulldog to help. Ask the patient to try heel-to-toe walking (for cerebellar disease) and then try standing and then walking on toes and heels (for an S1 or L4/L5 lesion, respectively). Ask him to squat and stand (for proximal myopathy).

HINT BOX

Specific testing of gait should help you decide whether there is an ataxic or high stepping gait (cerebellar or proprioceptive problems) or muscle weakness (proximal or distal, or both).

2. Note the patient's general appearance. Especially look for upper limb girdle wasting and the presence of a urinary catheter. Look for pes cavus. Look around the room for a walking stick or frame and special shoes.

3. Have the patient lie in bed with the legs entirely exposed. Place a towel over the groin. As the patient gets back into bed look at the back for scars.

4. Look for muscle wasting and fasciculation. Note any tremor. Feel the muscle bulk of the quadriceps and run your hand up each shin, feeling for wasting of the anterior tibial muscles.

5. Test tone at the knees and ankles.

6. Test clonus at this time. Warn the patient first. Push the patella sharply downwards. Sustained rhythmical contractions indicate an upper motor neurone lesion. Also test the ankle by sharply dorsiflexing the foot with the knee bent and the thigh externally rotated. Always test both sides!

7. Assess power next.
   (a) Hip:
   - flexion (L2, L3): ask the patient to lift up his straight leg and not let you push it down (having placed your hand above his knee)
   - extension (L5, S1, S2): ask him to keep his leg down and not let you pull it up
   - abduction (L4, L5, S1): ask him to abduct his legs and not let you push them together
   - adduction (L2, L3, L4): ask him to keep his legs adducted and not let you pull them apart.
   (b) Knee:
   - flexion (L5, S1): ask him to bend his knee and not let you straighten it
   - extension (L3, L4): with the knee slightly bent, ask him to straighten the knee and not let you bend it.
   (c) Ankle:
   - plantar flexion (S1): ask him to push his foot down and not let you pull it up
   - dorsiflexion (L4, L5): ask him to bring his foot up and not let you push it down
   - eversion (L5, S1): ask him to evert his foot against resistance; loss of this may also indicate a common peroneal (lateral popliteal) nerve palsy
   - inversion (L5): ask him to invert his plantar flexed foot against resistance.

8. Elicit the reflexes:
   (a) knee (L3, L4)—quadriceps muscle
   (b) ankle (S1, S2)—calf muscle
   (c) plantar response (S1).

9. Test coordination with the heel–shin test, toe–finger test and tapping of the feet (p 388).

10. Examine the sensory system as for the upper limbs: pin prick, then vibration and proprioception, and then light touch (see Fig 15.52).

HINT BOX

Sensory changes can be variable. If sensory loss is not quite consistent but seems generally to fit a pattern, it may be a good idea to describe it confidently as 'patchy'.

Figure 15.52 **Dermatomes of the lower limb.**

11. If there is a peripheral sensory loss, attempt to establish a sensory level on the abdomen.
12. Examine the saddle region sensation (S3–5).
13. Ask to test the anal reflex (S2–4); if intact, there is brief contraction of the external sphincter of the anus to scratching of the perianal skin.
14. If you have not done this already go to the back. Look for deformity, scars and neurofibromata. Palpate for tenderness over the vertebral bodies and auscultate for bruits. Test straight leg raising.
15. It may be relevant to ask whether you can proceed to the upper limbs and cranial nerves.

Notes on the neurological examination of the limbs

Grading muscle power (Medical Research Council)

0. Complete paralysis
1. Flicker of contraction
2. Movement with *no* gravity
3. Movement with gravity only (any resistance stops movement)
4. Movement with gravity plus some resistance
5. Normal power

This grading is weighted towards severe weakness (grades 0–3 are all severe). A more sensible scale would be the following:

1. Complete paralysis
2. Severe weakness
3. Moderate weakness
4. Mild weakness
5. Normal

Signs of a lower motor neurone lesion

1. Weakness
2. Wasting
3. Hypotonicity
4. Decreased or absent reflexes
5. Fasciculation (prominent in anterior horn cell diseases unless far advanced)

Signs of an upper motor neurone lesion

1. Weakness in an 'upper motor neurone pattern'; all muscle groups are weak, but may be more marked in upper limb abductor and extensor muscles—shoulder abduction, elbow and wrist extensors—and lower limb flexor muscles—hip flexion, knee flexion, ankle dorsiflexion
2. Spasticity
3. Clonus
4. Increased reflexes and extensor plantar response

An approach to peripheral neuropathy

This may be sensory (glove and stocking) or motor, or both.

Causes of peripheral neuropathy

But remember: diabetes 30%, hereditary 30%, idiopathic 30%, all others 10%.

1. Drugs and toxins—isoniazid, vincristine, phenytoin, nitrofurantoin, cisplatinum, amiodarone, large doses of vitamin B_6, heavy metals
2. Alcohol (with or without vitamin B_1 deficiency); amyloidosis
3. Metabolic—diabetes mellitus, uraemia, hypothyroidism, porphyria
4. Immune-mediated—Guillain-Barré syndrome
5. Tumour—lung carcinoma
6. Vitamin B_{12} or B_1 deficiency or B_6 excess
7. Idiopathic
8. Connective tissue diseases or vasculitis—SLE, polyarteritis nodosa
9. Hereditary

Causes of a predominantly motor neuropathy

1. Guillain-Barré syndrome and chronic inflammatory demyelinating polyradiculoneuropathy (CIDP)
2. Hereditary motor and sensory neuropathy (Charcot-Marie-Tooth disease)
3. Acute intermittent porphyria

4. Diabetes mellitus
5. Lead poisoning
6. Multifocal motor neuropathy

> **HINT BOX**
> Motor neurone disease and neuromuscular junction disorders must always be considered in the differential diagnosis of distal motor weakness.

Causes of a predominantly sensory neuropathy (sensory neuronopathy)
This is unusual and results in sensory ataxia and pseudoathetosis. Causes include the following:
1. carcinoma (e.g. lung, ovary, breast)
2. paraproteinaemia
3. vitamin B_6 intoxication
4. Sjögren's syndrome
5. diabetes mellitus
6. syphilis
7. vitamin B_{12} deficiency (occasionally)
8. idiopathic.

Causes of a painful peripheral neuropathy
1. Diabetes mellitus
2. Alcohol
3. Vitamin B_{12} or B_1 deficiency
4. Carcinoma
5. Porphyria
6. Arsenic or thallium poisoning
7. Heredity (most are not painful)

> **HINT BOX**
> Burning soles of the feet can be caused by a painful peripheral neuropathy, tarsal tunnel syndrome or an S1 lesion. An S1 lesion will cause a decreased or absent ankle jerk.

Causes of mononeuritis multiplex
Mononeuritis multiplex refers to separate involvement of more than one peripheral or rarely cranial nerve (e.g. a common peroneal nerve palsy plus an axillary nerve palsy). Common causes include:
1. acute (usually vascular):
   (a) diabetes mellitus
   (b) polyarteritis nodosa or connective tissue diseases—SLE, rheumatoid arthritis
2. chronic:
   (a) multiple compressive neuropathies, especially with joint-deforming arthritis
   (b) sarcoidosis
   (c) acromegaly
   (d) leprosy
   (e) Lyme disease
   (f) carcinoma (rare)
   (g) idiopathic.

Causes of thickened nerves
1. Hereditary motor and sensory neuropathy
2. Acromegaly
3. Chronic inflammatory demyelinating polyradiculoneuropathy
4. Amyloidosis
5. Leprosy
6. Others—sarcoidosis, neurofibromatosis

Causes of fasciculation
Fasciculation is *not* always motor neurone disease. Causes include:
1. benign idiopathic fasciculation (by far the most common)
2. motor neurone disease
3. motor root compression
4. malignant neuropathy
5. any motor neuropathy (less commonly).

HINT BOX
Myokymia resembles benign coarse fasciculation of the same muscle group (e.g. eyelids). Electromyographic myokymia can occur in multiple sclerosis, brain stem neoplasm, Bell's palsy, radiculopathy or radiation plexopathy or chronic nerve compression.

Hereditary motor and sensory neuropathy (HMSN)
Charcot-Marie-Tooth disease: usually autosomal dominant

Clinical features
1. Pes cavus (short, high-arched feet with hammer toes)
2. Distal muscle atrophy owing to peripheral nerve degeneration, not usually extending above the elbows or above the middle one-third of the thighs
3. Absent reflexes
4. Slight to no sensory loss in the limbs
5. Thickened nerves
6. Optic atrophy; Argyll Robertson pupils (rare)

An approach to brachial plexus lesions
Complete lesion
1. Lower motor neurone signs affect the whole arm
2. Sensory loss (whole limb)
3. Horner's syndrome (an important clue, but only if the lesion is proximal in the lower plexus)

HINT BOX
Remember always to feel for axillary lymphadenopathy at the end of your examination for a brachial plexus lesion.

Upper trunk (Erb-Duchenne) (C5, C6) lesion
1. Loss of shoulder movement and elbow flexion—hand is held in the 'waiter's tip' position
2. Sensory loss is present over the lateral aspect of the arm and forearm, and over the thumb

Lower trunk (Klumpke) (C8, T1) lesion
1. True claw hand with paralysis of all the intrinsic muscles
2. Sensory loss along the ulnar side of the hand and forearm
3. Horner's syndrome

Cervical rib syndrome
1. Weakness and wasting of the small muscles of the hand (true claw hand)
2. Sensory loss over the medial aspect of the hand and forearm
3. Unequal radial pulses and blood pressures
4. Subclavian bruit and loss of the pulse on arm manoeuvring (this sign is often also present in normal persons)
5. Palpable cervical rib in the neck (uncommon)

Important peripheral nerves
Radial nerve (C5–C8) lesion
Clinical features
1. Wrist and finger drop (wrist flexion normal)
2. Triceps loss (elbow extension loss) if lesion is above the spiral groove
3. Sensory loss over the anatomical snuff box
4. Finger abduction *appears* to be weak because of the difficulty of spreading the fingers when they cannot be straightened

Median nerve (C6–T1) lesion
This nerve supplies all muscles on the front of the forearm except flexor carpi ulnaris and half of flexor digitorum profundus. It also supplies the following short muscles of the hand (LOAF):

Lateral two lumbricals
Opponens pollicis
Abductor pollicis brevis
Flexor pollicis brevis (this sometimes has ulnar innervation)

Clinical features
1. Loss of abductor pollicis brevis with a lesion at or above the wrist—pen touching test: with the hand flat, ask the patient to abduct the thumb vertically to touch your pen
2. Loss of flexor digitorum sublimis with a lesion in or above the cubital fossa— Ochsner's clasping test: ask the patient to clasp the hands firmly together—the index finger on the affected side fails to flex
3. Sensory loss over the thumb, index, middle and lateral half of the ring finger (palmar aspect only)

HINT BOX
Causes of carpal tunnel syndrome:
1. idiopathic
2. arthropathy—rheumatoid arthritis
3. endocrine disease—hypothyroidism, acromegaly
4. pregnancy
5. trauma and overuse.

Ulnar nerve (C8–T1) lesion
Clinical features
1. Wasting of the intrinsic muscles of the hand (except LOAF muscles)

2. Weak finger abduction and adduction (loss of interosseous muscles)
3. Ulnar claw-like hand (*Note:* A higher lesion causes less deformity, as an above-the-elbow lesion also causes loss of flexor digitorum profundus.)
4. Froment's sign: ask the patient to grasp a piece of paper between the thumb and lateral aspect of the forefinger with each hand—the affected thumb will flex (loss of thumb adductor)
5. Sensory loss over the little and medial half of ring finger (both palmar and dorsal aspects)

Wasting of the small muscles of the hand
Examine as for the upper limbs and make sure you feel the pulses and examine the neck, unless the cause is very obvious (e.g. rheumatoid arthritis).

Causes
1. Nerve lesions:
   (a) median and ulnar nerve lesions
   (b) brachial plexus lesions
   (c) peripheral motor neuropathy (in the examination, don't forget hereditary motor and sensory neuropathy)
2. Anterior horn cell disease:
   (a) motor neurone disease
   (b) polio
   (c) spinal muscular atrophies (e.g. Kugelberg–Welander disease)
3. Myopathy:
   (a) dystrophia myotonica—forearms more affected than the hands
   (b) distal myopathy
4. Spinal cord lesions:
   (a) syringomyelia
   (b) cervical spondylosis with compression of C8 segment
   (c) other (e.g. tumour)
5. Trophic disorders:
   (a) arthropathies (disuse)
   (b) ischaemia, including vasculitis
   (c) shoulder–hand syndrome

Femoral nerve (L2, L3, L4) lesion
Clinical features
1. Weakness of knee extension (quadriceps paralysis)
2. Slight hip flexion weakness
3. Preserved adductor strength
4. Loss of knee jerk
5. Sensory loss involving the inner aspect of the thigh and leg

---

HINT BOX

When distinguishing an ulnar nerve lesion from a C8 root/lower trunk brachial plexus lesion, remember that the sensory loss of a C8 lesion extends proximal to the wrist and the thenar muscles are involved with a C8 root or lower trunk brachial plexus lesion. Distinguishing a C8 root from a lower trunk brachial plexus lesion is difficult clinically, but the presence of Horner's syndrome or an axillary mass suggests that the brachial plexus is affected.

Sciatic nerve (L4, L5, S1, S2) lesion
Clinical features
1. Weakness of knee flexion (hamstrings involved)
2. Loss of power of all muscles below the knee causing a foot drop, so the patient may be able to walk, but cannot stand on the toes or heels
3. Knee jerk intact
4. Loss of ankle jerk and plantar response
5. Sensory loss along the posterior thigh and total loss below the knee

Common peroneal (lateral popliteal) nerve (L4, L5, S1) lesion
Clinical features
1. Foot drop and *loss of foot eversion only*
2. Sensory loss (minimal) over the dorsum of the foot
   Note: The reflexes are normal.

> **HINT BOX**
> If there is a foot drop, test foot inversion and eversion. *Inversion* of the foot will be normal with a peroneal nerve compression but *absent* with a L5 radiculopathy. (Eversion is absent with both lesions.)

Lateral cutaneous nerve of the thigh lesion
Meralgia paraesthetica is caused by compression of this nerve, which may result in sensory loss and/or hyperaesthesia over the lateral aspect of the thigh, but no motor loss.

Causes of foot drop
1. Common peroneal nerve palsy
2. Sciatic nerve palsy
3. Lumbosacral plexus lesion
4. L4, L5 root lesion
5. Peripheral motor neuropathy
6. Distal myopathy
7. Motor neurone disease
8. Precentral gyrus lesion

> **HINT BOX**
> Remember, if there is a foot drop, test the ankle jerk carefully. As a very rough rule of thumb, if it is absent, an S1 lesion should be suspected; if it is normal, a common peroneal palsy should be considered; if it is increased, an upper motor neurone lesion is likely.

Notes on spinal cord lesions
Assessment of the paraplegic patient
1. Is there also a sensory level? Patterns of sensory loss depend on the level and type of lesion. Consider:
   (a) cord compression, which causes a loss of all modalities bilaterally below the level involved (*note:* extrinsic compression may spare the perineum), and radicular pain and lower motor neurone weakness are present at the level of spinal compression

(b) transverse myelitis
(c) anterior spinal artery occlusion (posterior column function is spared)
(d) intrinsic cord lesion
(e) multiple sclerosis.
2. Back examination: for example, deformity, tenderness or bruits may provide clues about the underlying disease process.
3. Arm involvement? Consider:
(a) cervical spondylosis
(b) syringomyelia
(c) motor neurone disease
(d) multiple sclerosis.
4. Cranial nerve lesions? Consider:
(a) motor neurone disease
(b) multiple sclerosis.
5. Peripheral neuropathy? Consider:
(a) vitamin B_{12} deficiency
(b) Friedreich's ataxia
(c) carcinoma
(d) hereditary spastic paraplegia
(e) syphilis.
6. Cerebral lesions?

HINT BOX

Intracranial lesions (e.g. parasagittal meningioma) cause paraplegia in extension only, whereas spinal cord lesions cause paraplegia in flexion or extension (i.e. flexor reflexes are released with spinal lesions).

Important motor and reflex changes of spinal cord and conus compression

Lower motor neurone signs occur at the level of the root lesion and upper motor neurone signs occur below the lesion.

Upper cervical
1. Upper motor neurone signs in the upper and lower limbs
2. Paralysis of the diaphragm occurs with a lesion above C4

C5
1. Lower motor neurone weakness and wasting of the rhomboids, deltoids, biceps and brachioradialis
2. Upper motor neurone signs affect the rest of the upper and all the lower limbs
3. The biceps jerk is lost
4. The supinator jerk is 'inverted'

C8
1. Lower motor neurone weakness and wasting of the intrinsic muscles of the hand
2. Upper motor neurone signs in the lower limbs

Midthoracic
1. Intercostal paralysis (cannot be detected clinically)
2. Loss of upper abdominal reflexes at T7 and T8
3. Upper motor neurone signs in the lower limbs

T10–T11
1. Loss of the lower abdominal reflexes and upward displacement of the umbilicus on contraction (Beevor's sign)
2. Upper motor neurone signs in the lower limbs

L1
1. Cremasteric reflexes lost (normal abdominal reflexes)
2. Upper motor neurone signs in the lower limbs

L4
1. Lower motor neurone weakness and wasting of the quadriceps
2. Knee jerk lost

L5 and S1
1. Lower motor neurone weakness of knee flexion and hip extension (S1) and abduction (L5), plus calf and foot muscles
2. Knee jerk present
3. No ankle jerk or plantar response
4. Anal reflex present

S3–S4
1. No anal reflex
2. Saddle sensory loss
3. Normal lower limbs

HINT BOX
Look for a urinary catheter if suspicious of a spinal cord lesion.

Important syndromes
Subacute combined degeneration of the cord (vitamin B$_{12}$ deficiency)
Clinical features
1. Symmetrical posterior column loss (vibration and position sense), causing an ataxic gait
2. Symmetrical upper motor neurone signs in the lower limbs with absent ankle reflexes; knee reflexes may be absent or, more often, exaggerated
3. Peripheral sensory neuropathy (less common and mild)
4. Optic atrophy (occasionally)
5. Dementia (occasionally)

The combination of upper motor neurone signs causing an extensor plantar response plus peripheral neuropathy causing loss of knee and ankle jerks is a distinctive pattern.

Causes of an extensor plantar response plus absent ankle jerk include:
1. subacute combined degeneration of the cord (vitamin B$_{12}$ deficiency)
2. conus medullaris lesion
3. combination of an upper motor neurone lesion with cauda equina compression or peripheral neuropathy
4. syphilis (tabo-paresis)
5. Friedreich's ataxia
6. diabetes mellitus (uncommon)
7. adrenoleucodystrophy or metachromatic leucodystrophy.

Brown-Séquard syndrome (hemisection of the spinal cord)
Clinical features
1. Motor changes:
   (a) upper motor neurone signs below the hemisection on the *same* side as the lesion
   (b) lower motor neurone signs at the level of the hemisection on the *same* side
2. Sensory changes:
   (a) pain and temperature loss on the *opposite* side of the lesion (*note:* the upper level of sensory loss is usually a few segments below the level of the lesion)
   (b) vibration and proprioception loss on the *same* side
   (c) light touch is often normal
   (d) there may be a band of sensory loss on the same side at the level of the lesion (afferent nerve fibres)

Common causes
1. Multiple sclerosis
2. Angioma
3. Glioma
4. Trauma
5. Myelitis
6. Postradiation myelopathy

Causes of dissociated sensory loss (usually indicates spinal cord disease, but may occur with peripheral neuropathy)
Spinothalamic (pain and temperature) loss only
1. Syringomyelia ('cape' distribution)
2. Brown-Séquard syndrome (contralateral leg)
3. Anterior spinal artery thrombosis
4. Lateral medullary syndrome (contralateral to the other signs)
5. Peripheral neuropathy (e.g. diabetes mellitus, amyloid, Fabry's disease)

Dorsal column (vibration and proprioception) loss only
1. Subacute combined degeneration
2. Brown-Séquard syndrome (ipsilateral leg)
3. Spinocerebellar degeneration (e.g. Friedreich's ataxia)
4. Multiple sclerosis
5. Tabes dorsalis
6. Sensory neuropathy or ganglionopathy (e.g. carcinoma)
7. Peripheral neuropathy from diabetes mellitus or hypothyroidism

Syringomyelia (a central cavity in the spinal cord)
Clinical triad
1. Loss of pain and temperature over the neck, shoulders and arms ('cape' distribution)
2. Amyotrophy (weakness, atrophy and areflexia) of the arms
3. Upper motor neurone signs in the lower limbs
Note: There may also be thoracic scoliosis owing to asymmetrical weakness of the paravertebral muscles.

An approach to myopathy
Causes of proximal muscle weakness
1. Myopathic (see below)
2. Neuromuscular junction disorder—myasthenia gravis

3. Neurogenic—Kugelberg-Welander disease (proximal muscle wasting and fasciculation as a result of anterior horn cell damage—autosomal recessive), motor neurone disease, polyradiculopathy

Causes of myopathy
1. Hereditary muscular dystrophy (qv)
2. Congenital myopathies (rare)
3. Acquired (mnemonic PACE PODS):
   Polymyositis or dermatomyositis
   Alcohol
   Carcinoma
   Endocrine (e.g. hypothyroidism, hyperthyroidism, Cushing's syndrome, acromegaly, hypopituitarism)
   Periodic paralysis (hyperkalaemic or hypokalaemic or normokalaemic)
   Osteomalacia
   Drugs (e.g. clofibrate, chloroquine, steroids)
   Sarcoidosis
   Note: Causes of proximal myopathy and a peripheral neuropathy include:
1. paraneoplastic syndrome
2. alcohol
3. connective tissue disease.

Muscular dystrophies
1. Duchenne's (pseudohypertrophic) (sex-linked recessive disorder):
   (a) affects only males (or females with Turner's syndrome)
   (b) the calves and deltoids are hypertrophied early and weak later
   (c) early proximal weakness
   (d) tendon reflexes are preserved in proportion to muscle strength
   (e) severe progressive kyphoscoliosis
   (f) heart disease (dilated cardiomyopathy)
   (g) creatine kinase level markedly elevated
   (h) patients die in the second decade, usually from heart disease
2. Becker (sex-linked recessive disorder): same features as Duchenne's, but less severe, has a later onset and is less rapidly progressive
3. Limb girdle (autosomal recessive):
   (a) shoulder or pelvic girdle affected (onset third decade)
   (b) face and heart usually spared
4. Facioscapulohumeral (autosomal dominant): facial and pectoral girdle weakness with hypertrophy of the deltoids (normal pelvic muscles early)
5. Distal dystrophies:
   (a) autosomal dominant disease, which is rare and causes distal muscle atrophy and weakness
   (b) dystrophia myotonica (autosomal dominant)

Tests for myopathy
1. Creatine kinase (highest in Duchenne's)
2. EMG
3. ECG (particularly Duchenne's and dystrophia myotonica)
4. Muscle biopsy

Dystrophia myotonica

'This 67-year-old man has noticed some arm weakness. Please examine him.'

Method

Standing back to observe the patient, you fortunately notice the features of myotonic dystrophy. Proceed as follows.

1. Observe the face for frontal baldness (the patient may be wearing a wig), dull triangular facies ('hatchet' face), temporalis, masseter and sternomastoid atrophy, and partial ptosis. Note thick spectacles, as these patients develop cataracts and fine subcapsular deposits, which are virtually diagnostic.
2. Look at the neck for sternomastoid atrophy, then test neck flexion (neck flexion is weak, while extension is normal).
3. Go to the upper limbs. Shake hands (for grip myotonia) and test percussion myotonia. Tapping over the thenar eminence causes contraction then slow relaxation of the abductor pollicis brevis (see Table 15.55).

TABLE 15.55 Causes of myotonia

1. Dystrophia myotonica
2. Myotonia congenita (myotonia of the tongue and thenar eminence, the recessive form being more severe)
3. Paramyotonia congenita (episodic myotonia after cold exposure)

Note: Drugs (e.g. clofibrate) can also cause myotonic discharges on EMG, but do not cause clinical myotonia.

4. Examine the arm now for signs of wasting and weakness, especially of the forearm muscles. Sensory changes from the associated peripheral neuropathy are usually very mild.
5. Go to the chest and inspect for gynaecomastia.
6. Ask to palpate the testes for atrophy.
7. Examine the lower limbs if there is time.
8. Always ask to test the urine for sugar (diabetes mellitus is more common in this disease) and to examine the cardiovascular system for cardiomyopathy. Finally test mental status (mild mental retardation is usual).

HINT BOX

Remember the classic EMG finding in dystrophia myotonica of a 'dive bomber' effect with needle movement in the muscle at rest.

Gait

'Please examine this man's gait.'

Method *(see Table 15.56)*

1. Scan the room for a walking stick or frame or special shoes.
2. Make sure the patient's legs are clearly visible. Ask him to 'hop out' of his bed or chair (look carefully while he is doing so for focal disease), watch him walk normally for a few metres and then ask him to turn around quickly and walk back towards you.
3. Next ask him to walk heel-to-toe to exclude a midline cerebellar lesion.
4. Ask him to walk on his toes (an S1 lesion will make this difficult) and then on his heels (a lesion causing foot drop will make this difficult).

TABLE 15.56 Gait examination

Standing (legs fully exposed)

1. GENERAL INSPECTION

Deformity

Diagnostic facies (see Table 15.35)

Upper limb lesions

Focal neurological disease (e.g. wasting)

Fasciculation

Abnormal movements

2. ASK THE PATIENT TO:

Walk normally and turn around quickly (abnormal gait)

Walk heel-to-toe (cerebellar disease)

Walk on toes (S1)

Walk on heels (L4 or L5)

Squat (proximal myopathy)

Romberg's sign—feet together with:

  Eyes closed (posterior columns)

  Eyes open (cerebellar disease)

3. EXAMINE LOWER LIMBS

TABLE 15.57 Typical gaits

1. Hemiparetic—the foot is plantarflexed and the leg swung in a lateral arc

2. Paraparetic (scissor gait)

3. Extrapyramidal (e.g. Parkinson's disease)

    (a) hesitation in starting

    (b) shuffling

    (c) freezing

    (d) festination (the patient hurries forward, trying to catch up with the centre of gravity)

    (e) propulsion (pull the patient towards you gently—he or she will be unable to stop), retropulsion

4. Cerebellar (a drunken gait that is wide-based or reeling on a narrow base; the patient staggers towards the affected side)

5. Apraxic (prefrontal lobe) (feet appear glued to the floor when erect, but move more easily when the patient is supine)

6. Posterior column lesion (clumsy slapping down of the feet on a broad base)

7. Distal weakness (high-stepping gait)

8. Proximal weakness (waddling gait)

5. Test for proximal myopathy by asking the patient to squat and then stand up, or sit in a chair and then stand.

6. Look for Romberg's sign (posterior column loss causes inability to stand steadily when the feet are together with the eyes closed, whereas cerebellar disease causes difficulty when the eyes are open too).

7. Go on to examine the lower limbs depending on your findings. The typical gaits to recognise are listed in Table 15.57.

Cerebellum

'This 30-year-old man has noticed a problem with his coordination. Please examine him.'

Method

This patient is likely to have a cerebellar problem (see Table 15.58). The only other likely possibilities are posterior column loss or extrapyramidal disease. Proceed as follows for assessment of cerebellar disease.

TABLE 15.58 Causes of cerebellar disease

Unilateral

1. Space-occupying lesion (tumour, abscess, granuloma)
2. Ischaemia (vertebrobasilar disease)
3. Paraneoplastic syndrome
4. Multiple sclerosis
5. Trauma

Bilateral

1. Drugs (e.g. phenytoin)
2. Friedreich's ataxia
3. Hypothyroidism
4. Paraneoplastic syndrome
5. Multiple sclerosis
6. Trauma ('punch drunk')
7. Arnold-Chiari malformation
8. Alcohol
9. Large space-occupying lesion, cerebrovascular disease, rare metabolic diseases

Midline

1. Paraneoplastic syndrome
2. Midline tumour

Rostral vermis lesion (only lower limbs affected)

1. Alcohol (most common cause of a cerebellar lesion)

1. Test gait (the patient will stagger towards the affected side unless the problem is bilateral or involves the vermis).
2. Go on to examine the legs. Test tone here.
3. Ask the patient to perform the heel–shin test, looking for accuracy of fine movement when the patient slides his heel down the shin quickly on each side for several cycles.

HINT BOX
Subtle cerebellar changes may be obvious only if the test is made more difficult. Ask the patient to lift the leg in an arc before placing it back on the top of the shin.

4. Next ask the patient to lift his big toe up to touch your finger, looking for intention tremor. Ask him to tap each foot rapidly on a firm surface.

HINT BOX
If cerebellar testing seems normal but Romberg's test was positive, test position and vibration sense.

5. Look now for nystagmus, usually jerky horizontal nystagmus with an increased amplitude on looking towards the side of the lesion.

6. Assess speech. Ask the patient to say 'British Constitution' or 'West Register Street'. Cerebellar speech is jerky, explosive and loud, with irregular separation of syllables.

7. Go to the upper limbs. Ask the patient to extend his arms and look for arm drift and static tremor as a result of hypotonia of the agonist muscles. Test tone. Hypotonia is caused by loss of a facilitatory influence on the spinal motor neurones in acute unilateral cerebellar disease.

8. Next ask the patient to perform the finger–nose test—the patient touches his nose, then rotates his finger and touches your finger. Note any intention tremor (erratic movements increasing as the target is approached owing to loss of cerebellar connections with the brain stem) and past pointing (the patient overshooting the target).

9. Test rapid alternating movements; the patient taps alternately the palm and back of one hand on his other hand or thigh. Inability to perform this movement smoothly is called dysdiadochokinesis.

10. Test rebound—ask the patient to lift his arms quickly from the sides and then stop. Hypotonia causes the patient to be unable to stop his arms. Always demonstrate each movement for the patient's benefit, asking him to copy you.

11. Look for truncal ataxia by asking the patient to fold his arms and sit up. While he is sitting, ask him to put his legs over the side of the bed, and then test for pendular knee jerks.

12. If there is time, look for possible causes of the problem. If there is an obvious unilateral lesion, auscultate over the cerebellum, then proceed to the cranial nerves and look for evidence of a cerebellopontine angle tumour (fifth, seventh, eighth cranial nerves affected) and the lateral medullary syndrome.

13. Always look in the fundi for papilloedema.

14. Next examine for peripheral evidence of malignant disease and vascular disease (carotid bruits).

15. If there is a midline lesion only (i.e. truncal ataxia or abnormal heel–toe walking or abnormal speech), consider either a midline tumour or a paraneoplastic syndrome. If there is bilateral disease, look for signs of multiple sclerosis, Friedreich's ataxia (pes cavus being the most helpful initial clue) (see Tables 15.59 and 15.60) and hypothyroidism (rare). Alcoholic cerebellar degeneration (which affects the anterior lobe of the cerebellar vermis) classically spares the arms.

16. If there are, in addition, upper motor neurone signs, consider the causes in Table 15.61.

TABLE 15.59 Clinical features of Friedreich's ataxia (autosomal recessive)

Usually a young person with:

1. cerebellar signs (bilateral), including nystagmus

2. posterior column loss in the limbs

3. upper motor neurone signs in the limbs (although ankle reflexes are absent)

4. peripheral neuropathy

5. optic atrophy

6. pes cavus, cocking of the toes and kyphoscoliosis

7. cardiomyopathy (ECG abnormalities occur in more than 50% of cases)

8. diabetes mellitus

TABLE 15.60 Causes of pes cavus
1. Friedreich's ataxia or other spinocerebellar degenerations
2. Hereditary motor and sensory neuropathy
3. Neuropathies in childhood
4. Idiopathic

TABLE 15.61 Causes of spastic and ataxic paraparesis (upper motor neurone and cerebellar signs combined)
In adolescence
• Spinocerebellar degeneration (e.g. Marie's spastic ataxia)
In young adults
• Multiple sclerosis
• Syphilitic meningomyelitis
• Spinocerebellar degeneration
• Arnold-Chiari malformation or other lesions at the craniospinal junction
In later life
• Multiple sclerosis
• Syringomyelia
• Infarction (in upper pons or internal capsule bilaterally—'ataxic hemiparesis')
• Lesion at the craniospinal junction (e.g. meningioma)
• Spinocerebellar degeneration
Don't forget, common unrelated diseases (e.g. cervical spondylosis and cerebellar degeneration from alcohol) may occur together by chance.

Parkinson's disease

'This 80-year-woman has Parkinson's disease. Please assess the severity of the condition.'

Method

1. Look at her first. Note the obvious lack of facial expression ('mask-like') and paucity of movement.
2. Ask her to walk, turn quickly and stop, and restart. Note particularly difficulty starting, shuffling, freezing and festination. It is probably a little dangerous to look for propulsion or retropropulsion (see Table 15.57).
3. Ask the patient to return to bed and look for a resting tremor with the arms relaxed (see Table 15.62). The characteristic movement is described as pill rolling and may be unilateral early on.
4. On finger–nose testing, a resting tremor diminishes, but an action tremor may appear. Test wrist tone, feeling for cogwheel or lead pipe rigidity. Reinforce this by asking her to turn her head from side to side.
5. Test for abnormal rapid alternating movements. Look also for involuntary movements produced by medication use.
6. Go to the face. Note tremor, absence of blinking, dribbling of saliva and lack of expression. Test the glabellar tap: the sign is positive (Wilson's sign) when

TABLE 15.62 A classification of tremor
1. Parkinsonian—resting tremor
2. Action tremor—present throughout movement but resolves at rest:
(a) thyrotoxicosis
(b) anxiety
(c) drugs
(d) familial
(e) idiopathic (most common)
3. Intention tremor (cerebellar disease)—increases towards the target
4. Cerebellar outflow tract tremor ('red nucleus')—abduction–adduction movements of upper limbs with flexion–extension of wrists (usually associated with intention tremor, e.g. in multiple sclerosis or brain injury)
Note: Flapping (asterixis) is not strictly a tremor but rather a sudden brief loss of tone in hepatic failure, cardiac failure, respiratory failure or renal failure.

the patient continues to blink after the middle finger taps several times over the glabella from behind—it is important that your finger is out of her line of vision.

7. Test speech, which is typically monotonous, soft, poorly articulated and faint.
8. Look at the ocular movements for supranuclear gaze palsies. Feel for a greasy or sweaty brow (owing to autonomic dysfunction).
9. Ask the patient to write (looking for micrographia) and test the frontal lobe reflexes and higher centres (looking for evidence of dementia).
10. Ask to test for postural hypotension.
11. Present your assessment of the degree of disability and whether the main problem is rigidity or tremor. Is there evidence or autonomic dysfunction or gaze palsy?

Causes of Parkinsonism
1. Idiopathic (Parkinson's disease)
2. Drugs (e.g. phenothiazines, methyldopa)
3. Postencephalitis
4. Other—toxins (carbon monoxide, manganese), Wilson's disease, Steele-Richardson syndrome, Shy-Drager syndrome, syphilis, tumour
   Note: Atherosclerosis is controversial as a cause of Parkinsonism.

Chorea
'Please examine this man's arms.'

Method
Happily you notice an extrapyramidal choreiform movement disorder. Choreiform movements are non-repetitive, abrupt, involuntary, more distal jerky movements, which the patient often attempts to disguise by completing the involuntary movement with a voluntary one. The condition is caused by a lesion of the corpus striatum.
- *Hemiballismus* is unilateral and usually involves rotary movements of proximal joints. It is caused by a subthalamic nucleus lesion on the opposite side.
- *Athetosis* means slow, sinuous distal writhing movements at rest. It is caused by a lesion of the outer segment of the putamen.
  If the patient has chorea, proceed as follows.

1. First shake the patient's hand, for a lack of sustained grip ('milkmaid grip').
2. Ask the patient to hold his hands out and look for a choreic posture (finger and thumb hyperextension and wrist flexion as a result of hypotonia). Note any signs of vasculitis.
3. Go to the face and look at the eyes for exophthalmos, Kayser-Fleischer rings and conjunctival injection (ataxia-telangiectasia). Ask the patient to poke his tongue out and note a serpentine tongue (moving in and out). Notice any rash (e.g. SLE).
4. If the patient is young, examine the heart for signs of rheumatic fever.
5. Test the knee jerks (pendular) and the higher centres (for Huntington's disease).

The causes of chorea are summarised in Table 15.63.

TABLE 15.63 Causes of chorea

1. Huntington's disease (autosomal dominant)
2. Sydenham's chorea (rheumatic fever)
3. Senility
4. Wilson's disease
5. Drugs (e.g. phenothiazines, the contraceptive pill, phenytoin, L-dopa)
6. Vasculitis or connective tissue disease (e.g. SLE)
7. Thyrotoxicosis (very rare)
8. Polycythaemia or other causes of hyperviscosity (very rare)
9. Viral encephalitis (very rare)

Further reading

> You will find it very good practice always to
> verify your references, sir.
>
> *Martin Ruth (1755–1854)*

Candidates for any medical examination must read widely. This particularly applies to the postgraduate candidate who wishes to pass both the written and oral exams. It is very important to spend plenty of time on your weak areas, where you have had the least clinical experience.

We have listed below some of the texts that may be useful. For further suggestions, see the recommendations from the American College of Physicians entitled 'A Library for Internists' published every three years in the *Annals of Internal Medicine*. Although it is unlikely that even the hardest-working candidates will read all these books, we believe reference to some of them will be invaluable.

General texts

American College of Physicians 2010 Medical knowledge self-assessment program XV. ACP, Philadelphia. Available: www.acponline.org.

Goldman L et al (eds) 2008 Cecil textbook of medicine, 23rd edn. Saunders, Philadelphia.

Hannaman RA, Mitchell C, Cross TJ 2009/2010 MedStudy. Internal Medicine Review Core, 13th edn. Books 1–5.

Kasper DL et al (eds) 2008 Harrison's principles of internal medicine, 17th edn. McGraw-Hill, New York.

McPhee, SJ, Papadakis M 2009 Current medical diagnosis and treatment. Lange, Norwalk.

Wiener CM et al (eds) 2008 Harrison's principles of internal medicine. Self-assessment and board review. Pretest self-assessment and review. McGraw-Hill, New York.

Aids to physical examination

Afzal Mir M 2003 Atlas of clinical diagnosis, 2nd edn. Saunders, Edinburgh.

McDonald FS et al (eds) 2004 Mayo Clinic images in internal medicine: self-assessment for board exam review. CRC Press, Boca Raton.

McGee S 2007 Evidence based physical diagnosis, 2nd edn. Saunders, Philadelphia.

Springhouse (ed.) 2005 Auscultation skills: breath and heart sounds (book with 2 audio CD-ROMs), 3rd edn. Lippincott, Williams & Wilkins, Baltimore.

Talley NJ, O'Connor S 2010 Clinical examination: a systematic guide to physical diagnosis, 6th edn. Elsevier, Sydney.

Zatouroff M 1996 Physical signs in general medicine, 2nd edn. Wolfe, London. (*Note:* Useful colour guide.)

Subspecialty texts
Cardiology

Braunwald E et al (ed.) 2007 Heart disease: a textbook of cardiovascular medicine, 8th edn. WB Saunders, Philadelphia.

Respiratory

Fishman A, Elias J 2007 Fishman's pulmonary diseases and disorders, 4th edn. McGraw-Hill, San Juan.

Fraser RS et al 2005 Synopsis of diseases of the chest, 3rd edn. Elsevier/Saunders, Sydney.

Gastroenterology and liver disease

Feldman M et al 2010 Sleisenger & Fordtran's gastrointestinal disease, 9th edn. Saunders, Philadelphia.

Talley NJ, Martin CJ (eds) 2010 Clinical gastroenterology: a practical problem-based approach, 3rd edn. Elsevier, Sydney.

Haematology

Hoffbrand V, Moss P, Pettit JE 2007 Essential haematology, 5th edn. Blackwell, Oxford.

Rheumatology and immunology

Hochberg MC et al 2008 Rheumatology, 4th edn. Saunders, Philadelphia.

Hunder GG 2005 Atlas of rheumatology, 4th edn. Lippincott, Williams & Wilkins, Baltimore.

Klippel JH 2008 Primer on the rheumatic diseases, 13th edn. Arthritis Foundation, Atlanta, GA.

Neurology

Donaghy M 2009 Brain's diseases of the nervous system, 12th edn. Oxford University Press, Oxford.

Fuller G 2008 Neurological examination made easy, 4th edn. Churchill Livingstone, Edinburgh.

Greenberg DA et al 2009 Clinical neurology, 7th edn. Lange, Los Altos, CA.

Medical Research Council 1997 Memorandum no. 45. Aids to examination of the peripheral nervous system. Her Majesty's Stationery Office, London. (*Note*: Very clear photographs and illustrations make this an invaluable reference book.)

Patten J 1996 Neurological differential diagnoses—an illustrated approach, 2nd edn. Harold Starke, London. (*Note*: Refer to this book for the clear, useful illustrations.)

Rowland LP (ed.) 2009 Merritt's textbook of clinical neurology, 12th edn. Williams & Wilkins, Baltimore.

Nephrology

Johnson R et al 2007 Comprehensive clinical nephrology, 3rd edn. Mosby, St Louis.

Endocrinology

Larsen PR et al 2008 Williams textbook of endocrinology, 11th edn. Saunders, Philadelphia.

DeGroot LJ (ed.) 2006 Endocrinology, 5th edn. Saunders, Philadelphia.

Dermatology

Wolff K et al (eds) 2009 Fitzpatrick's color atlas and synopsis of clinical dermatology, 6th edn. McGraw-Hill, New York.

Pharmacology

Katzung BG 2009 Basic and clinical pharmacology, 11th edn. McGraw-Hill, New York.

Radiology
Hughes J 2000 Radiology for the MRCP. Churchill Livingstone, Edinburgh.

Infectious diseases
Mandell GL et al (eds) 2009 Principles and practice of infectious diseases, 7th edn. Churchill Livingstone, New York.

Journals
All postgraduate candidates must read journals because textbooks are always somewhat out of date by the time they are published.

The following journals are specifically recommended by the Royal Australasian College of Physicians:
1. *Lancet*
2. *New England Journal of Medicine*
3. *British Medical Journal*
4. *Annals of Internal Medicine*
5. *Internal Medicine Journal*
6. *American Journal of Medicine.*

Note: The excellent review articles and editorials should be studied. *The Medical Journal of Australia* is also worth a look. The consensus statements on management produced by the specialist societies are particularly useful. UpToDate (www.uptodate.com) is an excellent source of current management advice on all topics.

Remember, topics often crop up from these articles in the multiple-choice examination, particularly those published in the three years or so prior to the setting of the multiple-choice questions.

Index